BUS

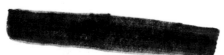

Ophthalmic
DISORDERS
SOURCEBOOK

Health Reference Series

Volume Seventeen

Ophthalmic
DISORDERS
SOURCEBOOK

Basic Information about Glaucoma, Cataracts, Macular Degeneration, Strabismus, Refractive Disorders, and More, along with Statistical and Demographic Data and Reports on Current Research Initiatives

Edited by
Linda M. Ross

Omnigraphics, Inc.

Penobscot Building / Detroit, MI 48226

BIBLIOGRAPHIC NOTE

This volume contains the following numbered publications produced by the National In-
stitutes of Health: 32-1183, 93-201, 93-2910, 93-3186, 93-3462, 93-3960; the following
numbered publications of the Department of Health and Human Services: (FDA) 92-1183,
(SSA) 05-10052; AHCPR publication numbers 93-0544, 93-0543, and Guideline Overview,
No. 4. Unnumbered publications from the *FDA Consumer* magazine, the National Eye
Institute, the National Eye Health Program, the National Institutes of Health, National
Institute on Disability and Rehabilitation Research, the National Library Service for the
Blind and Physically Handicapped. This volume also contains copyrighted documents from
the following sources: *20/20 is Not Enough* (Alfred A. Knopf), the American Academy of
Ophthalmology, the American Foundation for the Blind, the American Health Assistance
Foundation, The Lighthouse, and University of Illinois at Chicago (UCI) Department of
Ophthalmology/UIC Eye Center. All copyrighted documents are used by permission. Spe-
cific source citations are listed on the first page of each article.

Edited by
Linda M. Ross

Peter D. Dresser, Managing Editor, *Health Reference Series*
Karen Bellenir, Series Editor

Omnigraphics, Inc.
Matthew P. Barbour, *Production Manager*
Laurie Lanzen Harris, *Vice President, Editorial*
Peter E. Ruffner, *Vice President, Administration*
James A. Sellgren, *Vice President, Operations and Finance*
Jane J. Steele, *Vice President, Research*

Frederick G. Ruffner, Jr., *Publisher*

Copyright © 1997, Omnigraphics, Inc.

Library of Congress Cataloging-in-Publication Data

Ophthalmic diseases and disorders sourcebook / basic information about
   glaucoma, cataracts, macular degeneration, strabismus, refractive
   disorders, and more, along with statistical and demographic data and
   reports on current research initiatives / edited by Linda M. Ross.
     p.   cm. -- (Health reference series ; v. 17)
   Includes bibliographical references and index.
   ISBN 0-7808-0081-8 (lib bdg : alk. paper)
    1. Eye--Diseases--Popular works. I. Ross, Linda M. (Linda
   Michelle) II. Series.
   RE51.064 1996
   617.7'1--dc20   96-33451
                                                      CIP

∞

This book is printed on acid-free paper meeting the ANSI Z39.48 Standard. The infinity
symbol that appears above indicates that the paper in this book meets that standard.

Printed in the United States.

Contents

Part III: Diseases of the Eye

Part IV: Corneal and Retinal Disorders

Part V: Glaucoma

Part VI: Cataracts

Part VII: Macular Disorders

Part VIII: Other Ophthalmic Problems

Part IX: Ophthalmic Disorders Related to Other Diseases

Preface

About This Book

Nearsightedness, farsightedness, childhood strabismus, presbyopia—these are among the many ophthalmic disorders that will affect nearly every person in the United States sometime during his or her life. Beyond the common vision problems, more serious diseases such as glaucoma, cataracts, and retinal cancer will threaten the eyesight of millions. This book contains information compiled from a variety of sources to help those afflicted by ophthalmic diseases and disorders. Many of the articles are from government sources including the Food and Drug Administration (FDA), National Eye Institute (NEI), and other divisions of the National Institutes of Health. The material contained in this book was selected because it provides basic medical information to the layperson, patient, and concerned friends and family.

How to Use This Book

The information in this book is divided into nine sections.

Part I: General Resources offers information that will help anyone suffering from ophthalmic problems or vision loss. It contains a glossary of vision terms, an explanation of Social Security and SSI benefits, general eye exam procedures, information for selecting low-vision devices, a listing of eye health education resources, and information of federally-sponsored book and music programs for the blind.

Part II: Alignment and Refractive Disorders concentrated on common problems such as strabismus, myopia and amblyopia. It also contains information on Radial Keratotomy (RK) Surgery, and Photorefractive Keratotomy (PRK).

Part III: Diseases of the Eye covers inflammatory eye diseases, macular edema, and cancer of the eye.

Part IV: Corneal Retinal Disorders is concerned with such topics as corneal structure and function, infectious diseases of the cornea, retinal detachment, floaters and flashers, retinitis pigmentosa, and retinopathy in premature babies.

Part V: Glaucoma and Part VI: Cataracts provide well-rounded information on each of these common but serious conditions.

Part VII: Macular Disorders treats the subjects of macular pucker, macular degeneration, nutrition and the macula, and vitrectomy surgery as a treatment of macular disorders.

Part VIII: Ophthalmic Disorders Related to Other Diseases highlights the ophthalmic ramifications of diseases such as diabetes, sickle cell anemia, AIDS, and thyroid disease.

Acknowledgements

The editor wishes to thank the many people who have labored to produce this book. In particular, Margaret Mary Missar whose diligence in leaving no research stone unturned made this book possible; Karen, whose patience and sense of direction were essential in guiding the editor through a sea of codes that was sometimes nearly impossible to navigate; and of course, Pete—thanks, Dude.

Note from the Editor

This book is part of Omnigraphics' *Health Reference Series*. The series provides basic information about a broad range of medical concerns. It is not intended to serve as a tool for diagnosing illness, in prescribing treatments, or as a substitute for the physician/patient relationship. All persons concerned about medical symptoms or the possibility of disease are encouraged to seek professional care from an appropriate health care provider.

Part One

General Resources

Chapter 1

Glossary of Vision Terms

Accommodation. The ability of the eye to change its focus from distant to near objects; process achieved by the lens changing its shape.

Anterior Chamber. The space in front of the iris and behind the cornea.

Aqueous Humor, Aqueous Fluid. (A-kwe-us) Clear, watery fluid that flows between and nourishes the lens and the cornea; secreted by the ciliary processes.

Astigmatism. (uh-STIG-muh-tizm) A condition in which the surface of the cornea is not spherical; causes a blurred image to be received at the retina.

Blind Spot. (1) A small area of the retina where the optic nerve enters the eye; occurs normally in all eyes. (2) Any gap in the visual field corresponding to an area of the retina where no visual cells are present; associated with eye disease.

Central Vision. See VISUAL ACUITY.

Choroid. (KOR-oyd) The layer filled with blood vessels that nourishes the retina; part of the uvea.

Ciliary Muscles. The muscles that relax the zonules to enable the lens to change shape for focusing.

Ciliary Processes. The extensions or projections of the ciliary body that secrete aqueous humor.

NEI, Fact Sheet, August 1993.

Cones, Cone Cells. One type of specialized light-sensitive cells (photoreceptors) in the retina that provide sharp central vision and color vision. Also see RODS.

Conjunctiva. (KAHN-junk-TY-vuh) The thin, moist tissue (membrane) that lines the inner surfaces of the eyelids and the outer surface of the sclera.

Contrast Sensitivity. The ability to perceive differences between an object and its background.

Cornea. (KOR-nee-uh) The outer, transparent, dome-like structure that covers the iris, pupil, and anterior chamber; part of eye's focusing system.

Dilation. A process by which the pupil is temporarily enlarged with special eye drops (mydriatic); allows the eye care specialist to better view the fundus.

Fundus. The interior lining of the eyeball, including the retina, optic disc, and macula; portion of the inner eye that can be seen during an eye examination by looking through the pupil.

Hyperopia. (hy-pur-OH-pee-uh) Farsightedness; ability to see distant objects more clearly than close objects; may be corrected with glasses or contact lenses.

Intraocular Pressure. (IOP) Pressure of the fluid inside the eye; normal IOP varies among individuals.

Iris. The colored ring of tissue suspended behind the cornea and immediately in front of the lens; regulates the amount of light entering the eye by adjusting the size of the pupil.

Lacrimal Gland. (LAK-rih-mul) The small almond-shaped structure that produces tears; located just above the outer corner of the eye.

Lens. The transparent, double convex (outward curve on both sides) structure suspended between the aqueous and vitreous; helps to focus light on the retina.

Legal Blindness. In the U.S., (1) visual acuity of 20/200 or worse in the better eye with corrective lenses (20/200 means that a person must be at 20 feet from an eye chart to see what a person with normal vision can see at 200 feet) or (2) visual field restricted to 20 degrees diameter or less (tunnel vision) in the better eye.

Macula. (MAK-yoo-luh) The small, sensitive area of the central retina; provides vision for fine work and reading.

Myopia. (my-OH-pee-uh) Nearsightedness; ability to see close objects more clearly than distant objects; may be corrected with glasses or contact lenses.

Optic Cup. The white, cup-like area in the center of the optic disc.

Optic Disc / Optic Nerve Head. The circular area (disc) where the optic nerve connects to the back part of the retina.

Optic Nerve. The bundle of over one million nerve fibers that carry visual messages from the retina to the brain.

Peripheral Vision. (per-IF-ur-al) Side vision; ability to see objects and movement outside of the direct line of vision.

Posterior Chamber. The space between the back of the iris and the front face of the vitreous; filled with aqueous fluid.

Presbyopia. (prez-bee-OH-pee-uh) The gradual loss of the eye's ability to change focus (accommodation) for seeing near objects caused by the lens becoming less elastic; associated with aging; occurs in almost all people over age 45.

Pupil. The adjustable opening at the center of the iris that allows varying amounts of light to enter the eye.

Retina. (RET-in-nuh) The light-sensitive layer of tissue that lines the back of the eyeball; sends visual impulses through the optic nerve to the brain.

Retinal Pigment Epithelium (RPE). (ep-ih-THEE-lee-um) The pigment cell layer that nourishes the retinal cells; located just outside the retina and attached to the choroid.

Rods, Rod Cells. One type of specialized light-sensitive cells (photoreceptors) in the retina that provide side vision and the ability to see objects in dim light (night vision). Also see CONES.

Schlemm's Canal. The passageway for the aqueous fluid to leave the eye.

Sclera. (SKLEH-ruh) The tough, white, outer layer (coat) of the eyeball; with the cornea, it protects the entire eyeball.

Trabecular Meshwork. (truh-BEC-yoo-lur) The spongy, mesh-like tissue near the front of the eye that allows the aqueous fluid (humor) to flow to Schlemm's canal then out of the eye through ocular veins.

Uvea, Uveal Tract. (YOO-vee-uh) The middle coat of the eyeball, consisting of the choroid in the back of the eye and the ciliary body and iris in the front of the eye.

Visual Acuity. The ability to distinguish details and shapes of objects; also called central vision.

Visual Field. The entire area that can be seen when the eye is forward, including peripheral vision.

Vitreous. (VIT-ree-us) The transparent, colorless mass of gel that lies behind lens and in front of retina.

Zonules. (ZAHN-yoolz) The fibers that hold the lens suspended in position and enable it to change shape during accommodation.

Chapter 2

How Social Security and SSI Can Help You

Part I: General Information

If you are blind, there are a number of Social Security rules you should know about. Some of the rules apply only to people who are blind, while others apply to nonblind persons as well. But they're important to know because they can help you qualify for Social Security or Supplemental Security Income (SSI). Once you're getting benefits, they can help supplement your monthly payments and increase your chances of getting back to work on a regular basis or entering the workplace for the first time. In fact, many of the special rules are designed specifically to make it easier for people who are blind to work.

This chapter will help you understand the rules so you can use them to help meet your life goals. We also identify those services that are available to help you get the most out of the Social Security and SSI programs.

Two Disability Programs

You should start by understanding the difference between Social Security and SSI and how they work together to provide a floor of income protection for people with disabilities. You can qualify for Social Security if you have enough prior work. You qualify for SSI payments

DHHS, SSA Publication No. 05-10052, June 1993.

if your income and resources, even with Social Security benefits, fall below certain limits. The medical criteria we use to decide if you qualify for benefits because of blindness are the same under both programs. However, other rules are different under each program. For this reason, this booklet is generally divided into Social Security and SSI sections to clarify the different rules.

What Do We Mean By "Blind"

You also should know the medical definition of blindness under Social Security. You are considered blind under Social Security rules if your vision cannot be corrected to better than 20/200 in your better eye, or if your visual field is 20 degrees or less, even with corrective lens. Many people who meet the legal definition of blindness still have some sight and may be able to read large print and get about without a cane or guide dog. If you do not meet the legal definition of blindness, you still may qualify for benefits if your vision problems coupled with other health problems prevent you from doing substantial work.

Qualifying For Social Security Disability Benefits

To qualify for Social Security disability benefits, you must have worked long enough in a job where you paid Social Security taxes. Or, you must be the disabled child or disabled widow(er) of somebody who did. When you work, you earn "credits" up to 4 per year that count toward future Social Security benefits.

The number of credits you need depends on your age. As a general rule, you must have credits equal to the number of years between age 21 up to the year you stop working. Blind persons under 28 need no more than 6 credits of work. If you become legally blind at age 41, you need 20 credits. Nobody needs more than 40 credits.

Nonblind people must meet another requirement. They must have earned half of the credits they need in recent years. For example, people over 31 must have earned 20 credits during the past 10 years. If you are blind, you do not have to meet this recent work rule. Your credits can be earned anytime during your working years.

Even if you are working regularly, you might want to file for a Social Security disability "freeze" if you meet the legal definition of blindness. Under this procedure, you won't get benefits now, but your benefits will be higher if you do become eligible later.

Qualifying For SSI Disability Benefits

Regardless of whether you have enough work credits to qualify for Social Security, you may qualify for SSI disability benefits. To get SSI, you need not have worked under Social Security, but your income and resources must be under certain limits. The income limits vary from one State to another. For more information about SSI, ask your Social Security office about the income limits in your area and for a copy of the booklet, SSI (Publication No. 0511000). This booklet is also available in braille from Social Security offices and as part of a talking book from the Library of Congress.

How To Apply

You should apply at any Social Security office as soon as you become disabled. (You may file by phone, mail, or by visiting the nearest office.)

The claims process for disability benefits is generally longer than for other types of Social Security benefits from 60 to 90 days. It takes longer to obtain medical information and to assess the nature of the disability in terms of your ability to work. However, you can help shorten the process by bringing certain documents with you when you apply. These include:

- The Social Security number and proof of age for each person applying for payments. This includes your spouse and children, if they are applying for benefits.

- Names, addresses, and phone numbers of doctors, hospitals, clinics, and institutions that treated you and dates of treatment.

- A summary of where you worked in the past 15 years and the kind of work you did.

- A copy of your W-2 Form (Wage and Tax Statement), or if you are self-employed, your Federal tax return for the past year.

- Dates of any prior marriages if your spouse is applying.

9

Your Social Security disability benefits will not begin to arrive until the 6th full month of the disability. This "waiting period" begins with the first full month after the date we decide your disability began.

If you are applying for SSI, you also need to bring with you information about your living arrangements such as the name of your mortgage company or a copy of your lease with your landlord's name; and information about your income and the things you own, such as payroll slips, bank books, insurance policies, car registration, and burial fund records.

Your SSI disability check can be paid back to the date you filed your claim.

Do not delay filing for benefits just because you do not have all of the information you need. The Social Security office will be glad to help you.

Evaluating Your Medical Condition

You should be familiar with the process we use to decide if you are legally blind or otherwise disabled. After the Social Security office reviews your claim to make sure you meet the non-medical rules, your application goes to a State disability determination service (DDS) where the medical evaluation takes place. In the DDS, a team consisting of a physician and a disability evaluation specialist will decide if you are legally blind. This generally means reviewing medical evidence from your doctors or the hospitals, clinics, or institutions where you have been treated. If this information is not available or incomplete, you may be asked to see a doctor for an examination which we will pay for.

Once we decide that you are legally blind, we will notify you that your claim has been approved. If you do not meet Social Security's definition of blindness, then we decide if your visual impairment, plus any other impairment you may have, prevents you from doing the work you did in the last 15 years. If it does not, your claim will be denied. If it does, we look to see if you can do any other type of work. We consider your age, education, past work experience, and transferable skills. If you cannot do any other kind of work, your claim will be approved.

Part II: What Happens When You Work While Receiving Benefits

A number of rules make it easier for persons receiving disability benefits to work and supplement their benefits and eventually work full time. The provisions are called "work incentives." While these rules in general are not geared solely to persons who are blind, they do provide a means for persons who are blind to increase their income and work their way off the disability rolls.

The Social Security and SSI work incentives are different but they are designed to accomplish the same objectives: to continue cash benefits until you are earning enough to get by on your own; to continue health care assistance (Medicare and/or Medicaid) even when earnings are too high to allow cash payments; to exclude from earnings the cost of extra work expenses caused by your disability; and to help with rehabilitation and finding new work. We will briefly explain each of these special rules and provide an example of how they work under both Social Security and SSI.

For more information on these provisions, you should ask for the booklet, Working While Disabled How Social Security Can Help (Publication No. 05-10095). This booklet is available in braille from Social Security and as a talking book from the Library of Congress.

Working While Receiving Social Security Benefits

People getting Social Security disability benefits can continue to receive their benefits when they return to work as long as their earnings are not "substantial."

You Can Earn More. Under the Social Security disability program, persons who are blind can earn up to $880 a month in 1993 before their work is considered "substantial." This is higher than the substantial work level of $500 a month that applies to nonblind disabled workers. The level of earnings a person who is blind can earn changes each year to reflect changes in general wage levels.

If you're blind and self-employed, the $880 level becomes the sole criterion of substantial work. We do not make a separate evaluation of the time you spend in the business as we do for nonblind beneficiaries. This means you can be doing a lot of work for your business but still receive disability benefits as long as your net profit averages less than $880 a month in 1993.

11

Work Figured Differently After 55. If you are 55 or older, we figure your ability to perform substantial work differently. After age 55, even if your earnings exceed $880 a month in 1993, benefits are only suspended, not terminated, if your work requires a lower level of skill and ability than what you did before age 55. Thus, eligibility for Social Security benefits may continue indefinitely and benefits may be paid for any month your earnings fall below the substantial level.

The Trial Work Period. A trial work period provides a beneficiary up to 9 months to test his or her ability to work and earn any amount without fear of losing benefits. The 9 months need not be consecutive, and the trial work period does not end until 9 months are used within a 60-month period.

After the trial work period, your benefits will continue if your earnings are less than $880 a month in 1993. If your earnings are $880 or more, benefits continue for 3 more months and then stop.

The Extended Period Of Eligibility. For 36 months after a successful trial work period, your Social Security benefits may be reinstated without a new application for any month your earnings drop below $880.

Impairment-Related Work Expenses Rule. This rule permits you to deduct impairment-related work expenses resulting from your blindness (such as the expense of paying for a sighted reader) from your income before we decide if it is substantial.

Continuation Of Medicare Coverage. This rule removes the fear of losing health care benefits due to work by continuing Medicare's premium-free hospital insurance coverage for at least 39 months after the end of the trial work period.

Medicare Coverage For Disabled People Who Work. At the end of the 39-month period, people who continue to have a disability and who lose Medicare hospital insurance coverage because earnings are substantial are permitted to purchase Medicare hospital and medical insurance coverage.

Continued Payment Under An Approved Rehabilitation Program Despite Medical Recovery. Ordinarily, benefits stop when a person shows sufficient medical improvement. Under this rule, benefits may continue after medical recovery if the person is participating in an approved vocational rehabilitation program whose services are likely to enable the person to work permanently. A person involved in such a program who had a successful eye operation, for example, could continue to receive benefits and complete the program even though he/she was no longer blind.

An Example Of How Social Security Work Incentives Can Help You

Cathy Jones is 25 and receives $460 each month in Social Security benefits because she is blind. Cathy also has Medicare coverage. In December 1992, Cathy completes a secretarial training course and gets a job for the first time in January 1993. She is hired by a local hospital to work 35 hours a week as a medical transcriber trainee. Her starting salary is $750 per month.

Cathy reports her work and earnings to the Social Security office and learns that her benefits will continue during her 9-month trial work period regardless of how much she earns. Her monthly income during the 9-month trial work period, including her $750 in earnings, increases from $460 to $1,210.

Cathy recontacts the Social Security office in September to let us know that she is completing her ninth month of work. She also tells us that she has increased her hours to 40 per week and has received a pay raise. She is now earning $900 per month, which is more than the $880 substantial earnings level in 1993 at which benefits to blind persons generally stop.

However, in evaluating her earnings, we learn that Cathy is paying a co-worker $25 a week ($100 a month) to take her to and from work because she does not have access to public transportation. This $100 qualifies as an impairment-related work expense. After subtracting the $100 per month, we find that Cathy has countable earnings of $800 per month which is less than the blind substantial earnings level of $880. Consequently, Cathy's payments continue though she completed her trial work period in September. Her monthly income is $460 plus $900 or $1,360.

In December, Cathy contacts the Social Security office to let us know that she has received another pay raise because she has been promoted from the trainee position. Her monthly earnings beginning in January 1994 will be $1,100 per month, and her transportation costs (her only impairment-related expenses) remain at $100. Cathy's countable income is now $1,000 per month, more than the $880 blind substantial work level. For this reason, her Social Security disability benefit is stopped as of January 1994, but she will receive her check for 3 additional months—January, February and March despite her earnings.

If Cathy's earnings drop below the substantial level for any month during the 36 months beginning with October of 1993 (the month following the month the trial work period ended), she can be paid her

Social Security benefit. Additionally, Cathy's Medicare coverage will continue for at least 39 months after the end of her trial work period regardless of her earnings.

Working While Receiving Supplemental Security Income Benefits

There are different work rules for people receiving SSI. The $880 substantial earnings level does not apply to people receiving SSI. Instead, you are permitted to have earnings until you exceed the SSI income limits, which vary from State to State. As earnings rise, SSI benefits are reduced and eventually stopped.

However, not all income is counted and you may earn up to $953 a month in 1993 before your SSI stops if there is no income other than earnings. (This figure is higher for people who live in a State that adds money—or a "State supplement" to the SSI payment.) In addition, there are other deductions applied to working SSI recipients under the work incentives rules.

The Student Earned Income Exclusion. Unmarried persons under age 22 and regularly attending school may exclude up to $400 of earned income per month. The maximum annual exclusion is $1,620.

The Earned Income Exclusion. This rule means we don't count the first $65 ($85 in some cases) of earnings in a month plus one half of any earnings over $65 ($85) when figuring the SSI payment amount.

Blind Work Expenses. This rule permits a person who is blind to exclude earned income which is used to meet the expenses of working. The expenses need not be related to blindness. Examples include the portion of a person's earnings used to pay income taxes, meals consumed during work hours, transportation costs, or guide dog expenses.

Plans For Achieving Self Support (PASS). A PASS lets you set aside income and/or resources over a reasonable period of time under a plan designed to enable you to become financially self-supporting. The income and resources set aside under a plan do not count against you when we decide if you're eligible for SSI and how much you will get.

Property Essential To Self Support. This provision allows full or partial exclusion of certain income-producing property necessary for self-support when determining SSI eligibility and payment amount.

Continuation Of Medicaid Coverage. Under this rule, Medicaid coverage for most working SSI beneficiaries continues even when their earnings become too high to allow an SSI cash payment.

Continued Payment Under An Approved Rehabilitation Program Despite Medical Recovery. As is true for people receiving Social Security benefits, people receiving SSI may have payments continue even after medical recovery if they are participating in an approved vocational rehabilitation program whose services are likely to enable them to work permanently.

An Example Of How SSI Work Incentives Can Help You

John Smith is 20 years old and receives SSI payments because he is blind. He receives $434 each month and has Medicaid coverage.

In January 1993, John begins working part time during the evenings and on weekends for the veterinarian who cares for his guide dog. John is paid $400 a month to answer the phone, make appointments, and help with the care and feeding of animals boarded at the kennel. John reports his work and earnings to his local Social Security office and reports the following blind work expenses:

- $45.00   Transportation to and from work
- $30.00   Care and feeding of his guide dog
- $35.50   Taxes
- $110.50   Total blind work expenses

Here is how we calculate John's SSI amount based on his earnings and his blind work expenses:

We first subtract $85 from John's earnings. This exclusion applies to anyone who works and has no other income:

- $400 minus $85 = $315.00

Then we deduct half of the remaining $315: (This exclusion also applies to anyone who works)

- $315 divided by 2 = $157.50

From this amount, we subtract the $110.50 in blind work expenses:

- $157.50 minus $110.50 = $47.00

John has $47 in countable income which we subtract from his $434 SSI payment, leaving $387.

- $434.00 minus $47.00 = $387.00

This means that, even though John is earning $400 per month, he loses only $47 in SSI payments, and his Medicaid coverage continues. John's monthly income is $787.

In late March, John reports to us that his employer has asked him to work longer hours and is also giving him a pay raise. John begins earning $650 per month in April. He tells us that he likes working with animals so much that he would like to go to school to learn to be a dog trainer and groomer. He plans to save $200 per month from his increased earnings so that he will have $1,000 saved to pay for books and tuition by September when the course begins at a local vocational school. We help John to write a plan for achieving self-support (PASS) so that we can exclude $200 per month from the income we must use to figure his SSI payment for the months from April through August. Additionally, John reports that working longer hours and earning more will increase his transportation costs and his taxes. He reports the following blind work expenses beginning with April:

- $60.00   Transportation
- $30.00   Expenses for the care and feeding of his guide dog
- $67.50   Taxes
- $157.50   Total blind work expenses

Here is how we compute John's SSI payment beginning with April: $650 minus $85 (for the earned income exclusion) equals $565. We then exclude half of this amount:

- $565 divided by 2 = $282.50

From this amount, we subtract John's blind work expenses of $157.50 leaving $125.00 in countable income.

- $282.50 minus $157.50 = $125.00

Then subtract the $200 that John is setting aside each month under a PASS.

- $125.50 minus $200 = ZERO

Because we were able to deduct so many of his work expenses, we do not have to count any of John's income so he now receives $434, which is the maximum SSI payment he can make in his State. Even though John is earning $250 more each month than he did in January,

February, or March, his SSI check will increase from $387 to $434 because he has developed a PASS to allow him to go to school. His Medicaid coverage continues. John's total monthly income beginning in April is $1,084.

John begins a 4-month course to learn to be a dog groomer and trainer in September of 1993. His PASS ends in August because he has saved $1,000 to pay for books and tuition, but now that John is a student and is under age 22, he can use the student earned income exclusion to reduce his countable income. He can exclude earnings of $400 per month up to a maximum of $1,620 annually. Since he will be in school for only 4 months in the calendar year, he can use the exclusion for each of these months without exceeding the $1,620 annual maximum. John continues to work for the veterinarian and receives another pay raise which increases his earnings to $750 per month beginning in September. His blind work expenses for transportation and care and feeding of his guide dog are unchanged, but his increased wages cause his taxes to go up $10. His total blind work expenses beginning in September rise from $157.50 to $167.50 per month, including the $10 additional taxes.

Here is how we compute John's countable income while he is a student from September through December:

From the $750 of earnings, we subtract $400 for the student earned income exclusion:

- $750 minus $400 = $350.00

We then subtract the $85 income exclusion from this amount:

- $350 minus $85 = $265.00

We exclude half of this amount:

- $265 divided by 2 = $132.50

From this amount, we subtract $167.50 in blind work expenses, leaving zero countable income for September through December.

- $132.50 minus $167.50 = ZERO

John continues to receive $434 per month in addition to his monthly earnings of $750 and his Medicaid coverage continues. John's total monthly income is $1,184.

Part III: Special Services For People Who Are Blind

There are a number of services and products specifically designed to ensure that you are able to take advantage of your rights and exercise your responsibilities under the Social Security program.

Social Security Letters

You have the option of receiving letters and other correspondence from Social Security by certified mail, by telephone, or in person. Just let Social Security know your preference.

Radio Reading Service

Social Security provides special tapes of its publications to local radio stations that offer reading service for their blind and visually impaired listeners. To find out which stations in your area provide radio reading services, you should call the Social Security office.

Library Of Congress (LOC) Talking Book And Braille Booklet

The National Library Service for the Blind and Physically Handicapped of the Library of Congress (LOC) have prepared a "talking book" (a cassette recording) and a braille booklet for distribution to LOC's network of 160 libraries across the country. The talking booklet and the braille booklet each contain information about SSA's major programs: Retirement; Survivors; Disability; Medicare, and Supplemental Security Income (SSI). You can find out the LOC branch nearest you from your Social Security office or your local library.

Audio Cassettes

The booklet, A Summary Guide to Social Security and Supplemental Security Income Work Incentives for the Disabled and Blind (Publication No. 65-030), has been recorded on a cassette tape. This guide is designed to assist professionals in the public and private sectors who work with disabled or visually impaired people. Requests for these tapes should be directed to any Social Security office.

Publications Available In Braille

The following publications are available in braille. The first five are booklets that provide an overview of each of the major Social Security related programs.

- *Retirement* (Publication No. 05-10035)

- *Survivors* (Publication No. 05-10084)

- *Disability* (Publication No. 05-10029)

- *Supplemental Security Income* (SSI) (Publication No. 05-11000)

- *Medicare* (Publication No. 05-10043)

- *Understanding Social Security* (Publication No. 05-10024)—A general but comprehensive overview of the Social Security program.

- *Working While Disabled—How Social Security Can Help* (Publication No. 05-10095)—A simple explanation of the work incentives under Social Security and SSI for beneficiaries who want to work.

- *Working While Disabled* (Publication No. 05-11017)—A guide to plans for achieving self-support (PASS) while receiving SSI.

- *When You Get Social Security Disability Benefits—What You Need To Know* (Publication No. 05-10153)—A guide to your rights and responsibilities while receiving Social Security disability benefits.

- *When You Get SSI—What You Need To Know* (Publication No. 05-11011)—A guide to your rights and responsibilities while receiving SSI.

- *A Summary Guide to Social Security and Supplemental Security Income Work Incentives for People With Disabilities* (Publication No. 64-030)—Known as the "Redbook," it provides a more detailed and technical explanation of work incentives than the booklet *Working While Disabled—How Social Security Can Help*.

The Social Security Office can order these braille publications for you on request.

Chapter 3

Taking a Look at Eye Exams

Ask people which of their five senses they value the most, and almost everyone would say their sight. The visual images that dominate our lives are priceless treasures, and we would sacrifice much to preserve them.

One important way to preserve the precious gift of sight is regular checkups by an eye doctor. (For exactly what is meant by an "eye doctor," see below.) In most cases, of course, people get their eyes checked to see if they need glasses, or a change in their prescription if they already wear them. But thorough, regularly scheduled eye exams also can be vitally important in detecting serious diseases and disorders that affect the eyes. Often, early detection and treatment can control or correct problems that otherwise could lead to permanently impaired vision or even blindness.

Another benefit of an eye exam is that, while peering into the eyes—with the help of sophisticated instruments—a doctor can discern symptoms of serious diseases, such as high blood pressure, diabetes and cancer, that affect the entire body. In fact, it's sometimes the eye doctor who is the first to pick up clues to such conditions.

Here's a rundown of what to expect from a good eye exam.

Medical History

Eye exams generally start with a medical history. What problems or symptoms are prompting the patient to seek an exam? Is there a

FDA Consumer, May 1987.

family history of eye disorders that may be linked to heredity, such as glaucoma or retinitis pigmentosa (an inherited degenerative disease of the retina)? Is the patient taking any medication? These are some of the questions an eye doctor may ask.

Vision Testing

Vision testing ordinarily begins with the patient reading letters of the alphabet from a Snellen chart—the standard used in all eye exams.

Most people know that normal visual acuity is designated as 20/20—meaning that the smallest print on the eye chart that someone can read at 20 feet corresponds to the line for standard "normal" vision. Someone who can't read the 20/20 line is asked to look progressively higher up on the chart to bigger print until the letters can be read. The designation for that line then becomes the measure of visual acuity. For example, if someone can begin to distinguish letters from 20 feet only after moving to the line that can normally be read at 200 feet, that's 20/200 vision.

Three types of problems related to the eye's focusing ability can cause poor vision: nearsightedness, farsightedness and astigmatism. Nearsightedness, or myopia, is by far the most common. It arises when the lens of the eye brings images into focus in front of, rather than precisely on, the back of the eye's interior, the layer of light-sensitive cells called the retina. Concave (like two saucers placed back to back) lenses correct myopia.

In farsightedness, or hyperopia, images fall into focus beyond the retina. Convex (curving outward, like the outside of a ball) lenses are used to correct hyperopia.

Astigmatism is caused by irregularities in the curvature of the cornea, the protective covering over the lens of the eye. Astigmatism results in blurred vision, which can be corrected by specially ground lenses.

Another term eye doctors use in discussing vision is "accommodation." Accommodation is the ability to focus on things near the eye, and it makes reading possible. Impaired accommodation results in presbyopia, which is corrected with concave lenses for reading or with bifocals that have a reading prescription in the lower part of the lens and a prescription above for distant focus.

The doctor has two ways of arriving at a prescription to correct visual defects. With an instrument called a retinoscope, light is focused through the pupil onto the retina. By observing the movement of the light as it is reflected back through the eye from the retina, the doctor is able to measure optical flaws.

Then, with another instrument called a phoropter, the eye doctor moves corrective lenses into place in front of the eye. The effect of the lenses can be checked by shining the retinoscope's light into the eye through the corrective lenses or by having the patient read from the Snellen chart. The corrections are then fine-tuned by asking subjects which lens or lens combination enables them to read best and most comfortably. Finally, color vision is checked by asking the subject to read the numbers seen in patterns of colored dots on an Ishihara Color Identification chart.

Following these checks for visual acuity comes the medical part of the exam. Because of their training as doctors of medicine and state laws that regulate eye-care practices, ophthalmologists may be best equipped to conduct this part of the eye exam.

Glaucoma

Glaucoma is an eye disorder caused by excess pressure in the eye. It accounts for 12 percent of the cases of blindness in the United States. The incidence of glaucoma is higher in older people, affecting about 2 percent of the population over 40.

The pressure of eye fluids inside the eyeball is regulated by a delicate circulatory mechanism that is indirectly linked to the cardiovascular system. When this mechanism is impaired by conditions such as structural defects, eye injuries or aging, excess pressure may rise.

Too much pressure can damage the optic nerve. As glaucoma progresses, it increasingly impairs peripheral vision and, if untreated, can cause blindness.

Symptoms of glaucoma can be detected in several ways, such as by measuring the eye's internal pressure and by gauging the extent of peripheral vision.

Internal pressure is measured with an instrument called a tonometer. To make measurements with a traditional type, part of the instrument briefly touches the cornea, so eyedrops containing a local anesthetic are applied to keep the eyelids from flinching. A newer type of tonometer directs a puff of air at the eye, making eyedrops unnecessary. Glaucoma can usually be controlled by drugs, but sometimes corrective surgery is necessary.

Cataracts

An eye exam also includes a check for developing cataracts. A cataract is a gradual clouding of the eye's lens. In some cases, the lens finally turns an opaque white, shutting off vision entirely. Cataracts most often occur among the elderly. German measles in a mother during pregnancy may cause congenital cataracts in her baby. Eye trauma and glaucoma are other causes.

To treat cataracts, the clouded lens is removed surgically. It is then either replaced by glasses, contact lenses, or intraocular lenses.

"Lazy Eye"

In "lazy eye," which doctors call amblyopia, an individual's best vision corrected with glasses is still poorer than normal 20/20 vision. In young children with amblyopia, one eye may appear to be turned away from the line of sight—thus, each eye may point toward a different visual object. This causes two conflicting images to be sent to the brain. To compensate, the brain tends to ignore the image from the lazy eye. As a result, the unused eye doesn't develop normally, and the untreated condition may progress to serious vision impairment.

In almost all cases, lazy eye can be corrected. However, if neglected, by the age of 9 vision in the "lazy" eye may be reduced permanently.

Conjunctivitis

The conjunctiva is a thin, transparent tissue that covers the front of the eye (except for the lens and iris, which are covered by the cornea) and the inside of the eyelids. The conjunctiva is inspected for inflammation (conjunctivitis) and other problems. Inflammation may be caused by microorganisms such as bacteria or viruses, allergenic agents, or chemicals. One common form of annoying—and contagious—conjunctivitis is called red or pink eye for the way it discolors the eye.

Although rare in North America, trachoma, another form of conjunctivitis, is the leading cause of blindness throughout the world. An astounding 500 million people have, or have had this disease, according to Dr. Thomas Chalkey, author of a book on eye care titled *Your Eyes*. It is caused by a microorganism called chlamydia. The infection can cause scarring of the cornea, which can impair or completely destroy vision.

A more detailed examination of the conjunctiva and the other front parts of the eyes is done with an instrument called a slit-lamp, or biomicroscope. The cornea is inspected for signs of disease and when prescribing contact lenses, which fit over the cornea.

Other potential indicators of eye problems may also be checked during a thorough eye exam, such as eye reflexes and muscle balance (to make sure the eyes are properly aligned).

Windows Into the Body

While our eyes serve as our windows on the world, for physicians they can serve as windows on the internal workings of the human body. With the help of an ophthalmoscope—an instrument that focuses a thin beam of light on the retina—an ophthalmologist can examine the inside of the eye and uncover a variety of diseases that may affect the entire body.

After administering eyedrops that contain a drug to dilate the pupil, the physician can peer through the ophthalmoscope to inspect tiny blood vessels called arterioles and venules. Those in the eye nourish the retina as others throughout the body nourish all other parts. But in the living patient, it's possible to see these tiny blood vessels only on the retina.

Their condition can give clues about high blood pressure, diabetes, stroke, transient ischemic attacks (so-called "ministrokes"), hardening of the arteries, and blood diseases such as leukemia.

Microaneurysms, tiny balloon-like swellings of the blood vessels, may be a sign of diabetes. The doctor also can look behind the eye, so to speak, to view the optic nerve (which carries light impulses from the retina to the brain) and examine its shape and color for signs of neurologic diseases such as brain tumors.

Other changes that may be visible include hemorrhages, discolorations and tears of the retina. Other health problems that leave telltale signs include syphilis, sickle cell anemia, collagen diseases such as lupus, lead poisoning, endocarditis (a life-threatening inflammation of the lining of the heart), German measles, and multiple sclerosis.

There's clearly a wealth of medical knowledge to be found within our bodies' "windows"—knowledge important to our overall health, and especially to the most precious of our senses.

A Schedule for Eye Exams

For proper eye care, specialists recommend this schedule of visits:

• Infants with a family history of vision problems, particularly genetic eye diseases, should be examined as early as possible. (Basic eye checks are usually part of routine physicals performed by pediatricians.)

• Preschoolers should be checked by an eye-care practitioner for visual acuity, alignment of the eyes, and eye disease.

• Thereafter, children of school age should be checked once every 18 months to 2 years, nearsighted children more frequently.

• Adults should have an eye examination periodically (the American Optometric Association says once every two years is enough).

• Impairment of accommodation and other eye changes are part of the aging process, so eye-care specialists recommend an examination around age 40. Thereafter, more frequent examinations may be advisable.

Of course, a health professional should be consulted any time there is an injury, infection, or other disorder affecting the eyes.

Who's Who in Eye Care

A person seeking eye care can easily be confused by the names of the different specialists. Opticians, optometrists and ophthalmologists do not have the same training, nor can they provide all the same services. Here's some help in sorting them out.

Ophthalmologist. An ophthalmologist is an M.D.—a doctor of medicine—in the medical and surgical specialty of eye care. Ophthalmologists are trained to treat the eyes for functional problems and for diseases. They have completed four years of undergraduate premed studies, four years of medical school, one year of internship, and a three-year residency in ophthalmology. They must then pass an examination and be licensed by a state medical board to practice medicine. They can prescribe drugs for diagnosing and treating eye problems and can perform eye surgery.

Ophthalmologists are therefore the best prepared to treat eye injuries, pain, swelling, inflammation, and other health concerns connected with the eyes.

Optometrist. An optometrist is a doctor of optometry—but not a medical doctor. Optometrists complete a four-year course of study at an optometric college. They diagnose and treat functional problems and visual defects such as those corrected with glasses, contact lenses, or visual training. In 48 states and the District of Columbia they are licensed to administer diagnostic drugs, and in 12 of these states they may also prescribe therapeutic drugs to treat eye disease.

Many optometrists have an undergraduate college degree even though the prerequisite for admission to schools of optometry is two or three years of undergraduate training.

In order to be licensed, they must pass oral, written and practical examinations.

If glasses or a new prescription for glasses or contact lenses is needed, either an optometrist or an ophthalmologist may be consulted.

Optician. Opticians are technicians who fill prescriptions for eyeglasses. They do not perform eye examinations. Opticians may or may not grind lenses, but they fit them into frames and adjust the frames so that they fit comfortably and the lenses are properly positioned to correct vision defects.

Thirteen states have licensing requirements for opticians. In Virginia, for example, candidates must complete a two-year program of training after high school or a three-year apprenticeship. The other 37 states have no formal requirements.

—by Egon Weck

Chapter 4

Protocols for Choosing Low Vision Devices

Abstract

Protocols for Choosing Low Vision Devices, the fourth Consensus Conference sponsored by the National Institute on Disability and Rehabilitation Research (NIDRR), brought together a variety of disciplines in the field of low vision to arrive at consensus on the best practices for choosing low vision devices. This statement, a product of the Consensus Conference, is a part of NIDRR's ongoing commitment to synthesize available scientific information that can improve the services offered to people with disabilities.

The Conference's 10-member expert panel, which included consumers, commissioned a series of papers summarizing research in the field and listened to a full day of testimony from providers, consumers, family members, researchers, and others in order to determine the current knowledge in the field.

The panel deliberated on questions that define the population of adults who can benefit from low vision devices to improve independence at home and at work, and to enjoy activities that enhance the quality of life. The panel also determined the best standard clinical and functional assessment practices in low vision rehabilitation and the best practices for determining which low vision devices are most effective in maximizing visual function for adults with low vision.

Although a wide array of information, innovations, and best practices were identified at the conference, there remains a substantial

NIDRR, January 1993, Volume 1, Number 4.

number of research questions that await answers. This consensus statement and its identification of future research issues can move the field forward quickly and effectively to meet the needs of people who use low vision devices.

Introduction

Estimates of the numbers of people with visual impairments in the United States range from 6 to 11.4 million. The most prevalent causes of visual impairment in this country are age-related: macular degeneration, diabetic retinopathy, glaucoma, and cataract. Visual impairment is commonly related to other impairments, causing multiple handicaps for people of all ages. Approximately 60 percent of people with visual impairments who are not institutionalized have one or more additional impairments as well. Vision loss has been ranked third, behind arthritis and heart disease, among the most common chronic conditions causing a need for assistance in activities of daily living for people who are elderly. These estimates include younger adults who have congenital visual impairments (such as Retinopathy of Prematurity or Albinism) and who have acquired visual impairments in youth (such as Retinitis Pigmentosa or Stargardts Disease).

Approximately 90 percent of individuals with visual impairments have useful vision. For these people, low vision devices and rehabilitation offer opportunities to enhance visual capacity. Low vision devices—optical, non-optical, and electronic—and rehabilitation provide means of augmenting or restoring independent function for daily activities. The ability to take advantage of low vision devices may allow individuals with low vision to be independent at home and at work, and enjoy activities that enhance quality of life.

Professionals, and peers working closely with individuals with low vision, and their significant others comprise the interdisciplinary network. Case management and decision-making are accomplished by dialogue among network team members. Professionals in low vision are mandated to provide educational opportunities that insure consumer input, because individuals must set personal goals and make final decisions about the usefulness of their low vision devices.

The professionals and consumers who participated in this consensus conference collaborated to develop consensus on the best practices for providing low vision devices. This consensus includes evaluating needs for intervention and deriving the best decision making processes for determining appropriate device(s) for specific individuals who wish to perform specific tasks. Following the presentation of expert testimony, the consensus panel deliberated to synthesize this information with that contained in research summaries prepared for their use in order to formulate responses to the following six questions:

1. What clinical measurements and functional behaviors define the population of adults who can benefit from low vision devices (any optical or non-optical device or environmental modification that enhances visual performance)?

2. What are the best standard clinical and functional assessment practices in vision rehabilitation addressing the needs of adults with low vision? What assessment and referral services do primary health care specialists (MD, OD, DO) provide for adults with low vision?

3. What are the optical-functional characteristics of available low vision devices that meet the needs of adults with low vision?

4. What are the best practices for determining which low vision devices will be most effective in maximizing visual function for adults with low vision? (Factors for consideration should include cosmetic acceptability and other psychosocial issues, cost effectiveness, accessibility, user-friendliness, and maintenance/repair/durability issues.)

5. What instruction and guided practice currently best insures successful utilization of devices?

6. What future research is needed?

What Clinical Measurements and Functional Behaviors Define the Population of Adults Who Can Benefit from Low Vision Devices?

Low vision, a term which emerged in the 1960's and has since gained wide acceptance and usage, is a general term which describes a serious loss of vision which may be congenitally or adventitiously acquired. This condition may result from eye diseases or accidents,

31

or it may result from health-related conditions commonly associated with the aging process, and cannot be adequately corrected medically, surgically, or with conventional spectacles or contact lenses. The population of individuals with low vision is far from homogeneous. It includes people with widely differing degrees and types of visual loss. Definitions are left broad and loosely specified for a reason. A study by the World Health Organization found no less than 65 different definitions of the level of visual function at which a person could be declared legally blind. Approximately 90 percent of people with low vision have some degree of measurable residual vision.

While commonly defined clinically in terms of remaining visual acuity or reduced visual field, the widely accepted World Health Organization's definition divides low vision into three categories: moderate, severe, and profound visual impairment, involving best corrected visual acuities from 20/70 to 20/500 and less, or visual fields of 10 degrees diameter or less. The World Health Organization further provides functional descriptions ranging from performing visual tasks at reduced levels to difficulty with gross visual tasks.

As recognition accumulates that clinical data alone gives little practical information regarding functional performance or difficulties experienced or needs of the individual involved, there has been a steady increase in emphasis on defining low vision functionally. Best practice underscores the importance of functional behaviors. For example, an individual with only light projection may be able to utilize this vision to plan or execute a task such as avoiding obstacles when traveling.

Blindness and visual impairment in technically developed countries is largely an age-related problem. Studies indicate that approximately 70 percent of people with low vision are over age 70. Increased longevity, habits of an improved life style, and improved medical control of such diseases as diabetes and hypertension are producing a steady increase in demands for assistance, information and services by adults with low vision.

Many "normal" aging changes are exacerbated for people with low vision. A person with an optically-reduced visual loss resulting from irregularities in refractive surfaces or media usually suffers from a degradation of the visual image. This deficit results from excessive intraocular scatter, which causes lower visual acuity and reduced contract sensitivity. Such a person has greater difficulty with resolution tasks, and as the angular extent of scatter broadens, resolution and performance suffer.

In some people, visual acuity may remain unaffected, but contrast sensitivity of all objects within the visual field is diminished. Research has demonstrated that loss of contrast sensitivity and loss of visual field contribute significantly to impaired mobility because of decreased vision. Additionally, visual acuity has been found to be a relatively poor predictor of mobility performance and reading accuracy.

Other functional behaviors associated with severe visual impairment may include difficulties with:

- reading printed materials
- writing, particularly on a straight line
- face recognition
- color discrimination
- detail vision at near and far distances
- depth perception
- light and dark adaptation, and
- light and glare sensitivity

There are important psycho-social issues which should not be overlooked. Some people who have experienced a recent visual loss may still be seeking a "miracle" cure and many have difficulty coming to terms with visual impairment which is not reversible. In cases of rapid onset of visual loss, this problem may be exacerbated. Such people and their families may experience natural feelings associated with loss which require substantial support and counseling from optometrists, ophthalmologists, social workers, rehabilitation and employment professionals, and peers.

A person with low vision may experience problems in performing daily activities such as dressing, grooming, personal hygiene, eating, telling time, caring for clothes and personal effects—virtually every facet of daily life. He or she may need to relearn many routines. Social insecurities and communication difficulties may be experienced, independence may be reduced, and self-esteem may be affected. Thus, the cognitive and psychological states of people with low vision, their ability to perform daily activities, and their socioeconomic need should be assessed.

What Are the Best Standard Clinical and Functional Assessment Practices in Vision Rehabilitation Addressing the Needs of Adults with Low Vision?

In availability and practice, a variety of clinical and functional methods exist for assessing the vision of adults with low vision. Best practice dictates an integrative approach of clinical and functional components to address the holistic nature of each individual. While type of delivery method (sole practitioner or team approach) and setting of delivery (hospital, rehabilitation center, etc.), may vary, an interdisciplinary assessment involving professionals from eyecare and vision rehabilitation is recommended. For the sole practitioner, this interdisciplinary approach need not be site specific. It can be achieved through a coordinated set of interdisciplinary referrals aimed at soliciting assessment information upon which the best decisions can be made regarding appropriate low vision services.

Elements of a comprehensive clinical assessment include:

- History. Individuals' concerns and interests, goal setting, knowledge of vision condition, occupational information, task-specific vision requirements, visual and medical history, family/friends support, attitude toward visual impairment, previous and current use of optical devices, current visual performance, and response to different illumination.

- Ocular Health. External and internal eye examination.

- Refraction. Objective (retinoscopy) and subjective (patient interpretation).

- Visual Acuities. Single letter and continuous text; near, intermediate and distance; monocular and binocular, with and without current prescriptive lenses, under different conditions of illumination.

- Visual Fields. Central and peripheral, monocular and binocular, under different conditions of illumination.

- Contrast Sensitivity. Monocular and binocular, varying distances.

- Illumination and Glare. Assessment of the impact by illumination and glare reduction adaptation on visual performance.

- Binocularity. Objective and subjective degree [thereof.]

- Optical and Non-optical Device Evaluation. Near, intermediate and distant magnification; magnification; visual field enhancement systems; lighting and glare control and recovery testing; assistive non-optical devices such as large print, reading stands, filters, signature guides.

- Direction and degree of eccentric viewing for persons with macular loss.

- Color Evaluation. Using larger target sizes.

- Ancillary Assessment. Referrals to such services as electrodiagnostic testing, genetic evaluation, prosthetic device evaluation.

A number of instruments are used to assess visual acuity and visual field. For appropriate testing, a standard visual acuity chart should include:

- the same number of symbols on each size line

- standardized spacing proportional to the size of letters or symbols, and spacing between rows proportional to the size of letters

- logarithmic size progression (constant ratio)

- acuity discrimination tasks should be the same at each distance or with whatever magnification device is used.

In addition to single letter acuity, continuous text acuity is important in determining the necessary optical device for reading activities, especially for people with macular losses. Recent research suggests the benefits of assessing reserve acuity versus threshold acuity when evaluating and recommending magnification for reading.

Both central and peripheral field assessments are important parts of evaluation. The tangent screen measures the central 30 degrees of field primarily necessary for a near point task. While grids measuring the central 10 degrees are widely used, recent research has shown them to be less valuable tools than previously thought. The emerging search coil instruments and scanning laser ophthalmoscope technology are particularly useful for precise mapping of field loss and designation of eccentric viewing positions. In addition, the scanning laser ophthalmoscope affords the clinician a more complete assessment of visual acuity anywhere on the retina. Though not widely available, referral for this information augments a comprehensive clinical assessment.

Perimetry field tests measuring peripheral fields are performed especially for people with severely constricted fields or pathology suggesting irregular scotomas throughout the field. Evidence suggests that it is worthwhile for the clinician to use threshold-size targets to obtain more precise measurements of threshold fields, as well as targets increased in size 10 or more times to assess gross or substantial loss of field. In addition, bowl perimetry enables the manipulation of variables such as target size and luminance, which are critical factors in the everyday functioning of a person with low vision. Perimetry field assessments are critical in the eventual recommendation of visual field enhancement systems for people with severely constricted fields.

The functional assessment determines a person's understanding and use of vision with and without low vision devices. It is understood and guided by the needs and goals of the individual relative to enhanced vision functioning in daily activities and common settings such as home, work and community environments. Assessment results guide instructional strategies and provide information to discriminate what combination of visual and non-visual techniques most appropriately enable the individual to accomplish a desired or required task. Though functional assessments of vision are often conducted after the clinical assessment, it is a recommended pre-clinical activity, as information gained facilitates the clinical assessment and promotes greater success. Any member of the interdisciplinary team might perform the assessment, depending on the variables of time, location, etc. In addition, for optimal results, it is necessary to conduct the assessment with and without optical and non-optical tools. It is also necessary to consider the need for instruction in the use of devices as part of the ongoing assessment process. Finally, the assessment, if possible, should occur in the person's own home, work, or community setting, using materials specific to the person's desired goals.

Common elements of a comprehensive functional assessment include:

- Initial interview—with emphasis on knowledge of, and previous/ current use of vision and low vision devices, goals/needs, everyday activities and interests, expectations, family/significant other involvement, etc.

- Functional visual acuities at varying distances and under varying conditions of illumination. Threshold identification and optimum viewing distances are noted for discriminating and identifying common objects such as food can labels, television, indoor and outdoor signs, facial details, printed materials, etc.

- Functional visual fields including extent of everyday objects and information perceived in upper, lower and side fields, and at near, intermediate and distant view. These are performed in both static and dynamic mode and in both indoor and outdoor settings, under varying lighting and weather conditions.

- Color/Contrast—including ability to discriminate and identify a variety of materials, objects, colors, and shades under varying figure-ground and lighting conditions.

- Ocular motor skills—fixation, localization, scanning, tracing, and tracking of objects, reading materials, etc.

- Lighting—including type, amount, position, and angle of light source used while performing tasks.

- Glare—including effects of glare in various settings, amount of time necessary to adapt from indoor to outdoor lighting and vice versa, and effect of absorptive lenses and non-optical techniques on eliminating glare.

- Combined use of visual and non-visual cues including detection of a variety of objects, landmarks, depth (slopes, steps, curbs), glass doorways, terrain differences, etc.

- Use of vision for performance of specific tasks that comprise the individual's goals.

A comprehensive mix of the above components comprises an environmental assessment which can be tailored to meet the specific needs of each individual. In keeping with this approach, it is necessary to attend to what the individual brings to the process: values, beliefs, attitudes and life experiences. Understanding the importance of relevant cultural issues, using appropriate assessment materials and approaches, and incorporating family members and support systems into both the clinical and functional assessment process augment chances for greater success.

The assessment process culminates in a vision rehabilitation plan which is a summary of the information with the person being evaluated, and with emphasis on an educational as opposed to a prescriptive process. A comprehensive instructional program in the use of vision, both with and without low vision devices, and in combination with other sensory systems, is recommended if successful rehabilitation is the goal.

What Assessment and Referral Services Do Primary Care Specialists (MD, OD, DO) Provide for Adults with Low Vision?

Typically, the primary health care specialist examining an adult with low vision will assess ocular health status and the general integrity of the visual system including refractive error and a basic assessment of magnification needs. People with higher levels of acuity are usually treated for minimum magnification needs. Those with more severe vision impairments should be referred to clinicians (optometrists or ophthalmologists) specializing in low vision.

There are a host of potential referrals which will be based on the condition of the individual, on the thoroughness of examining practitioners, and on the setting within which they practice.

Just as a person who loses a limb is naturally referred to physical rehabilitation, an individual with low vision should experience the same referral flow to vision rehabilitation. Proper referral bridges the gap between health care and rehabilitation. Of primary importance is the immediacy of the referral, as delay may result in reduced independent functioning and psycho-social problems for the adult with low vision.

Additional referrals will depend upon other sensory, emotional, mental or physical conditions. Examples of possible referrals representing best practice include, but are not limited to:

- general practitioner for systemic conditions;
- genetic counselor for hereditary eye conditions;
- neurologist for unexplained vision fluctuations or field loss;
- rehabilitation counselors, orientation and mobility specialists, and rehabilitation teachers for vision rehabilitation services;
- physical and occupational therapists for physical/motor assessments;
- psychologist, social worker, or gerontologist for counseling and human services;
- speech pathologists and augmentative communication specialists; and
- specialists such as diabetologists, audiologists, etc. depending upon additional problems discussed or detected.

Comprehensive referrals to a network of diverse professionals further assures the interdisciplinary array of assessment information necessary to look beyond the eye toward the needs of the whole person.

What Are the Optical and Functional Characteristics of Low Vision Devices that Meet the Needs of Adults with Low Vision?

Most low vision devices are "task specific", that is, their optical characteristics do not allow individuals to use the same device for all visual tasks desired. This paper classifies low vision devices as optical (providing magnification, magnification, and perceived field expansion) or non-optical devices. The cognitive abilities of individuals with low vision is assumed to be equal to the task to be performed.

Magnification may be classified as of four types: relative size, relative distance, angular, and electronic. Relative distance magnification is provided by bringing the target to be viewed close to the eye. Spectacle magnifiers focus the image at ranges closer than the eyes can accommodate, and allow very close distances. Lenses must be prescribed by an eye care specialist experienced in low vision, in order to incorporate the refractive error of the individual. Spectacle magnifiers can be prescribed for bifocal, half-eye, full field, and for use with one or both eyes. Typically, devices require a close working distance and have a short depth of focus. Depending on power and focal distance, they can be used for near tasks such as reading, writing, viewing photographs, etc. Individuals need to maintain the focal distance, maintain fixation through the center of the lens (using eccentric viewing if necessary) and to scan the target, usually continuous text, with a well developed scanning pattern. Motor skills are required to hold the target at the correct distance and, in the case of reading, to move the target slowly to the left to see successive words on a line. Using all these skills at the same time can require both instruction and practice, because high magnification usually results in a small field of view, and because postural adjustments must be made to achieve success.

Magnification may also be provided by stand or hand-held magnifiers. These devices are often easier to use, they do not require a close eye to lens distance, and some are available with built-in illumination. Individuals who develop low vision later in life may have previously used these devices for tasks like map-reading, so they seem more familiar. These devices are used for reading, writing and other near tasks, and require the same visual skills as spectacle magnifiers. The distance from lens to eye may be wherever the individual feels most comfortable. Hand held magnifiers require a steady hand to maintain the focus, and may be fatiguing for long-term use. Stand magnifiers require the ability to accommodate, or the individual must wear an appropriately determined near prescription.

Telescopic devices provide angular magnification by the use of a positive and negative lens in a housing (Galilean) or by the use of two positive lenses with an erecting prism (Keplerian). Optical design of telescopes influences quality and brightness of image and field of view. They are commonly used by individuals with low vision for tasks that require arms length or further viewing, including such tasks as identifying street signs, or sustained viewing such as watching television. These devices are available in a wide variety of powers, types, and prescribing options. Mounting options for spectacle-borne telescopes include a center mount for watching TV or sports, a bioptic mount for alternate viewing through the carrier lens and the telescope, and a "surgical" mount for viewing at intermediate ranges. Recent advances in the design of such devices include variable focus, a short focus feature, smaller telescopes, and telescopes with less obtrusive appearances. The visual skills required for using telescopes include spotting, scanning, tracing, tracking and focusing. Holding a monocular or binocular to the eye while performing visual tasks can be challenging for some individuals, and mounted telescopes may overcome problems with motor coordination. Many individuals have used binoculars prior to the onset of visual impairment for sports, bird-watching, or other tasks, and will be able to transfer those skills to the use of a telescope. If the individual wishes to drive with a telescope, more instruction and practice is usually necessary. The telescope prescribed for driving will usually be a superior bioptic mount.

The closed circuit television system (CCTV), an example of electronic magnification, was introduced in the '60s as an option for providing low vision individuals with a method of performing near tasks such as reading or writing. Although the camera can be used at any distance, this system is often designed for creative use in home, vocational, and educational settings. The advantages of the CCTV include more magnification than any other device, a wider field of view, and contrast enhancement via reverse polarity. While the CCTV makes some visual skills easier, such as fixation with eccentric viewing, localization and scanning require other motor skills, and the ability to set the magnification, focus the camera, and move the material on the XY table can be challenging. A digital low vision magnifying device has been developed that provides an automatic computer-controlled scrolling mechanism for the individual and alleviates the need for this motor skill. Although overhead and rear screen projection are useful for some tasks, they are not routinely used as low vision devices. Electronic magnification, including the closed circuit television system, offers future promise for low vision devices that are not bound by the optical principle of "more magnification equals smaller field of view." Low vision researchers are studying electronic magnification as a means to provide new low vision devices that are miniaturized, headborne versions of the CCTV. These devices offer a mechanism for taking advantage of new computer technology such as contrast enhancement, image warping, and field remapping.

A variety of software and hardware packages have been developed that produce enlarged print on the computer screen. Computer use in conjunction with CCTV can utilize multiple camera sources to provide split screen images for designing a work station that simultaneously accesses computer, print viewing, typing, and distance viewing.

Devices that minify are helpful to individuals who maintain high acuity while experiencing decreased field of view. Minifying devices provide the ability to find targets by expanding the perceived field of view. Once the desired target is spotted, it can be viewed by an individual without the minifying device to obtain full detail. The minifier may be as simple as a low power telescope viewed in reverse, through the objective rather than the ocular lens, or as complicated as a pair of reverse telescopes mounted in a bioptic position. An "amorphic" lens is available that minifies in the horizontal meridian only. Perceived field expansion may also be obtained by the use of prisms attached to a pair of spectacles. The most commonly prescribed are Fresnel press-on prisms. This field expansion system requires individuals to become comfortable with the prism blur and displacement, and overcome problems with image confusion. As an individual practices with the prism, enough scanning ability is usually developed that the prism segment must be reduced in size. If a permanent prism system is to be used, the Fresnel prism can be used for instruction and loaned for practice. Special mirrors may also be prescribed for field enhancement with hemianopsia.

Non-optical devices may enhance visual function. Included in this category are illumination controls such as lamps, shades, sunglasses, typoscopes and colored filters. Some individuals require more illumination, especially for near tasks such as reading or sewing, but are susceptible to glare. Individuals who are photophobic may find that light filtering lenses, side shields, visors, caps or hats make them more comfortable. Custom filtering lenses can block a higher percentage of the total light spectrum or selectively filter the portion of the light spectrum causing sensitivity to glare. These devices also assist individuals who have long adaptation times when traveling from a bright environment to a dim one or vice versa. Some low vision devices require environments with appropriate illumination controls, reading stand, table, chair with arms, good back and neck support, etc. Environmental modifications that meet the needs of adults with low vision include changes in color, contrast, illumination and size and position of targets to be viewed in the environment. Recent research has shown that appropriate lighting can increase reading rates with optical low vision devices; unless individuals duplicate clinical lighting at home, reading rates drop. Sunlight, incandescent, fluorescent, halogen, and high pressure sodium lamps offer choices. Recent research has suggested that electroluminescent panels may provide lighting that is cool and glare-free. Although experts agree that individualized lighting systems are important to the successful use of low vision devices, there are no clinical guidelines that enable practitioners to evaluate and recommend the most appropriate lighting.

Recommendations are usually the result of individual selection after experimentation.

Improved contrast through the use of filters or reversed polarity can also enhance visual performance with and without devices, and has been shown to increase reading speed for individuals with cloudy media.

Large print books, large phone dials, felt tip pen, and bold line paper employ relative size magnification to allow individuals with low vision to read and write more comfortably. Reading stands assist by holding reading material so that the short or fixed focus of low vision devices is easier to manage. Signature guides and stencils assist in writing.

Device portability is an important feature. Most devices are fairly small and may be carried in pocket or purse, but larger devices such as headborne telescopes require their own carrying cases or may be hung around the neck. Many individuals with low vision find that more than one device is required to meet their viewing needs and so must carry all of them in order to enhance vision in a variety of environments. Some electronic low vision devices are portable and are provided with carrying cases, but most electronic low vision devices are meant for stationary use at home, work, or school. There are situations in which the optical/functional characteristics of the most appropriate low vision devices presently available still do not meet the needs of an individual (e.g. a certain reading rate); it is often advisable to evaluate non-visual techniques.

Although full scale studies of the use of low vision devices have not been done, researchers have shown that approximately 45 percent to 80 percent of individuals prescribed low vision devices continue to use them. Information from previous studies is difficult to extrapolate because of differences in definitions of success. The characteristics of low vision devices and the effects of service delivery models that relate to use or non-use have yet to be researched.

What Are the Best Practices for Determining Which Low Vision Devices Will Be Most Effective in Maximizing Visual Function for Adults with Low Vision?

Best practice includes several distinct components which need to be considered individually and in combination when determining the most effective low vision device(s) for any individual. This selection process is conducted through many models of best practice which typically include an interdisciplinary team approach and designated case management with an emphasis on the empowerment of the individual with vision loss. Opinions vary concerning the appropriate sequence in which the components are provided. The components include:

1. functional goal setting concerning distinct visual tasks required or desired;

2. holistic evaluation of the individual involving multiple considerations apart from vision such as lifestyle, other disabilities, and priority of need among functional goals. The formal and informal support systems of the individual should be understood;

3. discussion with the individual concerning the range of potential feelings about low vision and the use of low vision devices;

4. comprehensive clinical evaluation conducted by an optometrist or ophthalmologist who is knowledgeable in low vision rehabilitation to discover whether and how the patient's residual vision can be enhanced by use of aids and devices;

5. evaluation of functional abilities, in the individual's everyday environments, whenever possible, incorporating tasks related to established functional goals. Since devices are always used within an environmental context, any needs for environmental modifications should be considered. Assessments should be made by qualified professionals who have had extensive training in the functional use of vision. Additional team members may include professionals from other disciplines whose expertise is relevant to an individual's overall functioning;

6. discussion concerning strengths and limitations of potential low vision devices and, when appropriate, between visual and non-visual approaches to functional tasks. This discussion should include the stability of the ocular disease entity and the need for refractive correction. Concerning potential low vision devices, the discussion should address: the adjustability, availability, cost and cost-effectiveness, maintainability, safety, transferability, and portability. In addition, the individual

should be encouraged to consider when to use non-visual approaches to functional tasks;

7. meeting with a peer counselor and/or support group to reinforce personal aspects of successful use of devices;

8. thorough instruction in the effective use of prescribed/selected low vision devices. Members of the individual's support system may require orientation and instruction concerning the functional capabilities and expectations for use of devices;

9. a trial and instructional period with loaner devices during which potential low vision devices are evaluated in "real world" application;

10. when appropriate, referral to consultation with an electronic aids specialist for selection and training in the use of the most appropriate computer access system or related technology;

11. modifications to the environment that are required for successful use of the devices. These include adjustments to lighting, positioning of materials to avoid postural strain, glare reduction, contrast enhancement, and the addition of tactile and auditory modifications.

12. final selection of low vision devices based on the synthesis of experiences during training and trial periods;

13. thorough determination of financial resources and funding alternatives for the purchase of selected low vision devices and associated services; and

14. on-going follow up service to monitor the continued effectiveness of the device to enhance visual functioning and to determine if there are any changes in other factors that may affect visual functioning. Follow up services include the opportunity to repeat any of the other components as needed.

Selection of a low vision device is a dynamic, multi-factored, complex matter. Best practice is based on updated knowledge of demonstrated, effective clinical and instructional techniques, coupled with an intuitive and sensitive approach which develops understanding, acknowledges and supports feelings, inspires and harnesses motivation, and reinforces success. Many of these components are interpersonal rather than clinical.

What Instruction and Guided Practice Currently Best Insures Successful Utilization of Devices?

For the purpose of this document, successful utilization of devices refers to use of a device, for the tasks for which it was prescribed or provided, effectively and efficiently within the bounds of the device's limitations. Ultimately, success is based on the opinion of the individual using the device, with input from professionals about the device's capabilities and the performance-limiting factors of the level and type of available vision. Because no studies have documented long range utilization of devices, there is little research documenting the instruction and guided practice techniques that insure success.

Instruction and guided practice are planned after clinical and functional assessments are completed and are driven by the goals of the individual. The low vision instructor compiles all information from the clinical and functional low vision assessment, and other relevant records and information that help in planning and implementing the instruction.

Best practice in this area suggests that the instructor or therapist be knowledgeable and skilled, not only in rehabilitation instruction, but also in the nature of vision, visual impairment, functional use of vision, basic optical principles, and the optical and functional characteristics of low vision devices. The instructor or therapist must also be knowledgeable and skilled in teaching the use of basic non-visual adaptive equipment and techniques. The instructor or therapist must make knowledgeable referrals to other rehabilitation professionals such as occupational or physical therapists, reading specialists, orientation and mobility specialists, and rehabilitation teachers.

The instructor gives the individual a prediction of the scope and duration of instruction required to meet goals. The range of possible devices is presented tactually and visually, and the instructor describes the devices, their uses, advantages and limitations. Limitations such as a small field of view, speed smear, initial experiences of nausea, and acuity decrease with prism, can be daunting. Individuals may need reassurance that instruction and practice can overcome initial difficulty and that use of devices can become automatic. "Trade-offs" between device limitation and the individuals' ability to complete personal goals must be discussed.

Professionals have recommended a sequence of instructional procedures that cover several areas:

- use of visual skills without low vision devices,
- use of visual skills with low vision devices, and
- use of vision and low vision devices for individualized functional tasks.

Instruction in the use of visual skills without devices covers:

- fixation,
- spotting,
- localization,
- scanning,
- tracing, and
- tracking

Individuals with macular degeneration may require additional instruction in the development and maintenance of fixation using eccentric viewing.

Instruction in the use of visual skills with low vision devices includes integrating unaided abilities with the unique demands of a device, such as maintaining focal distance or focusing the device and adjusting eye and head movements to compensate for a restricted field of view. If the individual is using eccentric viewing, the instructor assures that the device selected allows the opportunity to maximize field and acuity in the eccentric position.

These skills are initially demonstrated in the clinical setting using targets that are selected by the instructor to ensure success. The instructor alters the environment to provide illumination and glare control, non-optical support devices such as reading stand or typoscope, to further ensure success. Frustration is minimized when an instructor can task-analyze in order to teach visual skills at the level of understanding and ability of the individual. Successively increasing the difficulty of the task until the individual achieves the task will maximize success. The pace of instruction is determined by the learning ability and style of the individual. If progress is slow, or reaches a plateau, the instructor or the individual may decide that using vision for the task is not feasible. Alternatives must be presented and experienced by the individual.

The use of vision and low vision devices must take place in the environment in which the task would usually be performed, or in a clinical or teaching setting that has been altered to resemble that environment. The instructor insures proficiency in goal-related tasks, or recommends additional instruction, and can assist with additional non-optical devices, including strategies for environmental modifications. If it is not possible to instruct in the actual environment, best practice dictates that the individual be loaned a device for practice in the actual environment. The instructor may provide on-site environmental analysis and suggest modifications. Modifications may include changes in illumination and glare control, color, contrast, size and distance of targets to be viewed, and changes that allow greater physical comfort of the individual for using vision. Modifications may be non-visual, such as tactile markings or audible outputs for clocks or appliance controls. Research has shown that duplicating clinically recommended lighting in the home environment increases reading speed with magnification. Studies have indicated that individuals who receive environmental modifications and on-site instruction with their low vision devices significantly improve their skills over those who receive clinical instruction only.

Best practice in instruction and guided practice with low vision devices includes:

1. the development of an individualized vision rehabilitation plan based on clinical and functional assessment for the goals identified by the individual;

2. guided instruction in the use of unaided visual skills, aided visual skills, and the use of the device for real world tasks;

3. instruction and practice which takes place in real environment and incorporates teaching the use of vision and devices for the actual task to be performed; and

4. follow-up by telephone, mail, or home visit that identifies possible vision changes, use and effectiveness of low vision devices, and need for further services.

What Future Research Is Needed?

Future basic and applied research should reflect the trend toward interdisciplinary and collaborative investigations, and include people with low vision as equal partners. Desired directions might include research under the following six headings:

Technology

- Design and development of new technology including optical and electronic systems as well as computer technology that are easier to use, and are less noticeable.

- Development of universal/accessible design criteria for existing and emerging technology in low vision.

- Development of technology to give people with visual impairments immediate access to electronic source materials for printed documents.

Environmental Issues

- Ergonomic design of living environments, including home, workplace, and related settings for individuals with low vision.

- Environmental design factors and standards relating to signage, industrial design, print legibility, contrast, proper illumination, glare control, and visual factors that facilitate independent travel.

- Public safety studies on needs of people with low vision (e.g., audible traffic signals, detectable tactile and visual warnings for curb cuts and hazardous vehicular ways).

- Develop technology which gives immediate access for individuals with low vision to electronic source material for printed documents.

Social/Cultural Applied Research

- Studies of social and cultural contexts in which low vision is experienced as a disability.

- Social and cultural and gender differences as they apply to service delivery, particularly the choice and use of low vision devices and environmental modifications.

- Development of strategies to identify needs and to cope with increasing demands for services by people who are aging and/or multiply disabled.

- Definition of elements of public policy that promote or limit the delivery of low vision services.

- International and cross-cultural research into alternative service delivery models.

- Identification of demographic factors in the selection and use of low vision devices.

Service Delivery

- Identify the most effective models of service delivery.

- Identify needed and effective comprehensive services for unserved and underserved populations, including ethnic minorities and individuals living in rural/remote areas.

- Gather data that will enable the formulation of national policy on equitable funding for providing low vision services and devices.

- Study the impact of the interaction between individuals with low vision and primary care physicians; how it affects functional assessment, management, and outcome of the low vision service.

- Prepare longitudinal studies of the effectiveness of low vision devices.

- Study existing curricular and instructional training materials to develop model curricular in low vision rehabilitation.

Basic and Clinical Sciences

- Evaluation of existing low-vision diagnostic procedures and the development of new methods that meet validation and reliability criteria.

- Basic research on the components of visual processing and their integration into effective visual function.

- Determination of visual criteria and training procedures for safe automobile driving by people with low vision.

- Validation of instructional procedures for the use of low vision devices.

- Development and validation of functional visual assessment instruments.

- Development and validation of measures of low vision rehabilitation outcomes.

Personal Preparation

- Studies of existing curricular and instructional materials to develop model curricular for preservice and inservice educational programs in low vision rehabilitation.

- Studies of effective strategies for team building and interdisciplinary communication and collaboration in vision rehabilitation.

Chapter 5

Music for Blind and Physically Handicapped Individuals

A special music collection for blind and physically handicapped individuals was authorized by Congress in 1962 as part of the free national library program of braille and recorded books and magazines administered by the National Library Service for the Blind and Physically Handicapped (NLS), Library of Congress. With the cooperation of composers and publishers who grant permission to use copyrighted works, NLS selects and produces music scores in braille and large-print formats and music magazines and books about music and musicians in large-print, braille, and recorded formats.

People interested in music materials receive them directly from NLS in Washington, D.C., rather than through the NLS network of cooperating libraries that circulates general reading materials and loans playback machines to eligible patrons. Music materials are sent to borrowers and returned to NLS by postage-free mail. Music patrons nationwide can call NLS toll free at 800-424-8567.

Eligibility

Anyone who is unable to read or use standard printed materials as a result of temporary or permanent visual or physical limitations may receive service. A survey sponsored by NLS found that two million persons with some type of visual impairment may be eligible and another million with physical conditions such as paralysis, missing

National Library Service for the Blind and Physically Handicapped Fact Sheet, January 1994.

arms or hands, lack of muscle coordination, or prolonged weakness could benefit from the use of reading materials in recorded form.

Magazines

Six music magazines are offered by direct mail to eligible readers. *Stereo Review*, containing reviews of audio recordings and equipment, and *Contemporary Sound Track: A Review of Pop, Jazz, Rock, and Country*, an NLS-compiled sampler of articles from national magazines, are available on flexible audio disc. The Quarterly Music Magazine Program, also on flexible audio disc, consists of four different and complete music magazine issues a year. The *Musical Mainstream*, another NLS-compiled sampler, is produced in large print and braille and on flexible audio disc, and includes current articles on classical music and music education reprinted from national magazines. The *Braille Music Magazine*, containing articles from British magazines about classical music and music criticism, is produced in braille by the Royal National Institute for the Blind. *Popular Music Lead Sheets* is published in braille by NLS. It contains melodies, lyrics, and chords to popular songs ranging from "golden oldies" to recent hits. The Collection The music collection, made up of some 30,000 books, scores, and instructional recordings, is a major resource for blind, partially sighted, and physically handicapped musicians, music students, and others who enjoy music.

Braille

Materials in braille make up the largest portion of the collection and include the standard repertoire for most instruments, vocal and choral music, some popular music, librettos, textbooks, instructional method books, and music periodicals. Braille is purchased comprehensively from international sources. The NLS Music Section also serves as an international clearinghouse for information about music that has been transcribed into braille and is available for individual purchase or for international interlibrary loan or purchase.

Large Print

Enlarged scores with a minimum of 14-point type size and a staff size of one inch are available for voice, piano, and other instruments.

Patrons can also borrow books about music, including opera librettos, biographies of popular and classical musicians, general music histories, and some music reference books.

Recorded

The material on audio discs and cassettes includes music theory, appreciation, and history; biographical sketches of musicians and examples of their art; interviews and master classes; and instruction for various instruments.

Courses for beginning guitar, piano, organ, accordion, recorder, and voice, and in modern harmony have been purchased or specifically developed for the NLS program. Musical recordings intended solely for entertainment, however, are not part of the free library program since these materials are readily available from stores and local libraries.

For Further Information

More information, including applications and catalogs of brailled, recorded, and large-print music materials, may be obtained by writing or calling NLS or by completing and mailing the attached preaddressed form. The toll-free number is 800-424-8567.

Chapter 6

Books for Blind and Physically Handicapped Individuals

A free national library program of braille and recorded materials for blind and physically handicapped persons is administered by the National Library Service for the Blind and Physically Handicapped (NLS), Library of Congress. With the cooperation of authors and publishers who grant permission to use copyrighted works, NLS selects and produces full-length books and magazines in braille and on recorded disc and cassette. Reading materials are distributed to a cooperating network of regional and subregional (local) libraries where they are circulated to eligible borrowers. Reading materials and playback machines are sent to borrowers and returned to libraries by postage-free mail. Established by an act of Congress in 1931 to serve blind adults, the program was expanded in 1952 to include children, in 1962 to provide music materials, and again in 1966 to include individuals with other physical impairments that prevent the reading of standard print.

Funding

The NLS program is funded annually by Congress. The fiscal year 1994 appropriation was $42,613,000. Regional and subregional libraries receive funding from state, local, and federal sources. Through an additional appropriation to the U.S. Postal Service, books and materials

National Library Service for the Blind and Physically Handicapped, Fact Sheet, January 1995.

are mailed as "Free Matter for the Blind and Handicapped." The combined expenditure for the program is approximately $120 million.

Eligibility

Anyone who is unable to read or use standard printed materials as a result of temporary or permanent visual or physical limitations may receive service. A survey sponsored by NLS found that two million persons with some type of visual impairment may be eligible and another million with physical conditions such as paralysis, missing arms or hands, lack of muscle coordination, or prolonged weakness could benefit from the use of reading materials in recorded form.

Book Collection

Books are selected on the basis of their appeal to a wide range of interests. Bestsellers, biographies, fiction, and how-to books are in great demand. Titles expected to be extremely popular are produced on flexible audio disc in several thousand copies and circulated to borrowers within several months of their publication in print form. A limited number of titles are produced in Spanish and other languages for readers whose primary language is not English. Registered borrowers learn of new books added to the collection through two bimonthly publications, *Braille Book Review* and *Talking Book Topics*. Through a union catalog available on microfiche and in computerized form, every network library has access to the entire NLS book collection and to the resources of several cooperating agencies.

Magazines

Over seventy magazines on audio disc and in braille are offered through the program. Readers may request free subscriptions to *U.S. News and World Report, National Geographic, Consumer Reports, Good Housekeeping, Sports Illustrated, Jack and Jill,* and many other popular magazines. Current issues are mailed to readers at the same time the print issues appear, or shortly thereafter. Magazines are selected for the program in response to demonstrated reader interest.

Equipment and Accessories

Playback equipment is loaned free to readers for as long as recorded materials provided by NLS and its cooperating libraries are being borrowed. Talking-book machines are designed to play disc books and magazines recorded at 8 rpm and 16 rpm; cassette machines are designed for cassettes recorded at 15/16 ips and the standard speed of 1-7/8 ips on 2 and 4 tracks. Readers with very limited mobility may request a remote-control unit; hearing impaired readers may be eligible for an auxiliary amplifier for use with headphones. A cassette machine designed primarily for persons with limited manual dexterity is also available.

Music Services

Persons interested in music materials may receive them directly from the Music Section of NLS. The collection consists of scores in braille and large print; textbooks and books about music in braille and large print; and elementary instruction for voice, piano, organ, guitar, recorder, accordion, banjo, and harmonica in recorded form.

Volunteer Services

Free correspondence courses leading to certification in braille transcribing (literary, music, and mathematics braille) and braille proofreading are offered. Voice auditions and informal training are given to volunteer tape narrators affiliated with local recording groups. A directory of volunteer groups that produce books for libraries and individuals is published frequently. Volunteers may call on NLS staff for their expertise in braille transcription and recording techniques.

Braille Competency

A free test is now available to demonstrate competence in reading and writing literary braille. It is designed primarily for classroom and rehabilitation teachers. It is available in both print and braille versions.

Information Services

Questions on various aspects of blindness and physical disabilities may be sent to NLS or to any network library. This service is available without charge to individuals, organizations, and libraries. Publications of interest to people with disabilities and service providers are free on request.

Consumer Relations

The consumer relations officer maintains regular contact with consumer groups and individual users of the program to identify and resolve service problems and to assure that users' needs are being met. Participating in surveys, evaluating new equipment, and serving on advisory committees are some of the ways in which consumers contribute to program development.

Research and Development

The NLS research program is directed toward improving the quality of reading materials and playback equipment, controlling program costs, and reducing the time required to deliver services to users. Current research activities include (1) the study of the centralization of storage and delivery of braille books and NLS audio playback equipment, (2) the development of new mailing containers for braille books, (3) the application of digital techniques to NLS recorded material, and (4) the thorough investigation of recent and potential audio technologies for possible use in the program.

Facts and Figures about Books for the Blind

From a beginning of 19 libraries, the network has expanded to 56 regional and 86 subregional libraries throughout the U.S.

About 77 percent of the NLS annual appropriation is budgeted for books, equipment, and related materials and 23 percent for support services.

More than 22 million recorded and braille books and magazines were circulated to a readership of 775,000 in 1994.

The international Union Catalog currently contains 231,800 titles (23 million copies). The average reader borrows 29 recorded books and magazines a year. Braille readers average 23 books and magazines a year.

A 4-track cassette recorded to play at 15/16 ips provides up to six hours of playing time. The average book consists of two cassettes.

The national music collection, the largest of its kind in the world, contains more than 30,000 items.

Telephone Pioneers and other volunteers repaired 147,200 talking-book and cassette machines in 1994.

Production costs average six dollars for a cassette book and three dollars for a book on flexible disc.

For Further Information

Ask your local public librarian for more information about the program and how to apply for service. Information is also available through the Internet and on computer diskette. To obtain publications, please use the attached preaddressed form.

Chapter 7

Playback Machines for Eligible Individuals and Institutions

Recorded materials provided on free loan by the National Library Service for the Blind and Physically Handicapped are available in recorded audio disc and audio cassette formats. Both disc and cassette recordings require specially designed playback equipment (see Part I, below), which is supplied on free loan to eligible individuals and institutions. Special accessories (see Part II, below) for these machines are also available on free loan. Disc players are designed to play at 8 1/3, 16 2/3, and the commercial standard 33 1/3 revolutions per minute (rpm); cassette machines play at either 15/16 or the commercial standard 1 7/8 inches per second (ips). Magazines are recorded at 8 1/3 rpm on flexible audio discs only. Books are recorded on either discs or cassettes or both.

To obtain any of the equipment and accessories described below, individuals or institutions must first be registered for the Library of Congress Talking Book Program. To receive an application for the free library service, write to the Reference Section, National Library Service for the Blind and Physically Handicapped, Library of Congress, Washington, DC 20542. All equipment and accessories are provided by the cooperating regional library serving eligible readers in their state of residence for as long as the reader is actively involved in the program.

National Library Service for the Blind and Physically Handicapped, Fact Sheet, January 1994.

Part I. Available Playback Machines

Talking-Book Machine

- plays recorded audio discs at 8 1/3 rpm, 16 2/3 rpm, and at the standard commercial speed of 33 1/3 rpm

- must be plugged into an electrical outlet; is not equipped with a battery

- has four controls; is simple to operate

- is needed to play flexible disc magazines

Cassette Machine

- plays audio cassettes at 15/16 ips and 1 7/8 ips, 2-track and 4-track

- is portable

- is equipped with a rechargeable battery and an electrical cord

- includes a variable speed control that permits speeding up or slowing down playback speed

- has ten controls

Easy Cassette Machine

- plays audio cassettes at only 15/16 ips, 4-track

- must be plugged into an electrical outlet; is not equipped with a battery

- does not include a variable speed control

- automatically rewinds cassettes; automatically changes tracks

- lacks the versatility of the standard cassette machine

- may be unsatisfactory unless disability (visual or physical) makes use of standard cassette machine difficult. Please contact your cooperating library to discuss the suitability of the Easy Cassette Machine.

Combination Machine

- has eleven controls; is fairly complex to use

- combines features of the cassette machine and the talking-book machine in a single unit

- has variable speed control for both cassettes and discs

- has fast forward and reverse features for both cassettes and discs

- has tone arm locator to assure correct placement on the playing edge of the recorded disc

- has battery option upon request

Part II. Special Accessories for Playback Machines

Headphones

- issued only to readers who require them for reading talking books where loudspeakers are not permitted, as in nursing homes and hospitals.

Amplifier

- for persons with a significant hearing loss requires a separate application with medical certification; the sound is boosted to a level that can cause permanent hearing loss to persons with normal hearing. Please contact your cooperating library about the application procedure for obtaining this accessory.

Remote Control Unit

- for persons confined to bed or with difficulty in mobility turns playback equipment on and off but will not control other functions such as volume and speed fits all playback equipment described in Part I, above requires a separate application. Please contact your cooperating library about the application procedure for obtaining this accessory.

Breath Switch

- for persons with little or no use of their extremities must be used with remote control unit

Extension Levers

- for persons who have difficulty manipulating the key controls on a standard cassette machine attaches to the key controls of the cassette machine

Pillow Speaker

- for persons who are confined to bed may be used with any playback machine is placed under the reader's pillow and is normally heard only by the reader

Individuals and institutions that wish to purchase their playback machines, that desire special features not included with NLS-provided machines, or that are ineligible for the free loan of NLS-provided equipment may consult a buying guide published by NLS entitled Facts: Sources for Purchase of Cassette and Disc Players Compatible with Recorded Materials Produced by the National Library Service (NLS). Request this free publication from the Reference Section, National Library Service for the Blind and Physically Handicapped, Library of Congress, Washington, DC 20542.

Chapter 8

Eye Health Education Resources

Introduction

The enclosed search is from the Eye Health Education (EY) subfile of the Combined Health Information Database (CHID). CHID is a computerized bibliographic database, developed and managed by health-related agencies of the Federal government. It contains references and abstracts for health information and health education resources, many of which are not referenced in any other computer system or print resource. CHID is intended to serve health professionals, librarians, and educators.

The EY subfile, coordinated by the National Eye Health Education Program (NEHEP), is a central and unbiased source of information about existing eye health education materials and resources. The subfile contains materials such as brochures, pamphlets, posters, journal articles, and program descriptions. Each search is updated twice a year.

Search Topics

- Age-Related Macular Degeneration
- Cataract
- Childhood Disorders
- Diabetic Retinopathy/Diabetic Eye Disease

Combined Health Information Database Search Series, July 1994.

- Eye Care and Eye Safety
- Glaucoma
- Inherited Disorders
- Low Vision
- Rehabilitation

If you are interested in other topics, please write to the NEHEP, CHID Search, 2020 Vision Place, Bethesda, Maryland 20892-3655.

Additional information on CHID and access to the database is attached at the end of this search.

The NEHEP has made every effort to provide accurate information in this search. Inclusion of an item does not imply endorsement by the NEHEP, the National Eye Institute, or the National Institutes of Health.

Anesthesia for Children: What to Expect.
American Academy of Ophthalmology. San Francisco, CA: American Academy of Ophthalmology. 1988. 2 p.

Available from American Academy of Ophthalmology, P.O. Box 7424, San Francisco, CA 94120-7424. (415) 561-8500. Price: Review copy free.

Anesthesia is necessary during eye surgery to eliminate pain. This fold-out brochure provides information about how anesthesia is used with children. Generally, anesthesia is given to children in two stages: a relaxing drug is given to induce sleep and then, another drug is delivered intravenously, rectally, or as gas through a face mask. The brochure tells parents how to prepare children for surgery and what may occur during the recovery period. It also describes the side effects of anesthesia and the risks associated with general anesthesia. Photographs are included. (EY0000131).

Blind Child in the Regular Preschool Program.
National Federation of the Blind. Baltimore, MD: National Federation of the Blind. 1990. 1 p.

Available from National Federation of the Blind, 1800 Johnson Street, Baltimore, MD 21230. (301) 659-9314. Price: Free.

The blind child can learn the same concepts that are taught the other children, the only difference is the method of learning. This fact sheet is an overview of common concerns about the education of visually impaired preschool children. Some of the issues discussed are specialized training for the teacher, material and equipment needed, discipline and reactions of other children. (EY0000308).

Bridges to Independence.
Braille Institute of America. (Insight Series). 1 videocassette (27 min.):½ in. (VHS). Los Angeles, CA: Braille Institute of America. 1991.

Available from Braille Institute of America, 741 North Vermont Avenue, Los Angeles, CA 90029. (213) 663-1111 or (800) 272-4553. Price: $25.00.

Vision plays an important role in finding out about the world around us. This videotape, introduced by actor Sidney Poitier, provides information to visually impaired teens, their parents, and the professionals that serve them. The videotape discusses visually impaired teens feelings of alienation and isolation and. suggestions to combat these feelings including the importance of building confidence and self-esteem, mainstreaming with sighted peers, and mastering living skills. Activities sponsored by the Braille Institute of America serve as examples of program activities that visually impaired teens can participate in. (EY0000429).

Bright Beginnings.
Braille Institute of America. (Insight Series). 1 videocassette (27 min.):½ in. (VHS). Los Angeles CA: Braille Institute of America. 1991.

Available from Braille Institute of America, 741 North Vermont Avenue, Los Angeles, CA 90029. (213) 663-1111 or (800) 272-4553. $25.00.

For visually impaired infants, it is important to stimulate as much of their existing vision as early as possible. This videotape, introduced by actor Robert Stack, helps parents of visually impaired children adjust to their environment. The techniques in the videotape include building on the child's interest, setting the stage for mainstreaming the child into sighted programs, and using playtime as an educational tool. Vision is developed like any other skill, and parents are encouraged to take their infants and preschool age children for eye examinations on a regular basis. (EY0000430).

Dancing Cheek To Cheek: Nurturing Beginning Social, Play and Language Interactions.
Meyers, L.; Lansky, P. Blind Children's Center. Los Angeles, CA: Blind Children's Center. 33 p.

Available from Blind Children's Center, 4120 Marathon Street, P.O. Box 29159, Los Angeles, CA 90029-0159. (213) 664-2153 or (800) 222-3566 or (800) 222-3567 (California).

There is a growing concern among researchers, therapists, teachers and parents of children with severe visual impairments, that lack of vision presents tremendous obstacles to the development of social, play and language skills. This booklet provides techniques and strategies that parents can use to successfully bypass some of these obstacles. (EY0000495).

Facts about Opportunities and Services for the Blind.
American Brotherhood for the Blind. Baltimore, MD: American Brotherhood for the Blind. 1990. 2 p.

Available from American Brotherhood for the Blind. 1800 Johnson Street, Baltimore, MD 21230. (301) 659-9315. Price: Free.

About 500,000 people in the United States are blind, and each year 50,000 more will become blind. This brochure describes services available to older Americans who have lost or are losing their sight as well as parents of visually impaired children. Some of these include braille calendars, a hot-line to the deaf-blind, rehabilitation, scholarships, civil rights, and products and aids. American Foundation for the Blind encourages use of their contacts and services. (EY0000309).

Getting in Touch with Play: Creating Play Environments for Children with Visual Impairments.
Lighthouse National Center for Vision and Aging. New York, NY: Lighthouse National Center for Vision and Aging. 1991. 44 p.

Available from Lighthouse National Center for Vision and Aging, 800 Second Ave., New York, NY 10017. (212) 808-0077. TDD (800) 334-5497. Price: Free.

This manual offers ideas that support more creative and satisfying play experiences for children who are blind or visually impaired, as well as for children with full vision. This manual demonstrates how outdoor play environments can be designed to provide stimulating activities through the manipulation of play elements, the organization of play spaces, and input from adults. (EY0000522).

Heartbreak of Being "A Little Bit Blind!"
National Association of the Visually Handicapped. New York, NY: National Association of the Visually Handicapped. 1989.

Available from National Association of the Visually Handicapped, 22 West 21st St. New York, NY 10010. (212) 889-3141. Also available from National Association for Visually Handicapped, 3201 Balboa St. San Francisco, CA 94121. (415) 221-3201. Memberships and contributions are tax deductible. Price: Review copy free.

There are approximately 14 million children and adults in the United States who see the world through blurred vision. The child who is "a little bit blind" frequently experiences rejection due to lack of understanding by peers, teachers and often, parents. This pamphlet outlines the problems faced by those who are unable to see images clearly. (EY0000253).

Learning to Play: Common Concerns for the Visually Impaired Preschool Child.
Blind Children's Center. Los Angeles, CA: Blind Children's Center. 11 p.

Available from Blind Children's Center, 4120 Marathon Street, P.O. Box 29159 Los Angeles CA 90029. (213) 662-2153.

Certain play situations seem to be especially difficult for children that are visually impaired. This booklet focuses on three areas of difficultly that many visually impaired children experience: exploring toys and materials, making transitions from one activity to another and playing with other children. (EY0000492).

Move With Me A Parents' Guide to Movement Development for Visually Impaired Babies.
The Blind Children's Center. Los Angeles, CA: The Blind Children's Center. 14 p.

Available from The Blind Children's Center, 4120 Marathon Street, P.O. Box 29159, Los Angeles, CA 90029-0159. (213) 664-2153. Price: $1.00.

Babies with serious visual loss often prefer their world to be constant and familiar, therefore, they tend to resist change. Visually impaired babies have the same potential to learn movements as sighted babies. This booklet describes a variety of ways to promote a visually impaired baby's movement development. Talking in a soothing voice, cuddling, and practicing exercises for a few minutes each day are some of the suggestions in the booklet to help the visually impaired infant through the first few months of life. This booklet is available in Spanish. (EY0000294).

My Fake Eye The Story of My Prosthesis.
Chernus-Mansfield, N.; Horn, M. Institute for Families of Blind Children. Los Angeles, CA: Institute for Families of Blind Children. 1991. 26 p.

Available from Institute for Families of Blind Children, 1300 North Vermont Avenue, Los Angeles, CA 90027. (213) 669-4649. Price: Free. Donations welcome.

It is sometimes difficult for parents to explain enucleation to their children. This book is written for children and uses colored photographs to illustrate ophthalmologist appointments, enucleation, and prosthesis fitting. (EY0000423).

My Friend Jodi is Blind.
Schwartz, N. New York: The Lighthouse, Inc. 1988. 39 p.

Available from National Center for Vision and Child Development, The Lighthouse, Inc. 800 Second Avenue, New York, NY 10017. (800) 334-5497 or (219) 808-0077. Price: $1.00 for single copy; discount for multiple orders.

This booklet, written for parents and teachers, is intended as a guide for introducing preschool children with impaired vision to computers. The booklet contains photographs of children learning to use computers at the Lighthouse Child Development Center. Center staff have been involved in the development of the CDC Computer Assisted Instruction program. The booklet addresses issues such as classroom environment, equipment considerations, and software assessment. Guidelines are offered on locating sources of funding and on eligibility, and a list of educational, health, and human service resources is included. (AA-M). (EY0000614).

Orientation and Mobility Primer for Families and Young Children.
Dodson-Burk, B.; Hill, E. W. American Foundation for the Blind. New York, NY: American Foundation for the Blind. 1989. 11 p.

Available from American Foundation for the Blind 15 West 16th Street, New York, NY 10011. (212) 620-2147. Price: $6.95 plus $3.00 shipping and handling.

People who are blind or have impaired vision need to learn other ways to become oriented and mobilized within their environment. This booklet is a guide for parents and families who have visually impaired children. Providing the child with a safe and stimulating environment will encourage the child to explore and learn. Frequently asked questions about the care of visually impaired children are answered. There are photographs throughout the book. A directory of resources is listed at the back of the booklet. A glossary of terms associated with orientation and mobility programs is also included. (EY0000264).

Parenting Preschoolers: Suggestions for Raising Young Blind and Visually Impaired Children.
American Foundation for the Blind. New York, NY: American Foundation for the Blind. 1984. 28 p.

Available from American Foundation for the Blind, 15 West 16th Street, New York, NY 10011. (800) 232-5463. Price: Single copy free.

Parents of blind or visually impaired children have many concerns and questions about how to raise their children. This book was written to respond to parents' commonly asked questions such as "What can I expect?" and "What does my child see?" This book offers suggestions to parents for raising their young blind and visually impaired children. (EY0000520).

Parents of Blind Children Division of the National Federation of the Blind.
National Federation of the Blind. Baltimore, MD: National Federation of the Blind. 1990. 2 p.

Available from National Federation of the Blind, 1800 Johnson Street, Baltimore, MD 21230. (301) 659-9314. Price: Free.

The real problem of blindness is the misunderstanding and lack of information that exists. Parents of Blind Children (POBC) is a national consumer organization designed to provide support, encouragement, and information to parents and friends of visually impaired children. This brochure describes the organization, and includes membership information and the goals of POBC. An application form is attached to the brochure. (EY0000310).

Pathways to Independence: Orientation and Mobility Skills for Your Infant and Toddler.
Lighthouse National Center for Vision and Aging. New York, NY: Lighthouse National Center for Vision and Aging. 1989. 14 p.

Available from Lighthouse National Center for Vision and Aging, 800 Second Ave., New York, NY 10017. (212) 808-0077. TDD (800) 334-5497. Price: Free.

Through simple games and activities easily integrated into daily routine, parents of visually impaired and blind children can help their children develop some basic orientation and mobility skills as early as the first year. This booklet discusses seven specific skills and offers game and activity sections for each. (EY0000518).

Problems of the Partially Seeing: See to Their Future.
National Association for Visually Handicapped. New York, NY: National Association for Visually Handicapped. 1900.

Available from National Association for Visually Handicapped, 22 West 21st St. New York, NY 10010. (212) 889-3141. Also available from National Association for Visually Handicapped, 3201 Balboa St. San Francisco, CA 94121. (415) 221-3201. Contributions in support of the National Association for Visually Handicapped services are tax deductible. Price: Review copy free.

There are many causes of low vision that affect 14 million people in the United States. The National Association for Visually Handicapped (NAVH) is a national health agency with a program devoted to the visually impaired. This pamphlet describes some of the causes of visual impairment and some of the programs the NAVH has established to aid those with vision impairments. (EY0000233).

Reaching, Crawling, Walking, Let's Get Moving: Orientation and Mobility for Preschool Children.
Blind Children's Center. Los Angeles CA: Blind Children's Center. 1992. 24 p.

Available from Blind Children's Center, 4120 Marathon Street, P.O. Box 29159, Los Angeles, CA 90029. (213) 664-2153. (800) 222-3566 (USA). (800) 222-3567 (California). Price: Free.

For visually impaired pre-school children, orientation and mobility means helping a child become independent through movement, exploration, the use of their senses, and gaining practical information about their world. This booklet helps parents of young children who are visually impaired or blind, understand what orientation and mobility is and how they can influence the independence of their child. (EY0000493).

Special Start: A Community Guide for Early Education and Child Development.
Lang M. A. Multimedia kit including manual (69 p.); ½ in VHS videocassette (17 min), col; poster-pamphlet. New York, NY: The Lighthouse. Inc. 1991. (multimedia information package).

Available from National Center for Vision and Child Development, The Lighthouse, Inc. 800 Second Avenue, New York, NY 10017. (800) 334-5497 or (212) 808-0077. Price: $25.00 (single kit); $40.00 (dual language). Available in English or Spanish and as an audiocassette. Individual pamphlets available at $0.25 each or $5.00 for 25 copies. Order Number: P217 for complete kit, P218 for pamphlet/poster.

This multimedia kit is designed to enable parents and service providers to help children make the most of their vision. It alerts parents to signs of vision problems in children, explains how vision problems affect children's early development, and suggest ways to help children compensate for vision loss. The kit outlines a program for mobilizing community resources and promoting cooperation among parents, teachers, vision-care professionals, and others who provide services to children. (AA-M). (EY0000611).

Technology for Tots: Using Computers with Preschool Children Who Have Visual Impairments.
Lighthouse National Center for Vision and Aging. New York, NY: Lighthouse National Center for Vision and Aging. 1992. 39 p.

Available from Lighthouse National Center for Vision and Aging, 800 Second Ave., New York, NY 10017. (212) 808-0077. TDD (800) 334-5497. Price: Free.

This book is a guide for teachers and parents who want to teach computer use to and create programs for young visually impaired or blind children. (EY0000521).

Touch the Baby Blind and Visually Impaired Children as Patients: Helping Them to Respond to Care.
Harrell, L. American Foundation for the Blind. New York, NY: American Foundation for the Blind. 1987.

Available from American Foundation for the Blind, 15 West 16th Street, New York, NY 10011. (800) AFBLIND (232-5463) or (212) 620-2147. Price: Free.

This illustrated pamphlet gives suggestions and general recommendations for the care of blind and visually impaired babies, neonates, blind preschool children, visually impaired preschool children and the newly blind child. Physical contact with the child, and dialogue to give them clues about their environment, are examples suggested activities for care takers of blind and visually impaired children. There is a list of other American Foundation for the Blind publications related to children with visual impairments. AFB regional offices also are included. (EY0000324).

Visual Impairments.
National Information Center for Handicapped Children and Youth. Washington, DC: National Information Center for Handicapped Children and Youth. n.d. 4 p.

Available from National Information Center for Handicapped Children and Youth, P.O. Box 1492, Washington, DC 20013. (703) 893-6061. Price: Free.

Visual impairments can include myopia, hyperopia, and astigmatism; problems in the visual field; and muscular problems that result in visual disturbances. This newsletter defines visual handicap, blindness, and low vision. It notes the incidence rate for visual impairments. It also notes the characteristics and educational implications in children with visual impairments. A resource list is provided. (19 references). (EY0000241).

You Seem Like a Regular Kid to Me!
American Foundation for the Blind. New York, NY: American Foundation for the Blind. 1988. 16 p.

Available from American Foundation for the Blind, 15 West 16th Street, New York, NY 10011. (800) 232-5463. Price: Single copy free.

This book is about Jane, an elementary school student who is blind. Jane answers some of the most common questions that people ask about how she handles situations that come up in school. She also responds to common concerns that people have of doing the "right" things for blind people. (EY0000519).

Your Baby's Eyes: A Good Start for Good Vision.
American Academy of Ophthalmology. San Francisco, CA: American Academy of Ophthalmology. 1993. 2 p. Available from American Academy of Ophthalmology. P.O. Box 7424, San Francisco, CA 94120-7424. (415) 561-8500. Price: Review copy free.

This fact sheet explains the importance of protecting the vision of infants as they grow. The fact sheet recommends that parents have their children's eyes examined by a pediatrician or family physician when the child is a newborn, at six months, and at three and one half years old. The fact sheet also lists circumstances that might contribute to higher risk for vision problems in infants. and includes signs that might indicate that a baby has an eye problem. (EY0000630) .

Your Child's Sight.
National Society to Prevent Blindness. Schaumburg, IL: National Society to Prevent Blindness. 1989. 10 p.

Available from National Society to Prevent Blindness, 500 East Remington Road. Schaumburg, IL 60173. (708) 843-2020. (800) 331-2020. Price: Review copy free.

Children that suffer from eye problems have a decreased ability to understand the world around them. This pamphlet discusses the stages of visual development and lists some eye problems in children. It describes some signs in behavior and appearance that can alert parents to possible eye problems in a child. It describes ways of testing infant vision and lists the treatments currently available to correct eye disorders in children. (EY0000217).

How to Access CHID and the EY Subfile

CHID is available through BRS Online, a division of InfoPro Technologies, a commercial database vendor. The database can be accessed via computer through medical libraries, university libraries, or any library service that subscribes to BRS Online. Individuals or companies that want to do their own searching can subscribe directly to BRS Online. Subscriber information is available from:

BRS InfoPro Technologies
Attn: CHID Database
8000 Westpark Drive
McLean, VA 22102
(800) 955-0906

For information about the EY subfile, please write to NEHEP, 2020 Vision Place, Bethesda, Maryland 20892-3655, (301) 496-5248.

Chapter 9

Selected Resources for People with Low Vision

The selected resources included in this list may help individuals with visual impairments make the most of remaining sight. Inclusion in this list does not imply endorsement by the National Eye Institute or the National Institutes of Health.

General Information

American Academy of Ophthalmology
P.O. Box 7424
San Francisco, CA 94120-7424
(415) 561-8500

- Provides brochures on low vision and other eye problems.

American Council of the Blind
1155 15th Street, N.W., Suite 720
Washington, DC 20005
(202) 467-5081

- Offers a wide variety of services to visually impaired persons with emphasis on employment opportunities. Publishes the Braille Forum.

NEI, Low Vision Resources, October 1994.

American Foundation for the Blind
15 W. 16th Street
New York, NY 10011
(800) 232-5463
(212) 620-2000

- Offers consultation services to eye care, rehabilitation, and education professionals. Serves as a national clearinghouse for information about blindness and visual impairment. Provides referrals to low vision centers. Maintains regional offices throughout the country.

   Regional Offices:
   (212) 620-2032 — New York
   (312) 245-9961 — Chicago
   (202) 457-1487 — District of Columbia
   (404) 525-2303 — Georgia
   (214) 352-7222 — Texas
   (415) 392-4845 — California

American Optometric Association
243 Lindbergh Boulevard
St.Louis, MO 63141
(314) 991-4100

- Provides brochures on low vision and other eye problems.

Council of Citizens with Low Vision International
5707 Brockton Drive, Suite 302
Indianapolis, IN 46220-5481
(800) 733-2258
(317) 254-1332

- Serves as an advocacy group for the visually impaired. Provides information on low vision technology. Publishes the CCLV News.

National Association for the Visually Handicapped
22 W. 21st Street
New York, NY 10010
(212) 889-3141

- Serves as a clearinghouse for information about all services available to the partially-sighted from public and private sources. Conducts self-help groups. Provides information on large print books, textbooks, and educational tools.

National Center for Vision and Aging
The Lighthouse, Inc.
111 E. 59th Street
New York, NY 10022
(800) 334-5497
(212) 821-9200

- Serves as a national clearinghouse for information on vision and aging.

National Center for the Blind
1800 Johnson Street
Baltimore, MD 21230
(800) 638-7518
(410) 659-9314

- Provides a wide variety of services to visually impaired people. Publishes the Braille Monitor and Future Reflections. Distributes a catalog of publications available in large print, braille, or audiocassette, and a catalog of aids and appliances.

Resources for Rehabilitation
33 Bedford Street, Suite 19A
Lexington, MA 02173
(617) 862-6455

- Offers training programs for public and professionals on coping with low vision. Distributes materials on coping with low vision.

Visions
120 Wall Street, 16th Floor
New York, NY 10005
(212) 425-2255

- Offers free services to anyone over age 55 with vision problems. Services include self-help study kits, counseling, professional support systems, consumer workshops, and an information center.

Aids and Devices

Anne Morris Enterprises, Inc.
890 Fams Court
East Meadow, NY 11554
(516) 292-9232

- Distributes a catalog of innovative products for the visually impaired.

Bossert Specialties, Inc.
3620 E. Thomas Road
Phoenix, AZ 85060
(602) 956-6637

- Distributes a catalog of low vision aids and devices.

Independent Living Aids
27 East Mall
Plainview, NY 11803
(800) 537-2118
(516) 752-8080

- Publishes a catalog of household, medical, communication, and recreation aids.

LS&S Group, Inc.
P.O. Box 673
Northbrook, IL 60065
(708) 498-9777

- Publishes an extensive catalog of products for the visually impaired.

Maxi Aids
P.O. Box 3209
Farmingdale, NY 11735
(800) 522-6294
(516) 752-0521

* Publishes an extensive catalog of products for the blind and people with visually impairments.

SpecialNet
GTE Educational Network Services, Inc.
5525 MacArthur Boulevard, Suite 320
Irving, TX 75038
(800) 927-3000

* Provides current information via network on special education and related fields.

Print and Audio Materials

National Library Service for Blind and Physically Handicapped
Library of Congress
1291 Taylor Street, NW
Washington, DC 20542
(800) 424-8567
(202) 707-5100

* Provides free library service to individuals with visual impairments. Offers braille and large print materials and recorded books and periodicals.

American Printing House for the Blind
1839 Frankfort Avenue
P.O . Box 6085
Louisville, KY 40206-0085
(800) 223-1839
(502) 895-2405

* Provides free subscriptions to *Reader's Digest, Newsweek* and other magazines on disposable audiocassettes. Provides *Reader's Digest* in braille.

Associated Services for the Blind
919 Walnut Street, 2nd Floor
Philadelphia, PA 19107
(215) 627-0600

- Provides subscriptions (for a nominal fee) to magazines such as: *Family Circle, Fortune, Smithsonian, Science News*, and others.

Braille Circulating Library, Inc.
2700 Stuart Avenue
Richmond, VA 23220
(804) 359-3771
(804) 359-3743

- Loans braille materials, talking books, audiocassettes, and large print Christian materials.

Choice Magazine Listening
85 Channel Drive
Port Washington, NY 11050
(516) 883-8280

- Offers selected articles from popular print magazines on special-speed, 4-track audiocassette. Free service nationwide.

Christian Record Services, Inc.
4444 South 52nd Street
P.O. Box 6097
Lincoln, NE 68506
(402) 488-0981

- Provides a lending library of books in braille, and large print materials, disks, and cassette tapes.

G.K. Hall and Co.
P.O . Box 159 Street
Thorndike, ME 04986
(207) 948-2962

- Provides direct sale of large print books.

Jewish Braille Institute of America
110 E. 30th Street
New York, NY 10016
(212) 889-2525

- Provides talking books, braille and large-print books, a circulating library and a public education program. Offers counseling and referrals to low vision care in the U.S.

John Milton Society for the Blind
475 Riverside Drive, Room 455
New York, NY 10115
(212) 870-3335

- Provides free Christian literature in braille, audiocassette, and large type.

New York Times/Large Type Weekly
229 W. 43rd Street
New York, NY 10036
(212) 556-1234
(800) 631-2500 (California only)

- Offers subscriptions to the New York Times.

Reader's Digest Large Type Publications
P.O. Box 241
Mount Morris, IL 61054
(815) 734-6963

- Offers subscriptions to *Reader's Digest* in large type.

Recording for the Blind — Headquarters Office
The Anne T. MacDonald Center
20 Roszel Road
Princeton, NJ 08540
(800) 221-4792 or 4793
(609) 452-0606

- Provides free cassette tapes, textbooks for students, and materials needed for occupational pursuits.

Recording for the Blind Regional Offices
(415) 493-3717 — California
(212) 557-5720 — New York

Talking Tapes for the Blind
3015 S. Brentwood Boulevard
St. Louis, MO 63144-2715
(314) 968-2557

• Provides textbooks on audiocassettes for students who are blind or visually impaired.

Vision Foundation, Inc.
818 Mt. Auburn Street
Watertown, MA 02172
(617) 926-4232
(800) 852-3029 (Massachusetts only)

• Publishes a catalog of materials available in large print and on audiocassette.

Xavier Society for the Blind
154 E. 23rd Street
New York, NY 10010
(212) 473-7800

• Serves as the National Catholic Lending Library and Publishing House. Publishes The Xavier Review in braille, large print, and audiocassette.

Employment

Job Opportunities for the Blind
National Center for the Blind
1800 Johnson Street
Baltimore, MD 21230
(800) 638-7518
(410) 659-9314

Occupational Information Library for the Blind
Greater Detroit Society for the Blind
16625 Grand River Avenue
Detroit, Ml 48227
(313) 272-3900

Blinded Veterans Association
477 H Street, NW
Washington, DC 20001
(202) 371-8880

Directories

Directory of Services for Blind and Visually Impaired Persons in the United States and Canada, 24th edition (1993), $75
American Foundation for the Blind
c/o American Book Center
Brooklyn Navy Yard, Building No. 3
Brooklyn, NY 11205
(718) 852-9873

Living with Low Vision: A Resource Guide for People with Sight Loss, 3rd edition (1993), $35
Resources for Rehabilitation
33 Bedford Street, Suite 19A
Lexington, MA 02173
(617) 862-6455

Rehabilitation Resource Manual: VISION, 4th edition (1993), $39.95
Resources for Rehabilitation
33 Bedford Street, Suite 19A
Lexington, MA 02173
(617) 862-6455

Part Two

Alignment and Refractive Disorders

Chapter 10

National Eye Institute Report on Strabismus, Amblyopia, and Refractive Problems

How do we see? This simple question does not have a simple answer. Vision is a complex series of events that begins when light enters our eyes and ends with perception. We are able to discriminate between objects of different size, contrast, and color, as well as track moving objects with precision. We routinely perform these tasks over an enormous range of light intensity. Our visual system easily out performs any manmade machine. We accomplish these impressive feats by integrating optical, metabolic, and neural processes with other brain systems that direct eye movement and enable us to focus on objects.

If any one of the many parts of the visual system is disrupted, our ability to see can be seriously impaired. Disturbances in neural and ocular development, metabolism, neural processing, and eye movements can lead to serious visual impairment such as amblyopia (reduced vision in one eye), strabismus (misalignment of the eyes), nystagmus (irregular eye movements), scotoma (regional blindness), myopia (nearsightedness), and other conditions requiring strong corrective lenses. More than 30 million people in the United States suffer from one or more of these visual disorders. While they seldom lead to legal blindness, these disorders cause substantial visual loss that interferes with learning, working, and the overall quality of life.

The Strabismus, Amblyopia, and Visual Processing Program of the National Eye Institute (NEI) supports both clinical and basic research on development, neural processing, eye movement, and associated

NIH Pub. No. 93-3186.

disorders involving the retina and those portions of the brain that serve vision. These studies on normal and impaired vision go hand in hand. Detailed knowledge of the normal visual system provides the foundation for understanding the causes of impaired vision and for developing corrective measures.

The Strabismus, Amblyopia, and Visual Processing Program supports research on a variety of species with the goal of understanding the human visual system and alleviating its disorders. Primates are the model system closest to the human, but species ranging from invertebrates, such as flies and horseshoe crabs, to nonprimate mammals, such as cats and rabbits, have yielded significant information on the fundamental mechanisms of vision common to all species including humans. Past research in vision demonstrates the wisdom of this approach: Key insights generally come from model systems that are well suited for exploring a specific research question. Past research also demonstrates the wisdom of using primates for investigations directly related to the human visual system.

Over the last three decades visual neuroscience has had a substantial impact on other fields of neuroscience. This is especially true for studies of central visual pathways, which have yielded results that have been generalized to the brain as a whole.

Now visual neuroscience is entering an exciting new era. Powerful techniques are emerging from the fields of molecular biology, neural imaging, and computational neuroscience to open up numerous opportunities for major advances in understanding basic visual mechanisms and visual disorders. Realizing the impact they can have on visual neuroscience, many outstanding investigators from these fields are now focusing their efforts on the visual system. Future research in vision with emerging technology holds great promise not only in understanding visual processing and associated disorders but in understanding the brain itself. Vision research will surely play a key role in the "Decade of the Brain."

The Strabismus, Amblyopia, and Visual Processing Program has made important new advances in both basic and clinical investigations of visual disorders that affect a major portion of the population in the United States. For example, myopia affects nearly one-quarter of the population at a yearly cost of $3 billion and reduces productivity and function as much as the common cold does. However, recent research with animal models casts new light on the etiology of myopia, and recent advances in instrumentation now allow longitudinal studies that will identify individuals with the highest risk for myopia.

Ecological studies have shown that the brain exhibits much greater flexibility in its control over eye movements than was previously thought. By allowing the use of both head and eye movements for viewing natural visual stimuli, visual scientists have discovered that the vestibulo-ocular reflex (VOR) is not fixed and immutable. Moreover, recent studies have revealed a major neural circuit in the brain that controls the visual pursuit of objects. The circuit begins with responses of retinal cells and ends with activation of extraocular motoneurons. Further studies promise to lead to the first complete understanding of the neural basis of visually guided behavior in primates. The excellent communication between basic and clinical investigators will continue to produce major advances in understanding and diagnosing ocular-motility disorders.

Major strides have been made in the treatment of strabismus. The recently completed Strabismus Prism Adaptation Trial has shown that correcting the angle of strabismus with prisms in patients with acquired esotropia preoperatively enhances motor and sensory alignment postoperatively. Also, the Food and Drug Administration (FDA) recently approved the use of botulinum toxin (Oculinum 'E') for the treatment of strabismus in patients ages 12 and older. Strabismus in much younger individuals (i.e., infantile esotropia) can be corrected early in life by corrective surgery.

Amblyopia is a multidimensional developmental disorder causing major visual loss in young children in the United States. Important new insights on its etiology have come from psychophysical studies of spatial vision. The reduction in vernier acuity in strabismic amblyopia points to an abnormally large spacing between cortical elements with which one analyzes the spatial features of fixated objects. The reduction of both vernier and grading acuity in anisometropic amblyopia indicates loss of the cortical mechanism that mediates our finest spatial resolution. Recent studies of excitatory neurotransmitters in central visual pathways suggest that the glutamatergic NMDA receptor (named after its specific agonist N-methyl-D-aspartate) could contribute directly to the changes that occur in strabismic and stimulus-deprivation amblyopia.

The Optic Neuritis Treatment Trial (ONTT), which was completed in 1991, has improved significantly our knowledge of this neuro-ophthalmological disorder and has provided a model for future neuro-ophthalmic clinical research. The ONTT indicated that oral corticosteriods were ineffective in treating optic neuritis and increased the rate of its recurrence. Intravenous corticosteriods however, had the opposite effect: They speeded recovery and did not increase the rate of recurrence. These results may prove useful in the treatment of multiple sclerosis.

New technology and increased interdisciplinary research over the last 5 years have yielded dramatic progress in our understanding of how the eye and brain process visual information. Neuroscientists, psychophysicists, computer scientists, and clinicians often working together on the same team delineate a visual problem, investigate its neural origins, develop testable models, and apply the results to the clinic. The wisdom of this approach may be best exemplified by the recent discovery of the parallel organization of the visual system. At least two major subsystems, operating largely in parallel, exist: (1) The M pathway (often called the motion pathway) and (2) the P pathway (often called the color and form pathway). Both pathways originate in the retina. The M pathway has many of the characteristics of achromatic vision, and the P pathway provides both color vision and high visual acuity. The segregation of visual information between the P and M pathways begins in the retina, continues through the thalamic relay station to the primary, visual sensory area in the cerebral cortex and on to higher visual pathways in the brain.

Although much remains to be learned about the parallel organization of the primate visual system, remarkable progress has been made in understanding how the brain processes moving images. Combined psychophysical, physiological, and computational studies of awake, behaving primates have established a strong link between neural responses of the M pathway in the middle temporal visual area (MT) of the brain and the perception of motion. These animal studies serve as valuable guides to clinical investigations of motion processing, which is highly abnormal in certain types of strabismus, particularly in infantile esotropia.

A wealth of powerful new imaging techniques are now allowing investigators to localize and analyze specific visual functions in the human brain. Positron Emission Tomography (PET) has revealed regions of brain activity analogous to those that segregate motion and form vision in nonhuman primates and is rapidly improving our understanding of the neural mechanisms underlying amblyopia in humans. Future use of PET, magnetic resonance imaging (MRI) magnetoencepholography (MEG), and visually evoked potentials (VEP) will greatly extend our understanding of the human cortex in health and disease.

Powerful techniques of cell and molecular biology have given us a new view of how the visual system develops. The environment of developing cells of the brain rather than their lineage determines their fate in the visual system. Dynamic processes involving transient cell types determine in part how growing neuronal processes find and select their targets in the visual system. Orderly mapping of the visual field in central pathways in mammals requires patterned neuronal activity both before and after birth. It is now clear that the environment within the developing brain is different than in the adult brain, indicating that conditions for neuronal growth and synapse formation may be absent in the adult brain. A major challenge for the future is to determine the molecular environment of the developing brain and learn how to recreate that environment following injury in the adult.

The Strabismus, Amblyopia, and Visual Processing Program has made significant progress in both basic and clinical studies involving the central pathways of vision. For example, recent research with animal models has cast new light on the etiology of juvenile onset myopia, which affects nearly one-quarter of all children in the United States after the age of 5. Animal research shows that emmetropization (i.e., proper growth of the eye) requires feedback within the eye to reduce focusing errors and may involve the retinal neuromodulator, dopamine. Significant advances in instrumentation now allow rapid measurement of refractive error and thus will encourage longitudinal studies of ocular growth in infants, children, and adults that will reveal the candidate risk factors for acquired myopia.

Ecological approaches to the investigation of eye movements have provided important new insights into the function of the oculomotor system. Studies that allow the use of both head and eye movements for viewing natural visual stimuli have shown that the VOR is not fixed and immutable. Instead, the brain exhibits much greater flexibility than was previously thought in its control over eye movements. Collaborative investigations among visual and oculomotor scientists have revealed a major control circuit for visual pursuit from responses of retinal cells to activation of extraocular motoneurons. Further studies promise to lead to the first complete understanding of the neural basic of visually guided behavior in primates. The excellent communication between basic and clinical investigators will continue to produce major advances in understanding and diagnosing disorders of ocular motility.

Recent quantitative studies of the eye movement pathway, which plays a major role in eye alignment, point to the brain as the primary cause of infantile esotropia. Such strabismic conditions are permanent in adults but can be modified early in life by corrective surgery.

The Clinical Amblyopia Classification Study has just completed its pilot phase. Its goal is to develop a functional classification of amblyopia. Scanning the brain of amblyopic patients with imaging techniques such as PET has helped improve our understanding of the neural mechanisms of the visual parts of the brain.

The ONTT, which was completed in 1991, has significantly improved our knowledge of this neuro-ophthalmological disorder and provided a model for future neuro-ophthalmic clinical research.

National Eye Institute Program Goals

- To determine the etiology of myopia and identify the risk factors associated with this and other refractive errors to prevent their occurrence or progression.

- To understand the neural and motor mechanisms that control eye movements under natural environmental conditions and the mechanisms that provide plasticity to the oculomotor system.

- To investigate the development of visual function in young children (< 3 years) with the high risk of amblyopia and strabismus and to determine the effectiveness of prompt therapeutic intervention to restore normal vision.

- To analyze visual performance in normal and dysfunctional states and develop clinically useful diagnostic tests for assessing visual performance, particularly in infants and young children.

- To understand how the brain processes visual information and how neural activity is related to visual perception.

- To understand how the visual system is assembled during development, how its assembly is influenced by endogenous and exogenous factors, and the factors involved in its regeneration.

Chapter 11

National Eye Institute Report on Refractive Problems and Contact Lenses

Introduction

An estimated 120 million people in the United States have correctable refractive errors. Although spectacles provide the cheapest, easiest, and safest method to correct a wide range of refractive problems, they may not enable wearers with high refractive errors to achieve the vision levels required for normal function. Approximately 24 million Americans wear contact lenses, either (1) to achieve superior correction of such high refractive problems as high myopia, anisometropia, and keratoconus or (2) to enjoy their convenience and cosmetic result. With the introduction of disposable soft lenses and improved technology of gas-permeable lenses, it is likely that the number of contact lens wearers will increase substantially in the next decade.

Considerable progress has been made in the contact lens field during the past decade, including the development of lenses that some patients can wear for extended periods of time. Unfortunately, many poorly understood side effects and changes in corneal physiology accompany extended lens wear. Until these effects are explained more fully and strategies are introduced to prevent their occurrence, overnight contact lens wear may be suitable for only a limited segment of the population. Despite the lack of information on extended wear effects, many individuals nevertheless are choosing to wear contact

NIH Pub. No. 93-3186.

lenses overnight. And the number of such individuals is expected to increase.

Intraocular lenses are being used increasingly for the visual correction of aphakia following cataract removal. They provide nearly optimal correction because they replace the eye's natural lens. Lens implants may be contraindicated in some aphakic patients because of such ocular conditions as glaucoma, endothelial dystrophy, diabetic retinopathy, and corneal edema.

The term refractive keratoplasty applies to several different surgical procedures that modify the surface of the cornea in order to correct refractive errors. Theoretically, surgical correction provides a permanent cure and is therefore appealing to both patients and practitioners. In fact, some results have been encouraging. Patients with high refractive errors, who would otherwise require thick glasses and who cannot or do not wish to wear contact lenses, are particularly good candidates for this type of visual correction. Surgical correction of the high hyperopia that occurs subsequent to cataract surgery offers an additional option to the aphakic patient. However, because these procedures require surgery on the healthy cornea, they involve a risk that must be weighed against the potential benefit. Present scientific evidence is insufficient to allow full evaluation of the long-term safety and efficacy of refractive keratoplasty. Until more information on the complications, expected magnitude of refractive change, and predictability of wound-healing results has been gathered, these procedures should be carried out within a randomized clinical trial.

Research on the correction of refractive error by contact lenses or surgery is related to portions of other NEI programs. For example, contact lenses are a principal method of correcting vision in the aphakic patient. They also are prescribed for children suffering from high anisometropia, amblyopia, or other sensorimotor defects and provide an important means of delivering normal imagery to the retina. More recently high-plus contact lenses are being used as part of a telescopic system to aid patients suffering from permanently decreased vision.

It is clear that we must gain a more fundamental knowledge of the biomechanical and structural properties of the cornea in order to understand both its normal function and its wound-healing response to pathologic situations. We lack basic information on the anatomical parameters of the human cornea. For example, the standard deviation of the thickness of Bowman's layer is not known nor whether it is age or sex dependent. Yet this parameter is very important for planning laser keratomileusis. In addition, understanding the refractive effects of keratotomy requires more exact data on the length, number, and direction of stromal lamellae.

Subprogram Objectives

- To understand the biologic effects of contact lenses on the cornea.

- To understand the corneal topographic and biomechanical properties that result in normal refraction.

Current Level of National Eye Institute Support

In FY 1992 the NEI supported 15 research projects in the area covered in this subprogram at a cost of $2,805,151. Supported studies include those that seek to evaluate the safety and efficacy of radial keratotomy, to examine wound healing following keratotomy, to improve and develop methods for measuring the optical and physiologic properties of the cornea, and to develop contact lens designs and materials.

Recent Accomplishments

Several important developments in the contact lens field have occurred since the last report. These include improvements in lens materials, acquisition of additional information on the biologic effects of contact lens wear, and modest success toward the development of improved lens design for the correction of high refractive errors.

The most significant advancement in contact lens materials has been the development of highly oxygen-permeable rigid (RGP) lenses. Chemists have been able to reformulate lens matrices and alter oxygen transmissibility by using either a combination of silicon, acrylate, and fluorocarbon or a pure fluorocarbon. With these materials, it is possible to manufacture lenses that can transmit sufficient oxygen to meet the metabolic requirements of the cornea during closed-eye wear. The Food and Drug Administration has approved several of these materials for up to 1 week of overnight wear. Several clinical studies have shown that people who wear these lenses often have a better ocular response over that to soft lenses during extended wear. Unfortunately, these hard lenses are not without problems for some patients. For example, they may adhere to the cornea overnight, which may result in peripheral corneal keratitis, conjunctival redness, and alterations in corneal topography. Also, for many wearers, the comfort of these lenses is not comparable to that of soft lenses. Finally, RGP lenses are more difficult to fit than are soft lenses; therefore, many clinicians have chosen not to offer these RGP lenses to prospective patients. There is a need for understanding of the lens mechanics that leads to adherence.

Important accomplishments also have been made in our understanding of the biologic effects of contact lenses on the cornea. Several studies have demonstrated clearly that contact lens wear causes corneal hypoxia and morphological changes in the corneal endothelium and epithelium. Apparently, the epithelial changes are reversible after approximately 1 month; however, the endothelial cell changes seem to be permanent. Other investigators have used a modified slit lamp as a pH-sensitive fluorophotometer and have shown that contact lenses that produce corneal hypoxia cause a reduction in stromal pH (corneal acidosis). It is thought that the changes in extracellular pH may be in part responsible for the changes in cell morphology (endothelial polymegethism and epithelial microcysts) that may accompany contact lens wear.

Clinical studies have demonstrated that ulcerative keratitis may result from contact lens wear. This infection is vision threatening and represents an important public health problem. Some progress has been made in defining the relationship between lens deposits and bacterial adherence. Unfortunately, this research does not provide the information needed for an understanding of why some contact lens wearers with bacterial deposits develop infection while others do not.

Other studies have analyzed the permanent effects of contact lens wear on corneal function. Apparently, some individuals who have had long-term hypoxic contact lens wear demonstrate reduced corneal hydration control and changes in endothelial morphology with time. Such disturbances to the epithelial and endothelial cells of the cornea that are sometimes found in long-term wearers cannot be ascribed to an acid environment on the tissue surface.

Finally, there has been some improvement in contact lens design for the correction of other visual conditions. Presbyopia affects almost everyone older than age 50, and this population has great interest in contact lens wear. Several lens designs have been introduced to correct presbyopia; however, most have resulted in vision that is not equal to spectacle correction. Many highly motivated patients are wearing contact lenses that correct one eye for distance vision and the other eye for near vision. This configuration reduces binocular vision and could conceivably increase the difficulty associated with visual tasks such as driving and machinery operation.

Several keratorefractive procedures were introduced in the early 1980s. Methods for analyzing the effects of keratorefractive techniques on corneal topography and corneal optical function have been improved. The information derived from these studies will affect the direction of future research. Clinical studies of common keratorefractive techniques (radial keratotomy and epikeratoplasty) and of recent investigational procedures (excimer laser photoablation) have sought to determine their safety, reliability, refractive accuracy, refractive stability, and optical performance. To date, these procedures have not shown an accuracy, stability, or optical quality as good as spectacle or contact lens wear.

The NEI-funded Prospective Evaluation of Radial Keratotomy (PERK) study has followed patients for 5 years and is the main source of information regarding the long-term results of radial keratotomy [see Chapter 19]. The procedure was most accurate for the correction of mild to moderate degrees of myopia, but even within this group, refractive accuracy was unpredictable. Five-year data from the PERK study show that 64 percent of patients were within one diopter of emmetropia. Three percent of patients lost two or more lines of best corrected visual acuity. Twenty-three percent of patients had changes of more than one diopter between the 6- and 4-year visits. Thus stability and predictability of this procedure remains a problem. Even if all the above factors could be controlled to produce an exact and predictable outcome of refractive surgery, the problem of adjusting the cornea to adapt to future changes in refraction or to presbyopia would still exist.

Epikeratoplasty has been most promising for the correction of aphakia in the pediatric patient with contact lens intolerance. In the adult aphakic population, epikeratoplasty is best restricted to contact lens–intolerant patients at high risk for intraocular procedures. The indications for epikeratoplasty for keratoconus remain controversial. The results of trials of epikeratoplasty for myopia have been disappointing and further evaluation is needed.

Treatment of a corneal surface with a 193-nm excimer laser allows for controlled ablation of corneal tissue with no thermal damage. Testing of systems for excimer laser photoablative keratectomy for the correction of refractive error have reached the clinical trial stage.

Primate studies show that individual variability in the wound-healing response (migration of activated fibroblasts, type III collagen production, dynamic changes in corneal epithelial hyperplasia, and corneal scarring) adversely affects refractive accuracy and stability. Initial clinical studies suggest these secondary biologic responses cause regression of the refractive effect in humans as well.

These findings from clinical studies demonstrate that keratorefractive procedures do more than correct refractive error. They irreversibly alter the physiologic optics of the eye as well, often in a highly individual and dynamic fashion. The goal of keratorefractive research is the development of procedures with excellent refractive accuracy and optical performance. The emergence of topographic analysis systems that can describe the degree and patterns of corneal irregularity has been an important advance. Topographic systems that provide accurate, reproducible measurements allow comparison of the topographic quality of competing technologies for the correction of refractive error. Dynamic changes in topography caused by secondary biologic responses to surgery can be evaluated. However, the ability of commercially available topography systems to describe irregular surfaces accurately must be validated.

The finding of topographic irregularity after keratorefractive surgery has spawned research into the effects of keratorefractive surgery on the optical performance of the human eye and has exposed the inadequacy of applying conventional visual-acuity testing methods to clinical trials of refractive surgery. Ray-tracing software that uses topographic data to model corneal optical performance is under investigation and should allow a better understanding of the effects of altered topography on the optical performance of the cornea. The optical importance of relative positioning of the pupil and the optical zone of the keratorefractive procedure has been explored. These studies suggest that changes in pupil size and decentration of the optical zone relative to the pupil have a significant effect on glare and refraction.

Important Research Questions to Be Addressed

Many challenging opportunities for research promise to advance the understanding of contact lens refractive correction of the eye and the effects of these corrections on corneal physiology. In general, the large body of industry-funded research has been concerned with materials rather than with understanding the basic principles of the

102

ocular and visual responses to contact lens wear. Questions that need to be addressed include the following:

What are the biologic effects of extended-wear contact lenses?

It is important to determine the mechanism of these effects and the factors that may make certain patients more susceptible to complications. This knowledge would help identify better contact lens materials or designs.

What new methods win allow improved and more accurate assessment of the optical performance of the human eye?

New methods are needed to measure the optical and physiologic properties of cornea. Improved techniques should allow more precise measurement of the topography of surgically altered corneas, with special emphasis on validating their accuracy. It also would be desirable to develop topography or other measurements to design the optimal surgical procedure before intervention.

What are the basic biomechanical properties of the cornea?

New approaches should be developed to investigate the stress-strain parameters of human corneal tissue and identify its load-bearing elements. We need studies that will add to our understanding of the basic macromolecular structure of collagen in order to determine the effects of corneal plasticity on light transmission. Stress-strain measurements should be made on the intact human cornea to determine such fundamental mechanical parameters as Young's modulus, Poisson's ratio, and nonlinearity coefficients. It is particularly important to know the interindividual variability and changes over time. These basic material constants should be the basis for microstructure-based models of the fundamental elements of the cornea. A baseline representation of the material characteristics of the corneal elements would bring the field together with a common base of properties and provide a technical platform for the approach to wound healing.

How is the corneal wound-healing process controlled?

One urgent need is to study cellular activity during corneal wound healing and remodeling. There is a lack of knowledge about where the cells originate, what factors attract them and cause proliferation and death, how old tissue is removed, and how these processes are modulated.

How do keratocytes respond to surgery?

It is important to devise techniques for determining how they are activated, how they migrate to wound sites, and if their behavior can be modified or controlled. The hierarchical structure of scar tissues should be investigated in order to devise ways to alter the refractive index imbalance between collagen and the ground substance in scars.

Chapter 12

National Eye Institute Report on Myopia and Refractive Problems

Introduction

In the United States less than 2 percent of all children beginning school (typically at age 5) are myopic. By the end of grade school (i.e., at approximately age 11 or 12) more than 15 percent of American children are myopic. By adulthood, about 25 percent of all Americans are myopic, thereby requiring some form of optical correction (i.e., glasses or contact lenses) to see clearly beyond an arm's length. About one-half of all nearsighted Americans developed their myopia during grade school years. Leaving aside college-bound young adults (a population that has an unusual incidence of myopia), the prevalence of myopia among Americans ages 14 to 64 remains relatively constant.

The cost of myopia to society is enormous. Because it affects one in four adult Americans, myopia has tremendous social, vocational, and public health implications. Vision Research—A National Plan: 1983–1987 reports that "...the loss of productivity and function due to refractive error may be said to rival that due to headache or the common cold." Refractive eye examinations cost consumers $1 billion annually, and more than $1.5 billion is spent each year on eyeglasses. Yet we still know very little about why a particular child becomes myopic, what the risk factors are, and exactly how the growth of the eye during grade school years leads to myopia in so many cases.

Excerpt from NIH Pub. No. 93-3186, *Vision Research: A National Plan, 1994–1998.*

Subprogram Objectives

- To elucidate, both from animal and human studies, the developmental mechanisms of emmetropization and refractive error.

- To establish the relationship between animal models of myopia and refractive error development and human myopia.

- To identify the biochemical mediators of eye growth and the way in which they are affected by characteristics of visual signals.

- To identify the risk factors, through longitudinal studies, for refractive error development in children and young adults.

Current Level of National Eye Institute Support

In Fiscal Year (FY) 1992 the NEI supported 10 research grants at a total cost of $1,970,181. Over the last 5 years, research accomplishments in this subprogram have furthered our understanding of myopia and refractive errors.

Recent Accomplishments

It has become clear that many infant animals have a "critical period" of eye development, during which the length of the eye (in particular the vitreal chamber) is very much affected by light exposure, patterned visual stimulation, light focus, and the introduction of particular chemicals to the retina. In chickens, and perhaps in other animals, these environmental variables trigger retinal mechanisms that help control the length of the developing eye. The effect, in chickens at least, is often reversible during the critical period. Accommodation (near focusing) is involved as a "fine tuning" mechanism in chickens and does not appear necessary in the modulation of avian eye growth. It may have a more important role in the development of myopia in other animals (e.g., primates).

By the age of 5 the human eyeball is very nearly adult size, and very few 5-year-olds are myopic. It is not clear exactly how the most common human myopia (i.e., juvenile onset myopia, which develops after most of our eye growth is completed) is related to the vision deprivation myopia that can be induced in animals during their critical period of ocular growth. Over the last 10 years, however, vision deprivation studies have demonstrated clearly that visual feedback is required for proper ocular growth. These studies of animal models have raised important considerations of the role the visual environment and local retinal factors may play in the development of human juvenile myopia. Animal experiments involving environmental manipulations have demonstrated that the growth of at least some of the optical components of the developing eye is modified to eliminate or reduce focusing error (i.e., they demonstrate emmetropization). Emmetropization itself is not a new discovery; it has been recognized in human development for many years. But the discovery in animal models of environmental and, possibly, local influences on emmetropization has caused a resurgence of research interest in the role these factors might play in human myopia. Furthermore, the animal studies that have examined the relationship between the size of eye components and optical focus have highlighted the need for similar measures in humans specifically the measure of human eye parts as they develop, especially in individuals who are developing refractive errors. At the same time, the development of sophisticated instrumentation for measuring eye components in very young children and infants has set the stage for aggressive studies on the development of myopia and other refractive errors.

Specific accomplishments over the last 5 years, in both animal and human vision research, point the way to further advances in understanding myopia and refractive errors.

Animal Studies

Some years ago vision researchers found that suturing the eyelid of a young animal affected the growth of the eye. This initial discovery of the connection between environmental effects and axial eye length has been extended with further animal studies. Specifically, emmetropization has been shown to be an active process; Some developing animals even overcome refractive errors caused by experimentally introduced lenses that create optical blurring. Through emmetropization, developing animals can recover from experimentally induced myopia or hyperopia (i.e., farsightedness).

Perhaps more surprising are the animal studies in which the optic nerve has been severed or ganglion cell activity blocked. These studies have shown that emmetropization can occur without activation of higher visual centers and without accommodation. Collectively these findings will accelerate the search for factors in the retina that influence emmetropization, with the outer retina receiving more attention.

A spectacular demonstration of the local retinal control of axial length comes from studies of chickens in which vision deprivation myopia is restricted to the deprived parts of the visual field. In the most recent experiments, retinal dopamine has been suggested as a candidate factor linking the control of ocular growth with vision. In chickens this may influence axial, but not equatorial, elongation of the vitreal chamber.

Experimental manipulation of developing collagen seems to alter vitreal chamber length in tree shrews but not in chickens. This interspecies difference still puzzles researchers. Equally puzzling is the question of whether the vitreal chamber elongation in animals with experimentally induced myopia is associated with passive stretching of the sclera or with an increase in sclerocytes and scleral substance.

Human Studies

The following significant advances in instrumentation now make it feasible to measure all components of refractive error in children and adults:

- Rapid measures of refractive error, both in infants (photo-refraction) and in children and adults (automated refraction) can be made in large populations.

- Techniques have improved for making ultrasonic measurements of the eye components (i.e., anterior chamber depth, lens thickness, and vitreal chamber depth) that contribute to the overall refraction and focusing in the eye. These improvements have grown out of the need to measure the power of intraocular lens implants following cataract surgery.

- The crystalline lens power, the most frequently omitted direct *in vivo* measure in studies of human refractive components, can now be measured relatively easily in young children using video ophthalmophacometry.

- Commercially available instruments can now document in detail corneal curvature and shape across the entire corneal surface. These instruments were developed along with surgical procedures for reshaping the cornea to reduce refractive error. This video keratography should rapidly replace the established, but more limiting, clinical keratometry measures, which typically provide a spherical approximation to curvature by sampling only the central 3 mm zone of the cornea.

These advances in instrumentation will encourage reliable and valid measures for longitudinal and cross sectional studies of ocular growth in human infants, children, and adults.

Studies have reported some treatment since the last review (e.g., bifocals for children, pharmacological paralysis of lens accommodation, fitting of hard contact lenses, drugs for lowering intraocular pressure), though all fail to provide clear or significant effects. Controlled studies are still needed. However, epidemiological studies and longitudinal studies identifying risk factors generally should precede human clinical trials of treatment.

Optical component studies show that some populations of school children do not exhibit a significant incidence of myopia. Consequently, risk factors will receive renewed interest, including environment (e.g., near work), genetics, and culture. The onset of myopia in college students is now well documented. Contrary to earlier reports that this adult onset myopia involved changes in the cornea or lens, it now appears to involve an increase in axial length. The candidate risk factors for adult onset myopia must now be identified with longitudinal studies. For example, a few studies of young adults suggest that accommodative behavior, particularly tonic accommodation after sustained near tasks, is different in groups exhibiting different refractive errors. Adult onset myopes appear to have lower tonic accommodation values than other individuals. How this might be related to myopia development or axial length elongation has not been demonstrated.

Studies of the prevalence of myopia and other refractive errors are still lacking, leaving us with very approximate figures from numerous flawed studies. Well-designed epidemiological studies of prevalence are needed to provide more insight into such association factors as gender, ethnicity, diet, educational level, extent of near work, climate, and culture. For context, the absence of well-designed, published studies made it very difficult for the National Academy of Sciences

109

National Research Council's Vision Committee to establish, with confidence, whether there had been significant trends in the prevalence of myopia among college-age individuals over the last 100 years. Conclusions about the progression of myopia in this same age group were even more difficult to make.

An objective of this subprogram is to understand how the eye changes as it grows in order to keep images clearly in focus on the retina and what goes wrong to produce nearsightedness or farsightedness. Studies of animals during their critical growth period have raised questions that were not even considered only 5 years ago about the exact nature of the visual environment and local retinal factors necessary for emmetropization. To investigate the important questions in myopia and refractive error research using animals, we will need to apply molecular and cellular biology, biochemistry, neurochemistry, neuropharmacology, and visual physiology. As apparent as this may seem, the idea of applying modern methods of neurobiology to these questions remains quite novel. We need to establish the relationship between deprivation myopia, which develops during the critical period of eye growth in animals, and the vast majority of human myopia, which develops after the critical period.

Many interesting findings in myopia research recently have come from the avian animal model. However, it is recognized that, in the absence of compelling reasons to use another species, the choice of the animal research model should closely resemble the human model, such as the nonhuman primate. In many cases it is appropriate that studies on avian or other nonprimate models and studies on primates that are directed toward cellular and biochemical mechanisms should proceed in parallel in order to facilitate the application of findings from the animal work to our understanding of human emmetropization and myopia.

The study of human ocular growth and refractive error in large populations of infant, child, and adult eyes is now feasible, thanks to new instruments that promise reliable and valid measures of the ocular components of refraction. In order to identify risk factors for myopia and other refractive errors, longitudinal studies of the ocular components of refraction in humans must parallel the already well-documented studies of changes in ocular components in animals. We need to identify risk factors if we are going to answer questions such as "Which child will become myopic?" and "Can myopia be retarded, prevented, or reversed?"

Important Research Questions To Be Addressed

The following research questions need to be addressed:

How do the ocular components change anatomically, physiologically, and biochemically to maintain a clearly focused image as the eye grows during emmetropization?

Studies of both animal models and humans will be necessary to elucidate the developmental mechanisms of emmetropization and refractive error development. It will be important to determine the relationship between animal models of myopia, such as those based on visual deprivation, and the human myopia that presumably develops during normal visual experience and after the eye is almost adult in size. Studies of biochemical mediators of eye growth appear particularly promising for the near future. Special attention should be given to local retinal chemistry and growth processes. The issue of scleral expansion from active growth mechanisms versus passive stretch also will have to be addressed.

Longitudinal studies of individual human eye growth are needed to identify risk factors for refractive error development. Such studies should include cycloplegic refraction, state clearly the target population and sample selection, define criteria for refractive error or change, and include confidence limits for all measures.

How do visual factors such as the nature of the stimulus and accommodation affect the development of myopia?

The characteristics of the visual signal detected by the retina and interaction with the optics of the developing eye (e.g., depth of focus, accommodative precision, and cornea and lens optics) may be important factors in regulating eye growth. The activity of populations of retinal cells needs to be related to the visual stimuli that experimentally produce myopia.

The role of accommodative factors in the development of myopia has long been controversial. There is a great need for studies of accommodation and convergence in the development of myopia in both juvenile and adult humans.

How do juvenile, adult onset, and pathological myopia differ in their risk factors and other characteristics?

The relative influence of heredity and environment needs to be assessed for each of these entities.

Are there effective means to prevent, retard, or reverse the development of myopia?

If biochemical mediators of ocular growth are identified, antagonists should be developed to intervene in the myopic process. Other noninvasive or medical interventions (e.g., bifocals, contact lenses, and topical drugs) also need to be evaluated.

Chapter 13

The Eye and Corrective Lenses

How the Eye Works

Light enters the eye through the cornea, the fluid-filled bulge at the front of the eyeball. The cornea slows down the light and bends it toward the center. The light now reaches the iris, which narrows or expands the dark hole at its center, the pupil, to regulate the amount of light that proceeds toward the retina. The pupil narrows in bright light, dilates when light is dim. The lens focuses the light when its shape is changed by the ciliary muscle; this sharpens the picture the lens has received from the cornea. To reach the retina, the image now passes through the ball of clear jelly that makes up the greater part of the eye. This "vitreous humor" exerts fluid pressure that maintains the eyeball's shape. (Occasional vague shapes we see before our eyes are dead blood cells floating in the jelly.) The retina is a thin membrane at the back of the eyeball. The macula, a small area near the center of the retina, is the region of greatest visual acuity. The sight is keenest of all at the center of the retina. When we turn our eyes toward what we want to look at, we are aligning them so that light falls directly on the fovea. The retina is where the image first recorded by the cornea and modified along the way is translated into electrical messages carried by the optic nerves to those parts of the brain where we interpret what our eyes record.

Excerpt from Seiderman, Arthur S., *20/20 Is Not Enough*. Alfred A. Knopf. New York: 1989, pp. 16-17. Used by permission.

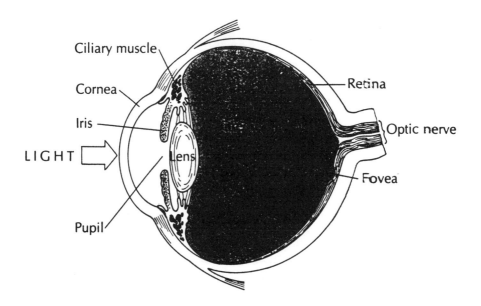

Figure 13.1. How the Eye Works.

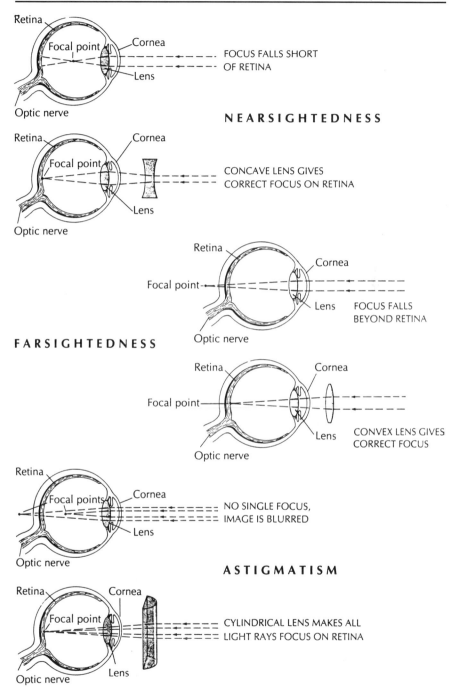

Figure 13.2. How Lenses Correct Refractive Error.

Chapter 14

Amblyopia

What is Amblyopia?

Amblyopia is poor vision in an eye that did not develop normal sight during early childhood. It is sometimes called "lazy eye."

When one eye develops good vision while the other does not, the eye with poorer vision is called amblyopic. Usually, only one eye is affected by amblyopia.

The condition is common, affecting approximately 2 or 3 out of every 100 people. The best time to correct amblyopia is during infancy or early childhood. Parents must be aware of this potential problem if they want to protect their child's vision.

How Does Normal Vision Develop?

Newborn infants are able to see, but as they use their eyes during the first months of life, vision improves. During early childhood years, the visual system changes quickly and vision continues to develop.

If a child cannot use his or her eyes normally, vision does not develop properly and may even decrease. After the first nine years of life, the visual system is usually fully developed and usually cannot be changed.

The development of equal vision in both eyes is necessary for normal vision.

American Academy of Ophthalmology ©1984. Used by permission.

117

Many occupations are not open to people who have good vision in one eye only.

If the vision in one eye should be lost later in life from an accident or illness, it is essential that the other eye have normal vision. Without normal vision in at least one eye, a person is visually impaired.

For all of these reasons, amblyopia must be detected and treated as early as possible.

When Should Vision Be Tested?

It is recommended that all children have their vision checked by their pediatrician, family physician or ophthalmologist (medical eye doctor) at or before their fourth birthday.

All children should have their vision tested at or before their fourth birthday Most physicians test vision as part of a child's medical examination. They may refer a child to an ophthalmologist (a medical eye doctor) if there is any sign of an eye condition.

New techniques make it possible to test vision in infants and young children. If there is a family history of misaligned eyes, childhood cataracts or a serious eye disease, an ophthalmologist can check vision even earlier than age three.

What Causes Amblyopia?

Amblyopia is caused by any condition that affects normal use of the eyes and visual development. In many cases, the conditions associated with amblyopia may be inherited. Children in a family with a history of amblyopia or misaligned eyes should be checked by an ophthalmologist early in life.

Amblyopia has three major causes:

Strabismus (misaligned eyes)

Amblyopia occurs most commonly with misaligned or crossed eyes. The crossed eye "turns off" to avoid double vision and the child uses only the better eye.

Unequal Focus (refractive error)

Refractive errors are eye conditions that are corrected by wearing glasses. Amblyopia occurs when one eye is out of focus because it is more nearsighted, farsighted or astigmatic than the other. The unfocused (blurred) eye "turns off" and becomes amblyopic. The eyes can look normal but one eye has poor vision. This is the most difficult type of amblyopia to detect and requires careful measurement of vision.

Cloudiness in the Normally Clear Eye Tissues

An eye disease such as a cataract (a clouding of the eye's natural lens) may lead to amblyopia. Any factor that prevents a clear image from being focused inside the eye can lead to the development of amblyopia in a child. This is often the most severe form of amblyopia.

How Is Amblyopia Diagnosed?

It is not easy to recognize amblyopia. A child may not be aware of having one strong eye and one weak eye. Unless the child has a misaligned eye or other obvious abnormality, there is often no way for parents to tell that something is wrong.

Amblyopia is detected by finding a difference in vision between the two eyes. Since it is difficult to measure vision in young children, your ophthalmologist often estimates visual acuity by watching how well a baby follows objects with one eye when the other eye is covered.

Using a variety of tests, the ophthalmologist observes the reactions of the baby when one eye is covered. If one eye is amblyopic and the good eye is covered, the baby may attempt to look around the patch, try to pull it off or cry.

Poor vision in one eye does not always mean that a child has amblyopia. Vision can often be improved by prescribing glasses for a child.

Your ophthalmologist will also carefully examine the interior of the eye to see if other eye diseases may be causing decreased vision. These diseases include:

- Cataracts;
- Inflammations;
- Tumors;
- Other disorders of the inner eye.

How Is Amblyopia Treated?

To correct amblyopia, a child must be made to use the weak eye. This is usually done by patching or covering the strong eye, often for weeks or months.

Even after vision has been restored in the weak eye, part-time patching may be required over a period of years to maintain the improvement.

Glasses may be prescribed to correct errors in focusing. If glasses alone do not improve vision, then patching is necessary. Occasionally, amblyopia is treated by blurring the vision in the good eye with special eye drops or lenses to force the child to use the amblyopic eye.

Amblyopia is usually treated before surgery to correct misaligned eyes, and patching is often continued after surgery as well.

If your ophthalmologist finds a cataract or other abnormality, surgery is required to correct the problem. After surgery, glasses or contact lenses can be used to restore focusing, while patching improves vision.

Amblyopia cannot be cured by treating the cause alone. The weaker eye must be made stronger in order to see normally. Prescribing glasses or performing surgery can correct the cause of amblyopia, but your ophthalmologist must also treat the amblyopia.

If amblyopia is not treated, several problems may occur:

- The amblyopic eye may develop a serious and permanent visual defect;
- Depth perception (seeing in three dimensions) may be lost;
- If the good eye becomes diseased or injured, a lifetime of poor vision may be the result.

Your ophthalmologist can give you instructions on how to treat amblyopia, but it is up to you and your child to carry out this treatment.

A common treatment for amblyopia is to patch the strong eye; the weak eye is strengthened because the child is forced to use it.

Children do not like to have their eyes patched, especially if they have been depending on that eye to see clearly. But as a parent, you must convince your child to do what is best for him or her.

Successful treatment mostly depends on your interest and involvement, as well as your ability to gain your child's cooperation. In most cases, parents play an important role in determining whether their child's amblyopia is to be corrected.

Loss of Vision Is Preventable

Success in the treatment of amblyopia also depends upon:

• How severe the amblyopia is;
• How old the child is when treatment is begun.

If the problem is detected and treated early, vision can improve for most children. Sometimes part-time treatment may have to continue until the child is about nine years of age. After this time, amblyopia usually does not return.

If amblyopia is first discovered after early childhood, treatment may not be successful. Vision loss from strabismus or unequal refractive errors may be treated successfully at a much older age than the amblyopia caused by cloudiness in tissues in the eye.

If you have additional questions or would like any further information, contact your ophthalmologist.

Chapter 15

Crossed Eyes

The eyes should work together as a team. When one eye is deviated (turned too far in one direction), we call the condition strabismus, or crossed eyes. Strabismus occurs most often in young children. A child with strabismus may have esotropia (one eye turning in), exotropia (one eye turning out), or hypertropia one eye higher than the other).

There are many causes for this breakdown in binocular vision. Most commonly, strabismus is inherited. In other patients, a deviation will result from a high degree of farsightedness. Strabismus also may occur after a loss of vision in one eye due to a disease process. (Esotropia is sometimes the first sign of a tumor in the eye of a child.) When there is a loss of vision in one eye, children under the age of four years will usually develop esotropia, whereas the older patient generally develops exotropia. Another cause of an eye deviation may be damage to one of the three nerves supplying the muscles that move the eye. In most cases, the muscles themselves are normal, but the coordination mechanism is defective.

If the eyes do not focus together, the patient has double vision (diplopia). To avoid this double vision, the child learns to ignore or suppress the picture in the deviating eye. Habitual suppression of one eye causes that eye to become lazy, or amblyopic. The vision becomes poor and cannot be improved with glasses. Amblyopia usually does not develop in children over the age of four years.

UIC Department of Ophthalmology, *Eye Facts*, April/May 1988.

Fortunately, strabismus can be treated. The earlier that treatment is instituted, the better the final result. While a certain amount of deviation may be considered normal in infants' eyes, a deviation still present at five months, and certainly by six months of age, must be considered abnormal, and the infant should be evaluated by an ophthalmologist. Similarly, any child who develops a deviation after six months of age should be brought promptly to an ophthalmologist for evaluation. Children do not outgrow strabismus.

The evaluation begins with a thorough eye examination. The eye movements are observed, and the fixation pattern (how the child uses each eye) is determined. In this way a lazy eye can be detected in infants. If the child is noted to prefer using one eye, occlusion therapy (patching of that eye) can be instituted. Using only the lazy eye helps the child develop better vision in that eye. A dilated examination of the back of the eye is of prime importance to verify that there is no eye disease responsible for the deviation. At the same time, it is possible to determine, even in the small infant or newborn, if the child is nearsighted or farsighted If a high degree of farsightedness is noted during the exam, the deviation may be corrected with the proper glasses. Glasses can be helpful in children as young as six months of age. They are most effective in treating the esotropic child, whose eyes turn in, and about one third of all such children will have their deviation corrected with glasses alone. Usually the child with exotropia or hypertropia will require surgery to correct the deviation. Eye exercises can be helpful once the eyes have been straightened with glasses or surgery. However, with the tendency toward early surgery, eye exercises have played a lesser role in the treatment of strabismus and are usually unnecessary. Furthermore, most children have to be at least four years of age before they can benefit from any type of eye exercises.

A great deal of progress has been made in the surgical treatment of strabismus. It is no longer the frightening experience it once was. The child is brought to the hospital on the day of surgery, is operated on, and is able to go home the same day. Parents are encouraged to be with their child as much as possible and are separated from the child only during the surgical procedure itself. As soon as the child starts to wake up in the recovery room, the parents are brought in.

The surgery consists of strengthening a muscle by cutting out a small piece of its tendon or weakening a muscle by moving the position where the muscle attaches. At no time is there an incision into the eyeball.

Because of newer techniques and a more accurate assessment of the problem, the treatment of strabismus is quite successful. Most deviations can be corrected with one surgical procedure.

Despite these excellent results, ophthalmologists are constantly striving to improve the success of strabismus treatment. The Pediatric Ophthalmology and Strabismus Service at the University of Illinois at Chicago is participating in a multicenter study, the Prism Adaptation Study, which is evaluating the importance of newer diagnostic modalities.

Note: Single copies of "Eye Facts" are available free upon request by contacting the Managing Editor. The publication is also available in Spanish. Readers are encouraged to reprint "Eye Facts" either in part or its entirety, with permission from the Managing Editor using the acknowledgment: "Reprinted from 'Eye Facts' with permission of the Department of Ophthalmology, the University of Illinois at Chicago."

The Department of Ophthalmology is located in the Eye and Ear Infirmary, 1855 West Taylor Street, Chicago, IL 60612. For eye appointments, call (312) 996-4356; for 24-hour emergency information, call (312) 1-TRAUMA.

—by Eugene R. Folk, MD, Professor

Chapter 16

Aligining Eyes:
Straightening Out Strabismus

"Why do you have that patch on? Did your eye fall out?" Kindergartner Kimberly May answered the jeer with a shrug. In 1974, it was Kim's first day of school in Gaithersburg, Md., and she and the boy harassing her were waiting with other children for the building to open. Standing nearby, Kim's 7-year-old brother Erik replied with gusto: "You dumb thing. She's got amblyopia, and she needs the eye patch so she can see better. So *there.*"

Although Erik couldn't explain how Kim's amblyopia (decreased vision) resulted from strabismus (eye misalignment), he defended his sister with the few terms and facts he's overheard at home. And although Kim couldn't find comfort in knowing that many other youngsters wear eye patches for amblyopia, she took heart from her brother's support.

Strabismus affects approximately 4 percent of U.S. children under age 6. Amblyopia occurs in about 2 percent of the general population.

Anne May, a registered nurse, discussed her daughter's condition with the teacher, emphasizing that strabismus would not hamper Kim's ability to do class work. May also spoke to the class.

"I told them one eye sometimes is weak but can often be strengthened by patching," May says. "We took the patch off to show them her eye was OK under there. After that, there were only one or two remarks, from students absent that day."

In Kim, strabismus occurred as crossed eyes. In others it may manifest as eyes that turn out, up or down. Its name can be traced to

FDA *Consumer*. November 1991.

the Greek word *strabismus*, to look obliquely or with unstraight eyes: some use the terms "squint" and "lazy eye." Strabismus can disable sight in one eye, yet leave the other with 20/20 vision. Strabismus can be acquired from diverse causes at any age. There are more than a dozen variations.

Sight: A Team Effort

Healthy eyes move together to send similar images along the optic nerve to the brain for fusion into a single 3-dimensional picture at the brain-vision junction, or visual cortex. Toward this end, six muscles attached to the outside of each eye contract and relax to move the eyes in perfect synchronization, permitting fusion, or binocular vision, across a large area of the visual field.

Strabismic eyes, on the other hand, do not move in unison. A muscle may pull too weakly or too strongly against its opposing muscle, creating an imbalance that causes one eye to drift from parallel alignment with its mate: more than one pair of muscles may be imbalanced.

Since each eye fixates on an object at a different point in space, the images received by the brain are dissimilar. The brain is unable to fuse the dissimilar images, resulting in double vision, which can be very disturbing. To avoid this disturbance, the brain may suppress vision in the deviating eye, allowing clear sight to develop solely in the straight eye. Decreased vision in the suppressed eye is called amblyopia. Prolonged amblyopia causes a loss in 3-dimensional viewing and depth perception.

The "squint" or turn usually is constant but may be intermittent and may occur in only one eye or alternate between the two eyes. Vision on people with alternating strabismus generally remains good in each eye individually.

While strabismus clearly stems from muscle imbalance, the causes of such imbalance are many and are not all completely understood.

"There's a strong genetic influence, but there are also many anatomic and neuromuscular reasons," says John F. O'Neill, M.D., and ophthalmologist (a physician who specializes in eye disease) and director of the Pediatric Ophthalmology and Strabismus Service at Georgetown University's Center for Sight in Washington, D.C. "One group of children may have eyes that turn, usually inward, from the day they are born. Another group may have perfectly healthy and straight eyes their first few years of life. However, as these children mature and start focusing more carefully on objects, the effort to see clearly causes their eyes to cross. Another group of children with neurologic conditions, such as cerebral palsy, not only may have poor movement of their arms and legs, but the eye muscle system is affected as well."

Strabismus can be associated with many other conditions that cause poor vision in one or both eyes—for example, cataract, Down syndrome, thyroid disease, eye tumor, damage to the fetal central nervous system from toxoplasmosis (a parasitic infection that can pass from the mother during pregnancy), damage the nerve supplying the eye muscle (perhaps from birth trauma), or eye disuse due to high refractive error (such as extreme farsightedness) or different refractive errors in each eye (such as nearsightedness in one eye and farsightedness in the other).

Is It Strabismus?

Maybe not. Some children have facial features that make the eyes look crossed when they aren't, and some normal newborns have a temporary outward drift.

Eye alignment is not fully mature at birth. A true developmental eye drift typically shows up from birth to 3 or 4 months of age, when normal eyes are straightening, but may occur through childhood or later. Misalignment that persists to age 5 or 6 months or occurs later should be assessed by an eye specialist. Early diagnosis is vital to detect and treat underlying causes and prevent severe vision disability.

"The first thing we do in examining children is to assess their vision, to determine the degree of visual attentiveness in each eye separately," O'Neill says. "We observe the child's ability to fixate on an object, and then we test how well each eye alone, and both eyes together, can follow that object in different directions and at different distances."

Many techniques are used to check the alignment and movement of the eyes to test for strabismus.

A quick screening method is the Hirschberg corneal reflex test, says Walter Sloane, M.D., an ophthalmologist with FDA's Center for Devices and Radiological Health, which regulates medical devices, including those used to test and treat the eye. The examiner directs an examining light onto the child's cornea (the transparent covering that admits light through the pupil) as the child looks at the light. In normal eyes, the light reflection appears in the center of pupils. An eye that reflects light from a different place may be strabismic and should be further examined, Sloane says.

Another corneal reflex tests is the Krimsky method. It compares the location of the reflected examining light in each pupil: again, light reflections that are dissimilar indicate strabismus. Prisms placed over one or both eyes align the reflections to estimate the amount of the turn.

The alternate cover test quickly spots misalignment. "The examiner rapidly covers and uncovers each eye, shifting back and forth from one eye to the other like windshield wiper," Sloane says. "If the child has any deviation, the eye will immediately move as the cover is shifted to the uncovered eye."

The cover-uncover test differentiates serious types of strabismus called tropias from latent drifts called phorias, which seldom require treatment.

"The brain immediately overcomes a phoria drift," Sloane says. "So when the drift is a phoria, we see movement immediately after the eye is uncovered as it responds to control by the brain. But when the eye with a tropia is covered, it becomes unhooked, so to speak, from the brain's control so that it drifts—in any direction—and remains turned in that position when uncovered until we cover its fellow eye, which has been staring at the object. When the fellow eye is covered, the turned eye is reconnected to the brain. The turned eye then moves to fixate on the object as if to say, 'Oops, I was facing the wrong direction.'"

One new method, a "preferential looking technique," uses Teller acuity cards. These devices are similar to educational flash cards, but instead of letters or numbers they have black and white stripes ranging in patterns from very broad to very narrow, simulating large to small pictures or letters.

"Vision is gauged," O'Neill says, "by how attentively a child, even a baby, looks at each pattern."

The use of drops to dilate the eyes allows inspection of the back of the eye to detect eye disease that may be contributing to the drift. Depending on the findings, other tests may be required.

Best Chance to See

Prompt attention to correcting eye misalignment will provide the most satisfactory outcome of treatment. Indeed, if some cases of strabismus are left untreated age 6, permanent visual impairment can result.

Treatment has three primary goals, O'Neill says: foremost, to obtain the best possible vision in each eye: second, to gain the best possible alignment of each eye alone and as a pair; and, finally, to provide the best opportunity for binocular vision. Corrective eyeglasses, patching, or both are the mainstay therapies, with about 30 percent of patients needing surgery, he says.

Corrective eyeglasses can help children as young as 6 months of age. They're most effective when there is significant farsightedness and the eyes turn in, and they're the only therapy needed in about a third of these patients whose eyes turn in. Prisms incorporated in eyeglasses may relieve double vision in some older patients.

To force use of a "lazy" eye while preserving vision in the preferred eye, patching is very effective.

"If a child doesn't develop vision equally in each eye early in life," O'Neill says, "it may never develop fully. For a 4-month-old child, patching might be used only an hour or two a day. A child that age probably takes 2 or 3 naps a day, so I'd patch for only one of those waking periods. But you have to be cautious. When you have a patch at this early stage of development, you inactivate the eye. If you cover the eye for too long a period at this time, the child can use sight in that eye, and the loss could be irreversible."

In 1969, when Kim May was first patched at age 6 months, doctors didn't have as much information about early development of vision.

"We were told to patch her straight eye 24 hours a day for an entire week, removing the patch only for changing it and for bathing," her mother says. "And then we were to patch the other eye. But at the end of that week, when I took the patch off and started covering her crossed eye, the straight one was basically blind. She couldn't see her baby bottle, I had to put it into her hand. Her brain had totally switched over to the crossed eye."

Sight did return to Kim's temporarily vision-disabled left eye. She had surgery on it in September 1970 and on the right eye in 1975 and 1980 to realign the imbalanced muscles. With corrective eye glasses, Kim today at age 22 has 20/30 vision in her left eye and 20/25 in her previously crossed right eye.

Surgery Can Help

Some 60,000 to 80,000 operations are performed each year to correct strabismus. When the eyes turn out, up or down, correction usually requires surgery. Sometimes as second operation is required. With current knowledge and techniques, it's uncommon for a patient (about 1 in 20) to need a third operation, O'Neill says. The need for further corrective surgery, he says, depends on the stability of the muscle system and the degree of muscle response (over- or under-response) to the surgical adjustment.

Complications related to strabismus surgery are infrequent. Besides general risks such as bleeding and infection that accompany any surgery, complications may include postoperative double vision, and—rarely—excessive tissue reaction with scarring.

By weakening or strengthening an eye muscle (or muscles), strabismus surgery alters the muscular pull on the afflicted eye in order to align its movements with the other eye. The ophthalmologist can weaken or strengthen a muscle function by repositioning the muscle on the outside of the eye (never cutting into the eyeball) and also can strengthen a muscle by cutting out (resecting) a small piece of its tendon. Techniques with adjustable sutures allow additional repositioning within the first following surgery. When the patient is a child, general anesthesia is always used. Some adults may have local anesthesia.

After surgery, bandages frequently are unnecessary and there are just redness in the eye. The parents are given an antibiotic ointment to print in the child's eyes, and the doctor generally will see the patient again in two or three days.

New Treatments

Following a number of years of investigations. FDA, in December 1989, licensed a therapy for strabismus patients age 12 and older: Oculinum, an injectable form of sterile, purified *Botulinum* toxin, type A. Before FDA granted approval, the agency's Center for Biologics Evaluation and Research reviewed safety and effectiveness data on Oculinum.

Wiley Chambers, M.D., an ophthalmologist with FDA's Center for Drug Evaluation and Research who contributed to this review, points out, "Oculinum can be used effectively to treat certain adults with strabismus, but its effect in children hasn't been adequately evaluated.

"We limited it to patients over age 12," he says, "because children under that age have a chance of developing amblyopia, and more information is needed to reliably assure muscle balance and prevent the risk of amblyopia. When amblyopia isn't a consideration, a lot of people think it's worth trying, to avoid an operation."

Unfortunately, effectiveness is unlikely in opposing-muscle weakness, severe misalignment, and certain other circumstances.

The toxin derives from *Clostridium botulinum* bacterial and is very potent. If accidentally eaten in contaminated foods, it can cause botulism poisoning that may result in paralysis, even death. In the treatment of strabismus, however, it is used in extremely dilute concentrations, and there have been no reports of botulism poisoning from Oculinum use in patients with strabismus or blepharospasm, an eye spasm disorder the product also is licensed to treat. In some 8,340 injections, nine accidental punctures and 16 instances of excess bleeding occurred. None resulted in vision loss. The most common side effects are eyelid droop and eye irritation.

Oculinum is injected into an eye-turning muscle, outside the eye, through an electromyographic needle that guides placement by recording the muscle's electrical activity. Anesthetic eye drops generally are used before the injection.

The toxin "turns off" the muscle by paralyzing it. Scientists theorize the paralysis affects muscle pairs by causing the injected muscle to lengthen, thus prompting the opposing muscle to shorten.

About half of patients require repeated treatments. In a recent study of 677 patients, 55 percent showed improvement six months later. Correction may be permanent, provided the injected muscle is paralyzed well enough and long enough and the opposing muscle is intact.

Another new therapy may benefit patients who acquire crossed eyes after age 6 months. It involves the use of eyeglasses overlaid with thin plastic prisms.

In September 1990, the University of Iowa Hospitals and Clinics in Iowa City announced the results of a six-year study led by William Scott, M.D., in which 14 medical centers tested the efficacy of treatment with prism eyeglasses before surgery in patients who had no previous eye surgery.

"By knowing the exact prism power that corrects the misalignment," Scott says, 'we can more accurately determine the surgical adjustment needed on the eye muscles, thus reducing the possible need for additional surgery." The eyes of about 83 percent of patients who used the special eyeglasses were straightened by the surgery, compared with 72 percent of patients without them.

Appropriate management offers strabismus patients the best possible circumstances for improvement.

"The key most often is early detection and treatment," says Georgetown's O'Neill. "Without proper care, strabismus in an infant or in a child early in life will generally get worse, not better. Children do not outgrow strabismus when the eyes are truly "crossed."

—by Dixie Farley

Chapter 17

Psuedostrabismus: Are Your Child's Eyes Really Crossed?

During the first few months of an infant's life, the eyes may drift in or out at times. Usually this misalignment lasts only for a few moments before the eyes straighten again. When a baby begins focusing on the environment, at about four months of age, the eyes are straight most or all of the time.

It is not uncommon for parents who notice their infant's eyes crossing to be concerned about the child's normal visual development. Misaligned eyes are indeed a cause of concern and if untreated can quickly lead to suppression of vision in one eye. However the appearance of crossed eyes can also be an illusion created by a wide, flat nose bridge. Prominent folds of eyelid skin (epicanthal folds) can cover the white part of the eye next to the nose and add to the illusion, especially when the child looks to the side.

The illusionary appearance of crossed eyes is called pseudostrabismus. Unlike truly misaligned eyes, which is called strabismus, the facial appearance causing pseudostrabismus improves with age as the bridge of the nose narrows and the folds of eyelid skin disappear.

True crossing of the eyes, a form of strabismus known as esotropia, is not outgrown and requires ophthalmological treatment to straighten the eyes and allow normal vision to develop in both eyes.

Less commonly, children may appear to have eyes that wander out, a condition known as exotropia. A form of pseudostrabismus (pseudoexotropia) may be caused by widely set eyes or there can be a real misalignment.

How Can You Tell The Difference?

If you shine a flashlight on the eyes, the reflection of the light can be seen as a spot on the front surface of the pupil. When the child is looking at the light, the reflection will be in the same location in each eye if the eyes are properly aligned. If the eyes are not properly aligned and the child has strabismus, the light reflection will not appear in the same location in each eye. The light reflection is in a normal position with pseudostrabismus since the reflection is not affected by the width of the nose or folds of eyelid skin. Parents often first notice an abnormal light reflection in flash photos of the child.

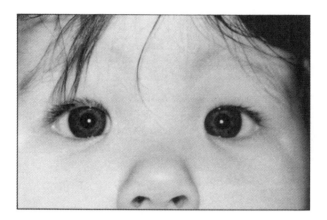

Figure 17.1. *Pseudostrabismus. Although the eyes appear misaligned, the light reflection is symmetrical in both eyes.*

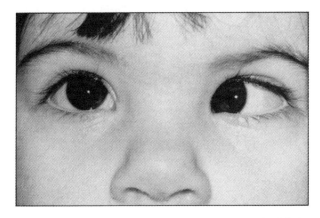

Figure 17.2. True strabismus. Notice the asymmetrical light reflection.

What Should You Do If You Think Your Child Has Strabismus?

If you have any questions as to whether your child's eyes are straight, ask your doctor to examine the child. Strabismus should not be ignored and a prompt examination may help avoid vision loss. Occasionally, strabismus may be caused by a cataract, a tumor in the eye, or a neurological problem. These conditions require immediate medical attention.

A child whose eyes are actually crossed will use only one eye at a time to avoid seeing double. The unused or crossed eye may not develop good vision and may become amblyopic (lazy) unless the child is made to use that eye by patching the good eye.

Early detection of amblyopia is important for successful treatment. The goals in treating strabismus are:

- Good visual development of both eyes;
- Straight eyes;
- Eyes that work together;
- Detection and treatment of any underlying eye problems.

How Can You Test Your Child's Vision At Home?

Older children can be tested for poor vision and amblyopia by using eye charts. The American Academy of Ophthalmology's Home Eye

Test for Children and Adults can be obtained from your ophthalmologist or by sending a business size, self-addressed, stamped envelope to the American Academy of Ophthalmology, P.O. Box 7424, San Francisco, CA 94120.

If you have any questions, contact your pediatrician, family doctor, or ophthalmologist.

Chapter 18

National Eye Institute Statement on Prospective Evaluation of Radial Keratotomy (PERK) Studies

After a decade of patient follow-up, a National Eye Institute (NEI)–supported study reported that radial keratotomy (RK) remained a reasonably safe and effective technique to improve distance vision.

However, the study found that more than 40 percent of RK-operated eyes continued to have a gradual shift toward farsightedness. This finding suggests that some people who have RK may need glasses at an earlier age for poor close-up vision, a common problem after age 40, than if they had chosen not to have the surgery.

"Based on these findings, it may be that some people will be pleased with their vision shortly after having RK, but their opinion may change five, ten, or fifteen years down the road," said Peter J. McDonnell, M.D., of the Doheny Eye Institute at the University of Southern California and the study's co-chairman.

[The] findings, published in Archives of Ophthalmology, were issued from the Prospective Evaluation of Radial Keratotomy (PERK). The PERK study is the first large, well-designed clinical study to evaluate the long-term effects of radial keratotomy on the eye and vision.

RK is performed to improve poor distance vision, called myopia, which affects millions of Americans. For some people with myopia, RK offers the prospect of good distance vision without the need for glasses or contact lenses.

NEI Press Release.

The surgery changes the shape of the cornea, the clear, rounded tissue at the front of the eye. It is performed by making spoke-like, partial-thickness incisions into the healthy cornea. These wounds cause the cornea to flatten, producing clearer distance vision.

Today, about 250,000 RK surgeries are performed annually in the United States, up from 30,000 operations just five years ago. However, eye care professionals still have little scientific information about the procedure's long-term effects on the cornea and vision.

To provide these data, PERK clinicians periodically examined the eyes of the 435 participants since the study began in the early 1980s. Based on these examinations, researchers have published occasional reports in medical journals, including the results issued today.

At the PERK's 10-year mark, researchers reported that RK effectively reduced but did not completely eliminate myopia in all patients. They found that 53 percent of the RK-operated eyes registered 20/20 vision, while 85 percent of the eyes had 20/40 uncorrected vision or better (required for a driver's license in most states). Approximately 70 percent of study participants said they did not wear corrective lenses for distance vision at the 10-year mark.

RK also had "a reasonable margin of safety," resulting in few vision-threatening complications. However, the researchers noted that 3 percent of operated eyes had poorer distance vision with glasses one decade after surgery, although none had corrected vision worse than 20/30.

Interestingly, the PERK scientists reported that 43 percent of the RK-operated eyes continued to have a gradual change toward farsightedness, called hyperopic shift. In fact, 36 percent of the eyes had become farsighted at the 10-year point.

"Typically, people who are myopic need reading glasses later in life than those who are not myopic," said Dr. McDonnell. "It may be that some people will reduce their need for glasses to see at a distance, but will need to wear reading glasses earlier than they otherwise would have needed to."

But the hyperopic shift was beneficial in some cases. In those who remained nearsighted after surgery, this gradual change caused an improvement in their vision, moving their sight closer to 20/20.

According to the researchers, this shift was detected in some affected patients as soon as six months after surgery and continued to progress a decade later. They said they do not know when and if this change will cease in the future. The scientists noted that the shift in vision was not related to the patient's age or post-surgical outcome.

They added that they could not predict based on the PERK data which patients will develop the hyperopic shift. They did note, however, that the shift was more common in those who had RK surgery using longer incisions in the cornea, a common technique in younger and/or more myopic patients.

"This clinical study provides ophthalmologists with scientifically validated information regarding the safety and effectiveness of radial keratotomy, said Carl Kupfer, M.D., director of the NEI, part of the National Institutes of Health. "With these results, prospective patients can have the best informed consent when considering radial keratotomy."

The National Eye Institute is the Federal government's lead agency for vision research.

Background

The PERK is a prospective clinical study involving 435 patients at nine centers nationwide. It was designed to evaluate the short and long-term safety and efficacy of one standardized RK technique. The procedure was evaluated by comparing each patient's refractive error and uncorrected vision before and after surgery.

The RK technique used in the study consisted of eight centrifugal, radial incisions made manually with a diamond micrometer knife.

All study participants were at least 21 years old and had myopia (two to eight diopters) that was correctable to 20/20 or better with glasses or contact lenses. Each patient agreed to have RK performed on one eye and wait one year before having surgery on their other eye.

Participants were examined before and after surgery at two weeks, three months, six months, annually for five years, and again at 10 years.

Chapter 19

Summary of PERK Studies

Purpose

- To determine if radial keratotomy is effective in reducing myopia.
- To detect complications of the surgery.
- To discover patient characteristics and surgical factors affecting the results.
- To determine the long-term safety and efficacy of the procedure.

Background

Approximately 11 million Americans have myopia that can be corrected with eyeglasses or contact lenses. Some of these people may also be candidates for radial keratotomy (RK), a procedure that aims to correct or reduce myopia by surgery that flattens the corneal curvature.

Keratotomy was first performed by surgeons in Europe and the United States m the late 1800's, and the basic optical and mechanical principles of the operation were defined in the 1940's and 1950's by the Japanese doctors, T. Sato and K. Akiyama, who used anterior and posterior corneal incisions. The posterior incisions damaged the cornea, and the procedure was modified in the Soviet Union by doctors Fyodorov and V. Dumev, to include incisions in only the anterior cornea. Since its introduction into the United States in 1978, numerous ophthalmologists have made technical and surgical improvements

NIH Pub No. 93-2910, August 1993.

in the procedure, such as ultrasonic methods to measure the thickness of the cornea and the use of diamond-bladed micrometer knives to make the incisions.

However, scientific assessment of RK lagged behind growing public and professional interest in the procedure. In 1980, in response to widespread concern about the long-term safety and efficacy of RK, a group of ophthalmic surgeons approached the National Eye Institute with a proposal for a multicenter clinical trial that would evaluate the potential benefits and risks of this procedure.

Description

The Prospective Evaluation of Radial Keratotomy study, involving 435 patients and 99 pilot patients, is a clinical trial designed to evaluate the short- and long-term safety and efficacy of one technique of radial keratotomy. The procedure is evaluated by comparing a patient's refractive error and uncorrected vision before and after surgery. The more myopic eye received surgery first. Patients were required to wait 1 year before having the second eye operated.

The surgical technique was standardized, consisting of 8 centrifugal radial incisions made manually with a diamond micrometer knife. The diameter of the central, uncut, dear zone was determined by the preoperative spherical equivalent cycloplegic refraction (-2.00 to -3.12 D = 4.0 mm; -325 to 4.3 D = 35 mm; 4.50 to -8.00 D = 3.0 mm). The blade length, which determined the depth of the incision, was set at 100 percent of the thinnest of four intraoperative ultrasonic corneal thickness readings taken paracentrally at the 3-, 6-,9-, and 12-o'clock meridians just outside the mark delineating the clear zone. The incisions were made from the edge of the trephine mark to the limbal vascular arcade and were spaced equidistantly around the cornea.

Patients were examined preoperatively and after surgery at 2 weeks, 3 months, 6 months, and annually for 5 years. Examinations in the morning and evening of the same day were done at 3 months, 1 year, and 3 years in a subset of the patients to test for diurnal fluctuation of vision and refraction.

The primary outcome variables measured at each visit are the uncorrected and spectacle corrected visual acuity and the refractive error with the pupil dilated and undilated. The corneal shape was measured with central keratometry and photokeratoscopy. Endothelial function was evaluated using specular microscopy. A slit-lamp microscope examination was made to check for complications from the incisions. Contrast sensitivity was tested in a subset of patients. Patient motivation and satisfaction were studied with psychometric questionnaires at baseline, 1 year, and 5-6 years.

Patient Eligibility

All men and women had 2 to 8 diopters of simple myopia and were correctable to 20/20 or better with glasses or contact lenses. All patients had the stability of their myopia documented by previous records. Patients were at least 21 years of age and lived in the metropolitan area of the study centers. Each patient agreed to have surgery on one eye and to wait 1 year for surgery on the other eye. Patients with systemic diseases that might affect corneal wound healing and patients with high corneal astigmatism were excluded from the study.

Patient Recruitment Status

Recruitment began in April 1981 and was completed in October 1983.

Current Status of Study

Ongoing. The investigators are involved in a 10-year follow-up examination of patients with the following timetable:

- In 1992, coordinators contacted patients to solicit their participation in the 10-year follow-up examination. As of November 1992, 96 percent of the 528 patients have been contacted, almost all of them agreeing to return for the 10-year follow-up examination.

- In 1993, each patient will undergo a complete follow-up examination, testing not only the variables in the original 5-year protocol, but also factors such as videokeratography and more modem methods of contrast sensitivity and glare testing.

- In 1994 and 1995, the data will be analyzed and the results published for both the main study and the sub-studies.

Results

In the PERK study it was found that radial keratotomy reduced myopia, but that the effectiveness of the outcome varied among patients. At 5-year follow-up (757 eyes—95 percent follow-up rate), the active change ranged from a 0.38 diopter increase in myopia to a 12.88 diopter decrease in myopia with an average 3.98 diopters (SD=1.69). For 64 percent of eyes, the refractive error was within 1 diopter of emmetropia, 19 percent of eyes were undercorrected and 17 percent were overcorrected by more than 1 diopter. At 5 years, 60 percent of eyes saw 20/20 or better, 88 percent of eyes 20/40 or better, and 2 percent of eyes saw 20/200 or worse. The surgery was more effective for patients with a preoperative refraction between -2 and -4.37 diopters.

Serious complications were relatively rare. Twenty-five (3 percent) eyes lost 2 or more lines of spectacle-corrected visual acuity, but only 10 eyes saw worse than 20/20. Twelve eyes experienced mild vascularization of the incisions, 2 eyes had delayed bacterial keratitis, both recovering their pre infection visual acuity, and 4 eyes had transient recurrent epithelial erosions. Fifteen percent of the eyes had an increase in refractive astigmatism of 1 diopter or more.

The primary factors affecting the surgical outcome were the age of the patient, the diameter of the clear zone, and the depth of the incision. An estimate of the variation in the refractive change among patients with the same age, clear zone, and depth of incision is +2 diopters.

The refractive error continues to change in some patients. Between 6 months and 5 years after surgery, 76 percent of eyes were relatively stable with a refractive change less than 1 diopter. Two percent of eyes had an increase in minus power of 1 diopter or more. However, 22 percent of eyes had a decrease in minus power of 1 diopter or more; that is, a change in the direction of a continued effect of the surgery. Among unoperated control eyes, none had a decrease in myopia of 1 diopter or more during the 4-year follow-up.

It is this continued hyperopic shift that is the major focus of study in the 10-year follow-up examination, which will determine the number of eyes that change in the hyperopic direction by a diopter or more and the extent of that change. In addition, diurnal variation will be studied in an extensive number of eyes at 10 years.

Changes in Unoperated Eyes in the PERK Study. Information on the stability of refraction in adult myopic eyes is a valuable reference standard when assessing the stability of refractive corneal surgery. We examined the unoperated eye of 82 patients in the PERK Study during 5 years. Spectacle corrected visual acuity: The change in spectacle-corrected visual acuity was zero Snellen lines for 37 of 77 eyes (48 percent), and one line for 34 eyes (44 percent). Only one eye (1 percent) lost 2 lines, and 5 (7 percent) gained 2 lines. Refractive Error: Of 37 non-contact lens wearing eyes, 5 (13 percent) became more myopic by at least 1.00 diopter; one (3 percent) became less myopic by 1.00 D; 31 eyes (84 percent) changed by less than 1.00 D. Of 45 contact lens wearing eyes, 17 (38 percent) became more myopic by at least 1.00 D, one (2 percent) became less myopic by more than 1.00 D, and 27 (60 percent) changed by less that 1.00 D. Therefore, the wearing of contact lenses can confound the results of stability studies.

Lens Wearing of PERK Patients After Surgery. The ability of a patient to function without spectacles or contact lenses after radial keratotomy is a partial indicator of the success of the surgery. Self-administered questionnaires were used to assess the lens-wearing behavior of patients in the PERK study an average of 6 years after surgery. Of the total 435 patients in the study, analyses were done on 328 patients who had surgery on both eyes, who completed a questionnaire, and who had refractive and visual acuity data available. For 328 patients with both eyes operated at 6 years, 170 (52 percent) stated that they wore no correction on either eye, 48 patients (14.6 percent) wore lenses for reading and dose work only, 59 patients (18 percent) wore lenses for distance only, and 51 patients (15.5 percent) wore lenses for both near and distance vision. Eighty-six percent of lens wearers wore only spectacles. Fourteen percent of lens wearers wore contact lenses only (7 patients) or wore contact lenses and spectacles (16 patients). The four lens-wearing groups differed in age, uncorrected visual acuity and cycloplegic refraction. The no lens group was the youngest (37.8 years), and the group wearing lenses for dose vision only was the oldest.

Although refractive error and uncorrected visual acuity are the most common measures used to assess the effectiveness of refractive corneal surgery, in some cases these two measures give conflicting evidence. Therefore, a visual function score combining refractive error and uncorrected visual acuity was devised that classified patients into excellent, good, fair, and poor visual function outcomes. Patients in the excellent category had a refractive error of -1 to +0.50 diopter and uncorrected visual acuity of 20/25 or better. Patients in the poor category had a refractive error with more than 3 diopters of myopia or more than 2 diopters of hyperopia and an uncorrected visual acuity of 20/100 or worse. Patients in the good and fair categories had intermediate values of refractive error and visual acuity. For PERK patients 5 years after surgery, the values of the visual function score were: excellent—48 percent, good—32 percent, fair—13 percent, and poor—7 percent.

Impact of the PERK Study. In the past, PERK provided scientific information about radial keratotomy, especially at a time when carefully done prospective trials were few. In the present, the results of the PERK study serve as a benchmark by which changes and advances in radial keratotomy and other types of refractive surgery can be measured. In the future, the PERK study will be one of the few sources of information about the long-term stability of radial keratotomy.

Publications

From 1983 to 1992, the PERK Study has published 32 original articles in peer reviewed journals, 15 ancillary communications, and 24 abstracts. The original articles are listed here. A textbook based largely on the experience and results of the PERK Study has also been published: Waring GO: Refractive Keratotomy for Myopia and Astigmatism. Mosby-Yearbook, St. Louis, MO, 1-1326, 1991.

Clinical Centers

California

Peter J. McDonnell, M.D.
Ronald E. Smith, M.D.
Doheny Eye Institute
University of Southern California
1450 San Pablo Street
Los Angeles, California 90033
Telephone: (213) 342-6426

Florida

William Culbertson, M.D.
Bascom Palmer Eye Institute
University of Miami School of Medicine
900 N.W. 17th Street
Miami, Florida 33136
Telephone: (305) 326-6364

Georgia

George O. Waring III, M.D.
Keith P. Thompson, M.D.
Department of Ophthalmology
Emory University School of Medicine
1327 Clifton Road, N.E.
Atlanta, Georgia 30322
Telephone: (404) 248-3244

Louisiana

Marguerite B. McDonald, M.D.
Bruce A. Barron, M.D.
Louisiana State University Eye Center
2020 Gravier Street, Suite B
New Orleans, Louisiana 70112
Telephone: (504) 568-6700

Michigan

Raymond R. Margherio, M.D.
Robert C. Arends, M.D.
John W. Cowden, M.D.
Robert L. Stephenson, M.D.
William Beaumont Eye Clinic
3535 West Thirteen Mile Rd, Suite 555
Royal Oak, Michigan 48073-2793
Telephone: (810) 551-2137

Minnesota

Donald J. Doughman, M.D.
Edward J. Holland, M.D.
J. Daniel Nelson, M.D.
Department of Ophthalmology
University of Minnesota
Box 493, Mayo Building
516 Delaware Street, S.E.
Minneapolis, Minnesota 55455
Telephone: (612) 625-4400

New York

Penny A. Asbell, M.D.
Steven M. Podos, M.D.
Department of Ophthalmology, Box 118
Mount Sinai School of Medicine
One Gustave L. Levy Place
New York, New York 10029
Telephone: (212) 241-7977

Oklahoma

Thomas C. Wolf, M.D.
McGee Eye Institute
University of Oklahoma
608 Stanton L Young Drive
Oklahoma City, Oklahoma 73104
Telephone: (405) 271-6050

Pennsylvania

Peter R. Laibson, M.D.
Michael A. Naidoff, M.D.
Elisabeth J. Cohen, M.D.
Christopher J. Rapauno, M.D.
Wills Eye Hospital
900 Walnut Street
Philadelphia, Pennsylvania 19107
Telephone: (215) 928-3180

Resource Centers

Co-Chairmen's Offices

Peter J. McDonnell, M.D.
Doheny Eye Institute
University of Southern California
1450 San Pablo Street
Los Angeles, California 90033
Telephone: (213) 342-6426
FAX: (213) 342-6440

George O. Waring III, M.D.
Department of Ophthalmology
Emory University School of Medicine
1327 Clifton Road, N.E.
Atlanta, Georgia 30322
Telephone: (404) 248-3244
FAX: (404) 248-5145

Clinical Coordinating Center

Katherine K. Lindstrom, M.P.H.
Department of Ophthalmology
Emory University
1327 Clifton Road, N.E.
Atlanta, Georgia 30322
Telephone: (404) 248-4381
FAX: (404) 248-5145

Statistical Coordinating Center

Michael J. Lynn, M.S.
Michael H. Kutner, Ph.D.
Portia Griffin, B.A.
Division of Biostatistics
Emory University
1599 Clifton Road, NE
Atlanta, Georgia 30329
Telephone: (404) 727-7695
FAX: (404) 727-8737

Psychometric Testing Center

Linda B. Bourque, Ph.D.
School of Public Health
University of California
10833 LeConte Avenue
Los Angeles, California 90024-1772
Telephone: (310) 825-4053
FAX: (310) 825-4440

NEI Representative

Donald F. Everett, M.A.
National Eye Institute
Executive Plaza South, Suite 350
6120 Executive Boulevard
Rockville, Maryland 20892
Telephone: (301) 496-5983
FAX: (301) 402-0528

Data Monitoring and Oversight Committee

John W. Chandler, MD.
University of Illinois
Chicago, Illinois

Robert J. Hardy, Ph.D.
University of Texas
Houston, Texas

Walter I. Stark, M.D.
The Johns Hopkins University
Baltimore, Maryland

Chapter 20

Photorefractive Keratectomy

On October 20, 1995, the Food and Drug Administration (FDA) approved for marketing the first laser to be used to correct mild to moderate nearsightedness—the ability to see nearby objects but needing corrective lenses for distance vision—in a procedure called photorefractive keratectomy (PRK). The laser, manufactured by Summit Technology, Waltham, Mass., is the SVS Apex Excimer Laser System. It uses computer controlled laser or light energy to rapidly pulse the cornea (the clear structure in front of the iris), vaporizing part of its surface layer and thus flattening the cornea so it focuses light more directly on the retina, so that spectacles or contact lenses may not be needed for distance vision.

FDA's approval is based on a review of clinical, engineering, and statistical data submitted by the manufacturer and on the recommendation of the Ophthalmic Devices Panel of FDA's Medical Devices Advisory committee which met on October 20, 1994 to review the marketing application. The company has agreed to conduct post-marketing studies on the long-term safety of the device. Details of these studies are being finalized.

Alternatives for correcting nearsightedness include eyeglasses, contact lenses, and a surgical procedure known as radial keratotomy (RK) which uses a precision scalpel to create radiating incisions in the cornea edge which flatten the cornea. The following can be used to answer questions.

Unnumbered FDA Publication dated October 20, 1995. Originally "Excimer Laser for Correction of Mild to Moderate Nearsightedness."

Clinical Studies

In the studies used to evaluate the safety and effectiveness of this PRK laser, the surgery was performed on more than 1600 healthy eyes. Surgeons first removed the outer layer of cells on the surface of the cornea with a special surgical tool, and then used an excimer laser programmed to deliver bursts of ultraviolet light to vaporize corneal tissue and alter the corneal curvature. The effect of the tissue removal is to flatten the cornea.

The firm submitted data on more than 1200 eyes upon which laser surgery was performed with a 5 mm treatment zone and on 398 eyes with a 6 mm treatment zone. Because of better results, FDA approved only the 6.0 mm treatment zone and the laser has been modified to lock in only this treatment zone. Almost all of the patients studied before the laser treatment were correctable to 20/20 vision or better if they used glasses or contact lenses.

With the 6.0 mm treatments, 65% of the 398 eyes had—without glasses—vision of 20/20 or better. In 95% of eyes, vision after laser treatment was 20/40 or better. About 5% of patients continued to need glasses all of the time for distance, and up to 15 percent needed glasses occasionally, such as when driving. Results were best in younger patients with lower degrees of nearsightedness.

About 63 percent of patients treated experienced mild but noticeable corneal haze after surgery, and 10 percent experience glare and halos around lights. These symptoms diminished or disappeared in most patients in the six months following surgery, but were still there at one year in 4% of patients. Longer term persistence of these symptoms has not been evaluated.

Although an uncommon occurrence, corneal scarring could occur and cause poor vision even with glasses. Best attainable vision (with or without glasses) was slightly worse after surgery in about 5 percent of eyes, and significantly worse in less than 1 percent.

The PRK surgery takes about 30 minutes, overall, with actual laser time about three minutes under local anesthesia. Initial time for the surface to heal is about 3 days for most patients, but at least three moths are required for vision to stabilize. Thus, patients need to wait three months after the first procedure before getting the other eye treated. The procedure is only adequately studied for patients with low to moderate (-1.5 to -7.0 diopters) nearsightedness and with no more than a low degree of astigmatism, up to 1.5 diopters.

Post-Approval Studies

The manufacturer will be required to continue to follow the patients treated in the existing studies for at least 4 years after approval to assure that vision remains stable over long periods of time. Also, a larger study in the general population will be conducted to look for additional adverse events as well as to obtain further information on the problems with glare, halo, and loss of vision acuity that were seen in some patients in the pre-market study.

Contraindications and Risks

PRK should not be performed on people with uncontrolled diabetes, auto-immune disease, certain eye diseases such as glaucoma, or on pregnant women (due to corneal changes that occur during pregnancy). In the clinical trials, patients who had undergone previous RK experienced a greater loss of visual acuity than those who had not previously received this different procedure. PRK therefore is strongly discouraged in patients with previous radial keratotomy.

Risks associated with PRK include worsening of best corrected vision, return to nearsightedness over several years, and induction of farsightedness, astigmatism, glare, halo, or double vision. After PRK, patients may experience farsightedness (the need for reading glasses)—as occurs in essentially everyone with age—earlier in life. Long term risks of PRK beyond three years have not been studied.

Considerations for Prospective Patients

The Agency has reasonable assurance that this laser is safe and effective for the correction of mild to moderate nearsightedness (-1.5 to -7.0 diopters with ≤ 1.5 diopters of astigmatism) to improve distance vision. However, an individual's choice of laser surgery of the cornea to correct mild to moderate nearsightedness should be made only after careful consideration of alternative means of correction and the possible risks of this approach. Individuals considering PRK surgery should discuss fully with one or more ophthalmic surgeons the complications of PRK surgery, the risks and the time required for healing, and have a full eye examination before making a final decision. Refractive error must be stable for at least one year before surgery.

An individual electing PRK should take adequate time to weigh all the options before making a decision to have laser surgery, and carefully consider the following facts:

No one has to have this treatment. It is a personal choice. Alternatives to PRK include glasses, contact lenses, and RK.

PRK is an operation to the cornea and cannot be reversed. Persons considering PRK should carefully read the Patient Information Booklet.

Possible complications of PRK surgery include: worsening of best corrected vision, return to nearsightedness over several years, and induction of farsightedness, or astigmatism. Noticeable glare or halo occurred more commonly and it may take several months for these problems to settle down to their best residual level. Long term risks of PRK beyond three years have not been studied.

Only one eye can be treated at a time with PRK; the interval between the first and second eye is a minimum of three months, and there may be vision problems during this interval.

PRK is indicated to correct mild to moderate nearsightedness. It is not indicated correct high or severe nearsightedness (>-7D), or astigmatism, or farsightedness. Also, it is not indicated to treat even mild to moderate nearsightedness if the accompanying astigmatism is >1.5D.

People who currently require glasses to read will continue to need them for reading after PRK, and some patients will require reading glasses who did not wear them before surgery. Also, as some PRK patients age, they may need glasses to read earlier in life than if they did not have the procedure.

PRK is not a laser version of radial keratotomy (RK); they are quite different from one another. In PRK, an excimer laser is used to flatten the cornea; in RK, diamond knives are used to cut spoke-like slits in the cornea.

Some occupations, such as pilots, do not accept applicants who have had any refractive surgery.

Chapter 21

Light for Sight:
Lasers Beginning to
Solve Vision Problems

Although it happened more than a year ago, 68-year-old Ervin Chudnow of West Palm Beach, Florida, still marvels at how a laser gave him back good eyesight.

Several years after having a cataract removed from his left eye, Chudnow began having problems with hazy vision. "It was like looking through a window with soap on it," he says. His sight became so poor he had difficulty with daily tasks such as driving and reading the paper.

Chudnow went to see his ophthalmologist, who used about a dozen one-billionth-of-a-second blasts of infrared laser light to puncture the clouded membrane lining the back of the lens of his eye that was obscuring his vision.

"I went in there nearly blind in one eye, and after the half-hour walk home, I could see perfectly again," Chudnow recalls.

Many people tell dramatic tales of how lasers restored their sight. A versatile tool, lasers are commonly used to treat a variety of eye disorders such as retinal tears and glaucoma. In the not-too-distant future, moreover, a few zaps of laser light might bring back 20/20 vision to those who are nearsighted, farsighted, or have problems with astigmatism.

"Someday lasers may be routinely used to treat most things wrong with the eye," says Richard Weiblinger, a senior scientist in the Food and Drug Administration's ophthalmic devices division.

FDA Consumer, July-August 1990.

FDA's Center for Devices and Radiological Health regulates medical lasers to ensure they are safe and effective. Although surgical lasers must comply with stringent FDA safety standards, like any other surgical procedure, laser eye surgery is not completely without risk.

A laser (an acronym for "light-amplification by stimulated emission of radiation") is a simple device that usually combines electricity, a series of mirrors, and a crystal or gas to generate an extremely intense and narrow beam of a single type of light, such as infrared or ultraviolet. (Sunlight, in contrast, is composed of a jumble of different colors, spread out in different directions.)

The laser's usefulness in ophthalmology stems from the precision and ease with which it can be used to reach tissues deep within the eye. Unlike the smallest scalpel used in surgery, which makes cuts as wide as the tip of a pin and crushes neighboring tissue, a "laser scalpel" can slice as thin as the width of a cell without damaging surrounding cells. This precision allows eye doctors to target diseased blood vessels, for example, while sparing healthy ones, and fosters a speedy recovery with little resulting scar tissue.

Even minor amounts of scar tissue can pose major impediments to sight by blocking the pathway of light entering the eye. That pathway is what makes the laser so useful in treating patients with eye disorders; the pupil acts as a natural window through which laser beams can enter to mend tissues deep within the eye. Because the ophthalmologist doesn't have to cut open the eye during laser surgery, there are fewer risks of infection and less pain than with standard surgery. Laser surgery can be done in an ophthalmologist's office or hospital outpatient department, so it also is less expensive.

Membranes of the Eye

Approximately half of all patients who have cataract surgery need the type of laser surgery Chudnow had. A cataract is a clouding of the normally clear and transparent lens of the eye. [See the chapter titled "Lifting the Clouds of Cataracts" in Part VI of this volume.]

During cataract surgery, an ophthalmologist often replaces the natural lens of the eye with an artificial one. Several months later, however, the membrane in the back of the eye, which surrounds and supports the lens, may become cloudy, impairing vision.

Ophthalmologists counter this problem by using the intense infrared light of a neodymium: yttrium aluminum garnet (Nd:YAG) laser to create an opening in the membrane. During this procedure, called a posterior capsulotomy, each flash of the laser causes a microscopic explosion in the membrane. The miniexplosion is thought to vaporize cells.

Although the laser beam travels through other eye tissues before it reaches the membrane, it doesn't harm these tissues because only the highly focused tip of the beam has enough energy to cause a microexplosion. This tip touches only the membrane in the back of the eye, which has no nerve endings. Posterior capsulotomies, consequently, are painless. This quick procedure rarely has any serious complications.

Glaucoma

An Nd:YAG laser is also used to treat some cases of glaucoma. This disease, which affects at least two out of every 100 Americans over 35, according to the American Academy of Ophthalmology, is one of the leading causes of blindness in this country.

The hallmark of glaucoma is an excessive build-up of fluid pressure in the eye. The unhealthy pressure is caused by a blockage of the canals through which the clear inner eye fluid continuously flows. If left untreated, glaucoma eventually damages the sight (optic) nerve.

An Nd:YAG laser can relieve the fluid pressure by creating an opening, allowing the eye fluid to drain properly. Although a slight risk of bleeding accompanies this type of laser surgery, it rarely causes serious problems.

Macular Degeneration

A different type of laser—the argon laser—is used to treat some patients with the more severe form of an eye disorder called macular degeneration. Although this disease doesn't cause total blindness, it is a leading cause of loss of both central and reading, vision. Macular degeneration is particularly common in people over 65.

The macula is the portion of the light-sensing retina (see diagram) that light rays strike to provide the sharp, straight-ahead vision needed for driving and reading small print. In the less common but more severe form of macular degeneration, for no known reason, new blood vessels grow beneath the macula. These abnormal vessels leak fluid and blood, destroying nearby macula cells. If the leakage and bleeding continue, much of the macula may be damaged irreparably within a few weeks or months. The resulting dense scar tissue blocks out central vision, much like an opaque smudge does in the center of one's glasses.

With early detection, severe vision loss from this type of macular degeneration can usually be prevented with argon laser treatment. This relatively low-energy laser heats, rather than vaporizes, tissues, acting essentially like a welder. A study conducted by the National Eye Institute showed that argon laser treatment can slash by more than half the chances of experiencing severe vision loss from macular degeneration.

The green beams of the argon laser are only absorbed by red objects, so it selectively heats up and seals blood vessels (because they contain red blood cells) and leaves most other parts of the eye undisturbed. The narrowness of the beam enhances laser precision, allowing the ophthalmologist to target only diseased blood vessels.

This type of surgery generally takes only a few minutes and may be done with the aid of a local anesthetic to prevent discomfort. Soon afterwards, the patient is able to return home and resume normal daily activities.

A fungal disease called ocular histoplasmosis can cause faulty blood vessels to grow and damage the macula. This is a significant cause of vision loss in the southeast and midwest United States, where this particular fungus is prevalent. Experts estimate that laser treatment of the abnormal vessels can prevent up to 2,000 cases of serious vision loss due to the disease each year if treatment is given early, before extensive damage has occurred.

Diabetic Retinopathy

Ophthalmologists use a similar procedure to seal off leaky blood vessels or destroy diseased tissue in the retinas of patients with diabetic retinopathy, another leading cause of blindness. The hallmark of this disease is faulty blood vessels on or within the retina. These vessels bleed, scarring the retina. According to the National Eye Institute, nearly half of all diabetics have at least mild diabetic retinopathy. If used in early stages of the disease, laser treatment often halts the patient's loss of vision and sometimes even reverses it. The procedure is usually painless and without complications.

Retinal Tears

An argon or another type of tissue-heating laser called a krypton laser is also used to spot-weld retinal tears. These horseshoe-shaped holes in the retina may open small blood vessels and cause bleeding into the central cavity of the eye. Often caused by a blow to the head, retinal tears can cause flashes of color or black spots to appear in one's line of sight.

Laser Sculpting

Still experimental is the use of the laser on the eye's surface to treat people for nearsightedness, farsightedness or astigmatism.

When light rays enter the normal eye, they are bent by the transparent front covering of the eye (cornea) and the lens so that they are brought to a single, sharp focus on the retina. But in the nearly one-third of Americans who are nearsighted (have trouble seeing distant objects), the light rays bouncing off faraway objects come to focus in front of—instead of directly on—the retina. This happens because either the curve of the lens or cornea is too steep or the eye is too long. In farsightedness (trouble seeing objects close up), the eye is too short or the curve of the cornea or lens is not steep enough. The rays, consequently, merge in back of the retina. The end result in both conditions is blurred vision.

To counter these vision flaws, most nearsighted or farsighted individuals wear glasses or contact lenses shaped to bend the light rays so that they properly reach the retina. By precisely reshaping the cornea with the laser, ophthalmologists hope to achieve the same effect. Theoretically, once the laser surgery is done, the person could throw away the no-longer-needed glasses.

Nearsightedness

Corneal surgery to cure nearsightedness has been attempted with traditional surgical tools, but without reliable results. In this procedure, called a radial keratotomy, an ophthalmologist uses a scalpel to cut several small slits in the cornea. These slits slightly flatten the cornea by changing the pressure in the eye and weakening the cornea's structure.

But nearly half of all the eyes treated with this procedure are either undercorrected or overcorrected, according to a study published in the Feb. 22, 1990, Journal of the American Medical Association. Apparently, the surgery often fails because the depth and shape of cuts made by the hand-held scalpel are inconsistent, or because scar tissue alters the desired contour of the cornea.

When an ultraviolet excimer laser is used, however, preliminary studies show that exact uniform tissue removal cuts can be accomplished with minimum scarring. The high energy of this laser beam ejects cell-sized fragments from the surface of the cornea. Such precision has enabled several research groups to directly remove minute quantities of tissue from the center of the cornea to flatten it, thus restoring sharp vision. Investigators hope to use the excimer laser on farsighted individuals, in whom the curve of the cornea is steepened rather than flattened.

Researchers speculate that because the excimer laser damages such small amounts of tissue, it "fools the eye into not knowing it's been traumatized," says Weiblinger. "Once the body knows it's been invaded, it tries to heal itself. That healing process can alter the desired recontouring of the eye."

The total sculpting procedure with the excimer laser takes less than a minute to complete, although about 20 minutes are needed beforehand to train patients to keep their eyes steady. The cornea may ache for about a day following surgery, and patients need to wear an eye patch for one or two days.

Initial results of laser sculpting by researchers at Louisiana State University Eye Center in. New Orleans and Johns Hopkins University in Baltimore are encouraging. These investigators were able to improve one patient's 20/300 eyesight to 20/40 eight weeks after treatment.

Another woman, whose nearsighted eye was corrected nearly two years ago, still sees perfectly without glasses or contact lenses. More extensive and longer-term testing will have to be done, however, to ensure the safety and effectiveness of laser sculpting for nearsightedness.

Astigmatism

The excimer laser is also being used experimentally to correct astigmatism. This blurred vision is caused by bumps and pits on the corneal surface, which prevent light rays entering the eye from merging into a single, sharp focus. Preliminary tests on more than 50 patients in Berlin, Germany, indicate that a series of T-shaped incisions made by the laser may be effective in smoothing out corneal irregularities. Various researchers in the United States are trying the same procedure on persons with astigmatism, but have not yet reported results.

If more extensive tests show laser sculpting is a safe and effective method for correcting near- or farsightedness or astigmatism and it becomes an accepted practice, various laser companies estimate the procedure will probably cost between $1,000 to $2,000 per eye.

Even if laser sculpting continues to show promise in clinical trials, however, it will be several years before a patient will be able to enter the ophthalmologist's office wearing glasses, get a few zaps of laser light, and achieve perfect vision after a few weeks.* Though today it's hard to imagine such a scenario, several years ago it would have been just as hard to believe the quick and easy laser surgery Chudnow had would one day be possible.

—by Margie Patlak

*[*Health Reference Series* Editor's Note: The FDA recently approved a laser surgery procedure called Photorefractive Keratotomy (PRK) as a corrective measure for myopia.]

Part Three

Diseases of the Eye

Chapter 22

Uveitis: Inflammatory Diseases of the Eye

Introduction

Inflammatory disorders of the retina and choroid comprise a large number of disorders that often are referred to as uveitis. The inflammation can be localized to the front, middle, or back portion of the eye. The term uveitis, coined in the 19th century, denotes an intraocular inflammation but in no way suggests a cause. In addition, the term uveitis suggests that the uvea, a layer of the eye, is the center of inflammation. This is not the case, however, since other portions of the eye are affected as well, depending on the entity. Inflammatory diseases of the retina and uvea generally are divided into two major categories: infectious and noninfectious. Infectious agents that can destroy portions of the eye include viruses, bacteria, fungi, and protozoa. The noninfectious conditions are thought to be caused by a dysregulation in the immune system, perhaps genetically determined in some cases, and to be fueled at times by autoimmune reactions.

The retina and choroid can be involved in a large number of conditions termed posterior and intermediate uveitis. These disorders can be caused by a well-defined invading organism, such as *Toxoplasma gondii* or CMV (both of which initially affect the retina), or may be of putative autoimmune origin, such as birdshot retinochoroidopathy. Other posterior uveitic disorders may be local manifestations of systemic diseases such as sarcoidosis, Behcet's disease, and

NIH Pub No. 93-3186.

the Vogt-Koyanagi-Harada syndrome. Other conditions may affect the front portion of the eye and collectively are called anterior uveitis. Conditions involving the retina and choroid can cause a rapid drop in vision and are usually painless. The changes in vision can be severe, yet the loss of vision may be reversed if treated rapidly. However, in some conditions, destruction of the retina and choroid prevents a return to useful vision if the part of the retina responsible for central vision, the macula, is affected. This is the case in CMV retinitis, a condition seen in 10 to 25 percent of patients with AIDS. When the inflammatory disease affects the front portion of the eye, the attack may be painful and accompanied by a loss of vision. Problems resulting from the inflammation can themselves produce a decrease in vision. These sequelae include cataracts, corneal clouding, and secondary glaucoma.

These disorders particularly strike children and adults in their prime years. It has been estimated by the National Society to Prevent Blindness that intraocular inflammation (both uveitis and chorioretinitis) resulted in 1,300 new cases of blindness in 1978, or approximately 2.8 percent of the cases registered for that year. In 1972 approximately $10 million was spent on the medical care of the estimated 67,000 Americans who had severe visual impairment from uveitis, of whom 23,000 were legally blind. These figures certainly have increased over the ensuing years and will continue to do so, particularly with the increasing number of AIDS patients who are at high risk for contracting intraocular inflammatory disease.

Subprogram Objectives

- To establish the fundamental causes and etiologic factors responsible for uveitis.

- To develop improved methods for the diagnosis, therapy, and prevention of uveitis.

- To establish the clinical manifestations, epidemiology, natural course, and prognosis of various forms of uveitis.

Current Level of National Eye Institute Support

In 1992 the NEI supported 37 research projects at a total cost of $8,096,994 in this subprogram. These investigations included clinical trials in ocular complications of AIDS, as well as projects evaluating the role of fragments of uveitogenic antigens in the eye, the effect of viruses on the eye, the unique immune characteristics of the eye, and newer methods of immunomodulation.

Recent Accomplishments

Natural Immunoprotective Mechanisms

Several experimental observations have established that natural immunoprotective mechanisms exist within the eye. Presumably these mechanisms have evolved to minimize nonspecific bystander cell entry into an inflammatory process directed against an offending pathogen. These mechanisms have been demonstrated not only for infectious pathogens but also for alloantigens, haptens, and tumor cells. The experimental systems that display such an inhibition of the intraocular immune response have been termed anterior-chamber-associated immune deviation (ACAID). ACAID is the inhibition of the systemic immune response noticed after the introduction of antigen into the anterior chamber of the eye. It is characterized by the suppression of delayed hypersensitivity and the enhancement of cytotoxicity (T-cell mediated) and antibody production. These aberrations in the immune system are antigen specific. T cells have been shown to recognize antigen within the eye and then elaborate a factor that enters the serum (T suppressor/inducer factor) and homes to the spleen, where there is an elaboration of T suppressor/effector cells.

Mediators. Recent experimental evidence suggests that soluble mediators within the anterior chamber of the eye modify the immune response that follows intraocular antigen presentation. Three soluble mediators have been identified to date: (1) TGFß, (2) a molecule that solely inhibits proliferation, and (3) a molecule with a molecular weight greater than 10kd molecule that is secreted by resident ocular cells that are bone marrow derived (T200+) and resides in the iris and choroid.

Recently it has been demonstrated that visible light is critical for ACAID. Specifically, wavelengths in the range of 490 to 500 nm can suppress delayed hypersensitivity. It also has been demonstrated recently that visible light is essential for the development of contralateral herpes simplex viral retinitis with ipsilateral protection of the retina.

Resident ocular cells. The resident ocular cells are an important component of the natural immunoprotective mechanisms within the eye. To date, three specific cell populations that are important in regulation of the intraocular immune response have been identified.

Within the retina, the Muller cell has been demonstrated *in vitro* to modulate the immune response. Under appropriate conditions, this cell can be induced to either upregulate or downregulate the immune response to a specific antigen. The mechanism by which this is accomplished is not clear, although evidence exists to suggest that the interleukin-(IL-) 2 receptor may be important for the observed regulatory effect of the cell.

The RPE has been implicated as a resident ocular cell also involved in modulation of the immune response. In experimental autoimmune uveitis (EAU) as well as in clinical uveitis, human lymphocyte antigens (HLA) class II expression has been observed on the RPE and can be induced with interferon gamma. Recently it has been shown that the RPE can present antigen to lymphocytes.

Resident ocular cells within the iris and choroid have been demonstrated to downregulate the immune response. A bone marrow-derived subpopulation (T200+) as well as other populations that have not been phenotypically characterized can mediate this effect.

Resident ocular cells *in vitro* from the iris and choroid secrete a soluble factor TGFß that can mediate downregulation. The molecular structure of this (these) mediator(s) and the effect of visible light on its secretion and activity requires further investigation.

Autoimmunity: Uveitogenic Peptides

Molecules purified from the retina can induce uveitis in animals. The sequences of the two major uveitogenic retinal proteins—S-antigen (S-Ag) and the interphotoreceptor retinoid- binding protein (IRBP)—have been determined for both the human and the bovine antigens. Consequently, peptide determinants with uveitogenic activity have been identified. Only a small number of peptide determinants of S-AG and IRBM have been found to be uveitogenic in Lewis rats (approximately 5 for S-AG and 10 for IRBM). However, the majority of the uveitogenic peptides induce EAU at doses much higher than those of the whole proteins. In contrast, one determinant of bovine IRBM (sequence 1179-1191) and one of human IRBM (sequence 521-540) were found to induce EAU at doses compatible with those of the parent proteins. It is assumed, therefore, that these peptides are "immunodominant" and participate in initiating the immunopathogenic processes in animals immunized with the whole protein. Recently such a determinant of S-AG has been reported. One of the uveitogenic determinants of S-AG, peptide M, was found to show partial sequence homology with certain microbial proteins. Rats immunized with microbial protein-derived peptides recognized peptide M and even developed EAU, thus confirming the possibility of "molecular mimicry" as a cause of uveitis.

In studies of the responses of uveitis patients toward these peptide determinants of S-AG and IRBM, preliminary data showed that lymphocytes from certain patients reacted against multiple determinants, with a few of these peptides being recognized by the majority of the responding patients.

Uveitis

New animal models. EAU recently has been induced reproducibly in susceptible strains of mice by active immunization. EAU in mice shows several new features: association with certain major histocompatibility complex (MHC) haplotypes, relapsing of the inflammatory process, and neovascularization as a component of the pathologic process. Peptides derived from S-AG or IRBM also were found to be uveitogenic in monkeys. However, unlike the whole proteins, the peptides were active in only some monkeys, suggesting that the susceptibility is regulated genetically.

Mechanisms. Recent studies have shown that most CD4+ uveitogenic cell lines, as the lines that induce experimental autoimmune encephalomyelitis (EAE), use the Vß8 component of the T-cell receptor (TCR). Much less is known about the identity of the cells that act to initiate the EAU process. Since resident cells may express class II MHC antigens, they also may act as antigen-presenting cells at later stages of uveitis, whereas macrophages may play this role at the initial stage of disease.

As is the case in other inflammatory processes, EAU is assumed to be mediated by cytokines. Elevated levels of IL-1, IL-2, and IL-6 have been detected in uveitic eyes, and IL-1, IL-6, and IL-8 have been shown to induce inflammation when injected into normal eyes. Oxygen metabolites may play a role in damaging the retina.

Modulation of EAU. With our increased understanding of the mechanisms of this animal model for human disease, several new modalities have been found in recent years to effectively inhibit EAU development. These include the use of monoclonal antibodies directed against various cell surface markers, such as HLA-DR and the CD4 molecule, as well as the genetically engineered compound of IL-2 linked to PE40 (IL2-PE40), the exotoxin of *Pseudomonas*. Use of newer immunosuppressive agents such as FK506 has been successful, as have attempts to biologically modify the immune response with autoantigen feeding and vaccination of T-cell lines.

Clinical Uveitis

Infection with *Borrelia burgdorferi,* or Lyme disease, recently has been documented as a cause of uveitis. It has been associated with iritis, intermediate uveitis, and optic neuritis. Identification of Lyme disease as a cause of intraocular inflammation is important because this form of uveitis is one of the few that can be cured by treatment with antibiotics.

Multiple innovations have occurred in the treatment of uveitis of various etiologies.

Medical therapy. The most important addition to our therapeutic armamentarium within the past 5 years has been cyclosporin. Although it is clear that nephrotoxicity is associated with using cyclosporin alone in therapeutic doses, the combination of cyclosporin and other antiinflammatory and/or immunosuppressive medications has become a useful therapeutic tool. Additionally, high-dose corticosteroid therapy has been found to be useful in the treatment of various forms of uveitis associated with profound visual loss. Studies evaluating the usefulness of cyclosporin G (thought to be less nephrotoxic) as well as biologic modifiers such as autoantigen feeding have begun.

Surgical treatment. Although the role of the vitreous in recurrent and persistent intraocular inflammation still needs to be determined, a therapeutic role for vitrectomy in patients with chronic persistent posterior uveitis (with vitritis) has been shown. In addition to the relief of vitreous traction, which can be associated with retinoschisis or retinal hole formation leading to retinal detachment, removal of the vitreous is frequently associated with fewer episodes, and at a reduced intensity, of recurrent inflammation. It is now recognized that extracapsular cataract extraction with posterior chamber intraocular lens (IOL) implantation is well tolerated by many eyes with uveitis, if proper therapy is given.

Evaluation of ocular tissue. New techniques of retinal and chorioretinal biopsy promise to provide further insight into the mechanisms of uveitis. Light microscopy, electron microscopy, and immunohistology have been used with biopsy-obtained tissue to determine an underlying etiology. However, the minute amounts of tissue obtained limit the applicability of these conventional techniques. With the introduction of the polymerase chain reaction the potential for sophisticated diagnostic evaluation with small samples of tissue has been greatly amplified.

Acquired Immune Deficiency Syndrome

AIDS has made a dramatic impact on the field of ophthalmology as it has in other fields of medicine. The majority of patients with AIDS have ocular manifestations, the most common of which is a noninfectious microangiopathy. Before the AIDS epidemic, CMV retinitis was a rare disease. Now CMV retinitis has become a common disease. CMV retinitis has been estimated to affect up to 38 percent of patients with AIDS; however, the average of several reported series gives an estimation of 10 to 25 percent for the frequency of CMV retinitis in patients with AIDS. Given the projection of 80,000 new cases of AIDS in 1992, these estimates suggest that there also may have been 16,000 new cases of CMV retinitis in that year.

CMV causes a blinding, necrotizing retinitis. Untreated CMV is a progressive disorder that given enough time will ultimately destroy the entire retina. Thus, there is a possibility of an increasing number of AIDS patients suffering from visual impairment or blindness, thereby adding to the medical, social, and economic burdens of this disease.

In June 1989 ganciclovir was the first drug approved by the Food and Drug Administration for the treatment of CMV retinitis in immunocompromised patients. Various studies have reported efficacy of this drug in the treatment of CMV retinitis, with response in 80 to 100 percent of patients and remissions of 60 to 80 percent. Foscarnet is a newer agent that was approved by the Food and Drug Administration in September 1991 for the treatment of CMV retinitis.

Because of the desire to coordinate the NEI's resources in the study of AIDS, SOCA was funded in August 1988. Its charge was to determine the important clinical questions related to the ocular complications of AIDS, develop relevant protocols for clinical trials and epidemiologic studies to address these issues, and develop the rest of the structure for such studies, including the recruitment of clinical centers and other support centers (e.g., centralized pharmacy, centralized laboratory, and specimen repository). The initial activity of SOCA was a randomized, multicenter clinical trial, the Foscarnet-Ganciclovir Cytomegalovirus Retinitis Trial, that was designed to compare the efficacy and safety of foscarnet and ganciclovir for the treatment of CMV retinitis. This comparison was particularly important because ganciclovir cannot generally be taken with full doses of zidovudine (AZT), the antiretroviral drug used in the treatment of HIV infection, because both drugs act as a bone marrow suppressant.

In December 1991 the study investigators reported that, although both drugs appear to be equally effective in halting the progression of CMV retinitis and preserving vision in patients newly diagnosed with the eye disease, the patients treated with foscarnet lived longer than those who received ganciclovir. Patients taking foscarnet lived an average of 12.6 months compared to 8.5 months for patients taking ganciclovir. The difference in mortality between the two treatment groups could not be fully explained by the differential use of AZT. These findings suggest that for many patients with AIDS and CMV retinitis, foscarnet may be a better initial treatment than ganciclovir.

In addition, the intramural program of the NEI has conducted a randomized, controlled clinical trial of foscarnet in peripheral retinitis, in cooperation with the National Cancer Institute, the National Institute of Allergy and Infectious Diseases, and the Clinical Center, that has demonstrated the efficacy of foscarnet for the treatment of CMV retinitis.

Important Research Questions to Be Addressed

Significant advances in our understanding of intraocular inflammatory disease have been made. Key questions and specific strategies for the future are listed below as research opportunities in inflammatory diseases of the retina:

What are the unique characteristics of the ocular immune response?

For ACAID future studies need to involve the biochemical and molecular characterization of T suppressor/inducer factor and the putative T suppressor/effector factor. Furthermore, the mechanisms responsible for enhanced cytotoxicity and antibody production need to be defined.

The exciting observations concerning the mediators in the eye need to be expanded to identify the specific intraocular cells that release these mediators as well as to identify the molecular structure of these factors. The effect of visible light is apparently not dependent on retinal phototransduction. The mechanism by which visible light has an effect on ACAID needs to be further explored, and the precise intraocular cells and mediators need to be defined.

How can a better understanding of human disease be achieved through the study of animal models?

Continued development of new laboratory techniques for the elucidation of animal uveitis models and the application of many of these techniques to the human situation are necessary.

Questions related to the homing mechanisms in uveitis and the role of the TCR as well as other membrane markers need to be better formulated. The triggering mechanisms of disease and the cause of recurrences still elude our understanding. The fragments of the uveitogenic peptides to which patients with uveitis respond need to be defined and understood in the context of genetic susceptibility. The relationship between the environment and the immune system still needs to be fully explored.

The newer methodologies of molecular biology may have a significant impact on the studies discussed earlier. Large quantities of fragments of various antigens (S-AG, IRBM) should be made available to increase the feasibility of both human and animal studies, the TCR rearrangement and usage of certain components in lymphocytes that produce disease in both humans and experimental animals should be analyzed, and the cytokines involved in the inflammatory process of uveitis (both posterior and anterior) should be identified by means of a variety of methods including *in situ* hybridization.

How can patients with uveitis be more effectively treated?

The application of newer methods of immunomodulation in the treatment of patients with uveitis should be a major goal. These methods could include many different types of approaches to immunomodulation, including the use of mediators and their receptors, vaccination techniques, feeding of autoantigens monoclonal antibodies, and competing peptides.

How can techniques in transplantation immunology be used effectively as a tool in the treatment and study of patients with ocular disease?

Approaches to retinal and RPE transplantation are being pursued by many researchers in ophthalmology, and the development of transplantation methodologies should logically be a goal of the ocular immunologist. Progress in the technical and surgical aspects of retinal transplantation has been rapid during the past 5 years. Unanticipated success in transplanting not only single-cell suspensions of retinal cells, including RPE, but also intact photoreceptor cell layers raises the possibility of allotransplantation and xenotransplantation of intact retinas for the cure of blinding disease. Virtually no effort has been made to understand the immune barriers to transplantation of allogeneic and xenogeneic tissues, especially those derived from retina, into the posterior compartment of the eye. Animal studies aimed at understanding the immunogenetic and immunologic rules of transplantation into the posterior segment are critically important.

What aspects of AIDS research need to be amplified to address the problem of AIDS-related ocular disease?

It will be important to use the SOCA model to study aggressively the ophthalmic complications of AIDS. It also will be important to gather more epidemiologic data on CMV retinitis in AIDS patients. Currently only limited information is available on risk factors for the development of CMV retinitis in AIDS patients. Therapeutic strategies in the treatment of AIDS are focusing increasingly on the use of primary prophylaxis for opportunistic infections such as the use of TMP/SMX as primary prophylaxis for *Pneumocystis carinii* pneumonia. For example, although acyclovir has no therapeutic benefit when directed against CMV retinitis, it may be potentially useful as a prophylactic drug to prevent the development of CMV retinitis. Clearly, if a high-risk group could be targeted for such prophylaxis, CMV retinitis might be prevented or its incidence decreased. Because the current therapies for CMV retinitis involve long-term use of intravenous drugs, these therapies may have a variety of complications, are expensive, and require home nursing care. Thus, epidemiologic studies of risk factors for the development of CMV retinitis aimed at identifying high-risk groups and clinical trials of strategies for preventing the development and improving the treatment of CMV retinitis will be important goals. In addition, newer agents such as oral ganciclovir and foscarnet are being developed for the treatment of CMV infections. Continuing investigation into the use of these agents for the treatment of CMV retinitis is an important goal.

Chapter 23

Uveitis

Uveitis refers to a group of inflammatory conditions that occur in the eye. Often uveitis reflects diseases that are occurring elsewhere in the body. Sometimes uveitis is the first evidence that there is a disease going on in the body. Frequently the cause of uveitis is unknown.

Inflammation vs. Infection

Inflammation is a reaction in the body in which swelling, redness, and dilated blood vessels occur. Infection is when a germ is growing in tissue. Not all inflammation indicates an infection. Inflamed joints in arthritis are seldom infected. Scraped skin is inflamed but not infected. Infection (germs—bacteria and viruses) also causes inflammation. In uveitis the inflammation can be due to an infection or can be noninfective.

Symptoms

In acute uveitis, patients frequently have pain, red eyes, and light sensitivity (photophobia). In chronic uveitis, patients will complain of dull aches and/or blurring of vision.

UIC Department of Ophthalmology, *Eye Facts*, June/July 1987.

Treatment

Because many kinds of uveitis have no known cause, they are treated nonspecifically with corticosteroids (cortisone) to suppress inflammation and to prevent structural damage to the eye. Corticosteroids may be given as eyedrops, ointments, injections next to the eye, or pills. Corticosteroids in pill form (prednisone) can have serious side effects. Because of this, ophthalmologists try to treat most cases of uveitis with eyedrops or injections of corticosteroids next to the eye. Even these "local" corticosteroids have side effects, including cataracts, glaucoma, and the loss of ability to fight infections around the eye caused by bacteria, fungi, or viruses. Any patient on corticosteroids must be carefully monitored for side effects by an ophthalmologist.

Common Types of Uveitis

Acute iritis (inflammation of the iris) affects young adults. It begins abruptly with the symptoms of pain, redness, and photophobia (light sensitivity). Often patients have a genetic tendency to acute iritis, and other family members may have had iritis. This genetic tendency often predisposes these people to other diseases such as ankylosing spondylitis (arthritis of the lower back), inflammatory bowel disease (colitis), and psoriasis (scaling skin disease).

Attacks of iritis generally last two to six weeks and usually occur in only one eye. Some patients have only one or two attacks in a lifetime, and others have multiple episodes. Acute iritis is usually treated with eyedrops but occasionally pills or injections are necessary.

Chronic iridocyclitis affects the iris and ciliary body (glandlike structure) behind the iris. Chronic iridocyclitis often has few symptoms but can severely damage the eye. This is especially true in children who have juvenile rheumatoid arthritis. In these children, often girls aged 2 to 6 years, this is a potentially blinding condition. Many of these children do not complain about problems with their sight. Therefore, it is important for pediatricians to refer all children with juvenile rheumatoid arthritis to an ophthalmologist for evaluation. Since chronic iridocyclitis may start years after the juvenile rheumatoid arthritis began, children with this form of arthritis should have periodic checkups into their teenage years.

Pars planitis tends to occur in teenagers and young adults. The cause is unknown, and pars planitis is unassociated with any systemic disease (disease of the whole body). The frequent symptoms are those of blurred vision or floaters (spots before the eyes). Most patients with pars planitis have a good outcome, but a minority have severe visual problems.

Toxoplasmic retinitis is an infection of the retina caused by a protozoan parasite. Over 30% of the American population has been exposed to this parasite. If a pregnant woman acquires this infection, her infant is at risk for eye disease and even mental retardation. Besides acquiring this parasite at birth, people can also be infected by eating raw or undercooked meat or by handling cat feces. Infection of the retina by toxoplasmosis can be blinding. Antibiotics will control the infection and suppress the inflammation in most cases, but the infection rarely is cured and can be reactivated. The Uveitis Clinic at the University of Illinois was the first to use "quadruple antibiotic therapy" to treat toxoplasmosis. Because of this therapy's great success, many other centers now use it to treat this difficult infection.

Sarcoidosis is an inflammation of unknown cause. It can affect any part of the body but most commonly is found in the lungs, skin, and eyes. In the eyes it can cause iritis or chorioretinitis (disease of the retina and choroid). Usually the symptoms are decreased vision and mild discomfort around the eyes.

Most cases of sarcoidosis of the eye are treated with corticosteroids.

A final type of uveitis is **viral retinitis**. Herpes viruses, which are normally kept at bay by the patient's immune defenses, sometimes can destroy the retina. People who have weakened immunity from diseases such as cancer or AIDS (acquired immunodeficiency syndrome) or from chemotherapy are at greater risk than others for this type of infection. Until recently if the immunity of these patients could not be restored, there was little that could be done to prevent damage to their eyes. Fortunately new antibiotics have been developed that seem to work well against these viruses.

Note: Single copies of "Eye Facts" are available free upon request by contacting the Managing Editor. The publication is available also in Spanish. Readers are encouraged to reprint "Eye Facts" either in part or its entirety, using the acknowledgment: "Reprinted from 'Eye

Facts' of the Department of Ophthalmology, the University of Illinois at Chicago."

Department of Ophthalmology (M/C 648)
Eye and Ear Infirmary
1855 West Taylor Street
Chicago, Illinois 60612

—by Howard H. Tessler, M.D.,
Associate Professor of
Clinical Ophthalmology

Chapter 24

Efficacy and Safety of Intraocular Lens Implantation in Uveitis

Purpose

- To evaluate the safety and efficacy of intraocular lens implantation in patients with severe uveitis over a follow-up period of a least 1 year.

- To compare the postoperative inflammation following the implantation of a standard intraocular lens or a heparin surface modified lens.

- To determine which of two types of lens surfaces leads to less complications in patients with uveitis.

Background

Patients with uveitis are at high risk for significant complications following cataract surgery with an intraocular lens implant. These complications can be related to the surgery itself or can result from the lens material that is being implanted into the eye. The postoperative inflammation is often more intense and prolonged in patients with uveitis and may lead to the formation of iris to lens adhesions and an increased amount of flare. By *in vivo* specular microscopy of the lens surface, fibroblast-like cells and multinucleated

NIH Pub. No. 93-3960.

giant cells can be seen on the surface of all implanted lenses, but the number usually decreases rapidly within several weeks following surgery. In patients with uveitis, cell deposits tend to persist for a longer period of time and, on occasion, giant cells will coalesce to form membranes which can obstruct the central visual axis and require a YAG laser to remove them. These giant cells are an indication of poor lens tolerance and are evidence of a foreign body reaction.

Modification of the lens surface with a uniform layer of heparin has been suggested to provide a more biocompatible surface. The total amount of heparin bound to the surface of the lens is approximately 0.5 µg which corresponds to less than 0.1 USP unit of heparin. Preclinical studies have shown a reduction in the degree of postoperative complications as compared to unmodified lenses.

Several retrospective series have looked at the use of intraocular lenses in patients with uveitis. However, no prospective controlled study to date has evaluated the safety and efficacy of intraocular lenses in uveitis patients. Furthermore, the surface modified lenses have never been tried in this patient population. Thus, it is appropriate to conduct a randomized controlled clinical trial of lens implantation in patients with uveitis.

Description

Patients with a history of recurrent anterior or posterior uveitis and anterior segment manifestations of past uveitis (e.g., synechiae, chronic flare, old keratic precipitates) will be entered in this prospective, double-masked randomized study. Eighty patients with uveitis under control with or without medications for at least 3 months and in need of cataract surgery will be randomized to receive either a standard PMMA lens or one that has been surface modified with heparin. Patients will be officially entered into the study at the time of surgery, after the nucleus and cortex have been successfully removed by standard extracapsular extraction or by phacoemulsification. The patient will then be followed periodically for a minimum of 1 year. The use of antiinflammatory medications will be closely monitored. Ocular inflammation will be assessed by careful clinical examination and the use of laser photometry. The development of synechiae, lens decentration or lens capture by the iris will be carefully documented and photographed. Lens tolerance will be assessed by determining the number and persistence of cell deposits on the lens surface. These will be assessed by using indirect specular microscopy of the lens surface and by determining the cell density and type on the anterior lens surface using serial photographs. These pictures will be graded by an independent investigator who will remain masked to the implanted lens type. Corneal endothelial cell counts will also be performed prior to surgery and at the end of 1 year. Any recurrence of posterior pole pathology will be documented by clinical exam and, where appropriate, by fluorescein angiography.

Patient Eligibility

Men and women eligible for the study must be age 18 or older and have a cataract in need of surgery and a history of recurrent anterior or posterior uveitis which has been under control for at least 3 months. Patients can only receive steroids and/or cyclosporine at the time of surgery, and patients taking cytotoxic agents will have to discontinue their use prior to surgery. Other exclusion criteria include: monocular patients, corneal pathology which would preclude visualization of the implant, uncontrolled glaucoma, diabetes, and patients unable to be followed for at least 1 year.

Patient Recruitment Status

Ongoing. Recruitment began in January 1993.

Current Status of Study

Ongoing.

Results

None.

Publications

None.

Clinical Center

Marc D. de Smet, M.D.
Laboratory of Immunology
National Eye Institute
National Institutes of Health
Warren Grant Magnuson Clinical Center
Building 10, Rm 10 N112
Bethesda, Maryland 20892
Telephone: (301) 496-3123

Chapter 25

Cystoid Macular Edema

What is cystoid macular edema?

Cystoid macular edema, commonly called CME, is a painless disorder which affects the retina, the light-sensitive inner lining of the eye. When this condition is present, multiple cyst-like (cystoid) formations appear in the portion of the retina responsible for central or "straight-ahead" vision and cause retinal swelling or edema.

Although the exact causes of CME are not known, it may accompany a variety of diseases such as retinal vein occlusion, uveitis or diabetes. It most commonly occurs after cataract surgery. About three percent of those who have cataract extractions will experience decreased vision due to CME in the first year, usually from two to four months after surgery. If the disorder appears in one eye, there is an increased risk—as high as 50%—that it will also affect the second eye. However, most people recover their vision after some time.

What are the symptoms of CME?

The most common symptom of cystoid macular edema is blurred or decreased central vision (CME does not affect peripheral or side vision). There may also be painless retinal inflammation or swelling. However, the condition may be present even when no visual loss occurs. In these cases it is diagnosed by an ophthalmologist after a thorough medical eye examination, usually using a photographic test called a fluorescein angiogram.

American Academy of Ophthalmology, ©1990.

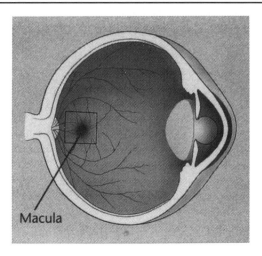

Macula

Figure 25.1. *Cross section of eye.*

How can CME be treated?

Since many factors can lead to CME, it is not possible to say which treatment, if any, will prove effective. After the diagnosis has been made and confirmed, the ophthalmologist may attempt several kinds of treatment. Signs of retinal inflammation are usually treated with anti-inflammatory medications, including cortisone-like drugs (steroid drops, pills or local injections) or anti-inflammatory drugs like indomethacin. Diuretics such as Diamox may help to reduce the swelling in some cases.

If the vitreous (the clear, gel-like substance that fills the center of the eye) is believed to be the source of the problem, laser surgery might be recommended. Another procedure called a vitrectomy can be used to suction the blood-filled vitreous out of the eye and replace it with a clear solution.

In some cases, the swelling and inflammation which accompanies CME can bring on glaucoma, a disorder which often occurs due to increased pressure within the eye. When this happens, the glaucoma must be treated with appropriate medications to reduce the pressure.

A great deal of research is presently being conducted to determine the causes of cystoid macular edema. Hopefully, this research will lead to more exact prevention and treatment measures in the near future.

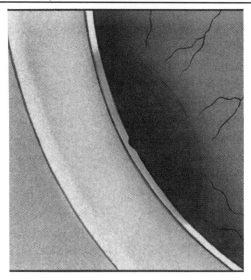

Figure 25.2. Enlarged detail of 1 Normal macula.

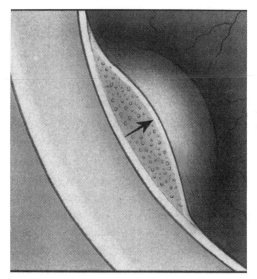

Figure 25.3. Swollen macula (edema).

Why are regular eye examinations important for everyone?

Eye disease can occur at any age. Many eye diseases do not cause symptoms until the disease has done damage. Since most blindness is preventable if diagnosed and treated early, regular medical examinations by an ophthalmologist are very important. Why an ophthalmologist? Because an ophthalmologist (MD or osteopath) provides total eye care: medical, surgical and optical.

Chapter 26

National Eye Institute Report on Retinal Cancer

Introduction

Cancer arising from the retina or choroid can cause loss of vision and loss of life in both children and adults. The most common intraocular malignancy of childhood is retinoblastoma, a tumor that is diagnosed in children from birth to age 7. The predisposition to retinoblastoma can be inherited as a dominant genetic trait, or the tumor can arise from the spontaneous transformation of a single cell in the retina.

Retinoblastoma is one of the best defined and understood of all the solid malignancies of childhood. The gene responsible for this tumor has been isolated, cloned, and sequenced. Understanding the role and function of the retinoblastoma gene is currently of major interest to research groups throughout the world.

There are between 300 and 400 newly diagnosed cases of retinoblastomas in the United States yearly. Approximately 60 percent of those children have only one eye involved, whereas the other 40 percent are affected bilaterally. Most commonly, successful treatment requires enucleation of at least one eye. As many as 25 percent of the children affected with bilateral retinoblastoma eventually lose both eyes. In developed countries, the overall survival of children with retinoblastoma approaches 90 percent; however, significant morbidity is associated with all the currently available treatment modalities. Enucleation, or surgical removal of the affected eye, causes the orbit to fail to complete normal growth, resulting in facial asymmetry.

NIH Pub. No. 93-3186, *Vision Research: A National Plan.*

External-beam irradiation increases the likelihood that a second primary tumor will develop in the radiation field. Chemotherapy is rarely effective for intraocular disease and carries its own significant side effects. The individual carrying the retinoblastoma predisposing mutation has a lifelong increased risk of independently arising second malignant neoplasms and as a result is rarely completely cured. Understanding the function of the retinoblastoma gene may hold the clue to more successful treatment and prevention of this blinding, life-threatening cancer.

The other malignancy arising in the eye is choroidal melanoma, a solid tumor arising from melanocytes or pigmented cells of the choroid and affecting adults. There are more than 1,500 new cases of choroidal melanoma diagnosed annually in the United States. The optimum therapy for this disorder is still unclear. The mortality rate of 5 years following diagnosis of ocular melanoma ranges from 35 to 90 percent, depending on the size and tumor cell type at the time of diagnosis. There is only scattered, scant evidence that genetic predisposition plays any role in the etiology of choroidal melanoma. As a result, there is unfortunately very little interest among basic scientists in working on understanding the etiology of this particular malignancy.

Subprogram Objectives

- To understand the role, function, and methods of regulation of the retinoblastoma gene and gene product in the development of retinoblastoma and in the embryology of the retina.

- To develop improved, cost-efficient technology that would allow the detection of a genetic predisposition to retinoblastoma in any individual.

- To improve treatment modalities and approaches to the management of retinoblastoma in order to increase survival without increasing the inherent risk of a second primary tumor in the genetically predisposed individual.

- To identify the activated oncogenes or mutant recessive cancer genes that play a role in the etiology of choroidal melanoma.

- To develop new approaches to the treatment of choroidal melanoma utilizing a multimodality protocol and emphasizing adjuvant hyperthermia and immunotherapy.

- To develop both diagnostic assessment modalities for the differentiation of small melanomas from choroidal nevi and vision-sparing treatment modalities for small choroidal melanomas.

Current Level of National Eye Institute Support

During FY 1992 the NEI supported 45 intraocular cancer-related projects at a total cost of $8,203,040. These projects involved research in the area of retinoblastoma and ocular melanoma and included both basic research projects and clinical trials, such as the Collaborative Ocular Melanoma Study (COMS).

Recent Accomplishments

Retinoblastoma

In perhaps one of the most significant accomplishments contributing to the understanding of human cancer, the retinoblastoma gene, the prototype of recessive cancer genes, has been successfully isolated, cloned, and sequenced. This gene is the prototype for a class of human cancer genes known as antioncogenes or recessive cancer genes. Loss or inactivation of both maternal and paternal copies of these genes is associated with the development or progression of malignancy. Success in understanding the structure and basic function of the retinoblastoma gene has been a major leap forward in cancer research.

The retinoblastoma gene is large, covering more than 200 kilobases and consisting of 27 exons. The mRNA, corresponding to the retinoblastoma gene, consists of 4.73 kilobases. Unique observations in the retinoblastoma gene were the findings that, within the transcribed DNA, there were multiple repeat and inverted repeat sequences. These multiple changes and the fact that this gene is present normally in organisms as old evolutionarily as the fruit fly provide strong evidence that this gene normally plays a major role in cell growth and development and also that the gene is ancient and has survived multiple changes during evolution.

The retinoblastoma gene product is a nuclear protein of 105 kd. The protein is regulated by cell cycle-specific phosphorylation with transient inactivation of the retinoblastoma protein (by the addition of phosphate groups), peaking just before the cell commits to DNA replication and cell division. The current theory is that the inactivation of the retinoblastoma protein is essential in normal cells to allow cell division to proceed. This theory is supported by the observation that the oncogenic proteins (i.e., large T, E1A, and E7) of animal viruses SV40, adenovirus 12, and HPV16 have been shown to bind and presumably inactivate the retinoblastoma protein.

The precise function of the retinoblastoma gene is currently the subject of extensive investigation. There has been demonstration of tumor suppression by replacement of the retinoblastoma gene. Whether growth suppression caused by the addition of a single normal copy of the retinoblastoma gene is specific for tumor cells or a generalized phenomenon is currently under investigation. Studies have indicated that retinoblastoma originates from cone photoreceptors. The availability of the molecular probes for the red and green cone pigment genes has been of help in making this determination. Recently a mouse model of retinoblastoma was created using gene "knock-out" or embryonic stem cell homologous recombination technology. This newly developed technique allows scientists to obliterate genes and see how the loss or mutation of a gene affects the development of the organism. Using these techniques, NEI-supported scientists replaced the normal gene in a developing mouse with a mutated retinoblastoma gene. This replacement was devastating and resulted in developmental arrest of the mouse. This newly created animal model will allow the role of the gene product to be investigated in normal development and cancer. The key to successful treatment and prevention of retinoblastoma lies in understanding the function of the retinoblastoma gene.

The availability of the retinoblastoma gene has led to the use of intragenic DNA polymorphisms for genetic diagnosis in rare, selected families. Unfortunately polymorphisms are not useful in more than 90 percent of retinoblastoma families where only a single individual is affected. Improvement in the current technology to allow rapid, accurate detection of point mutations and small deletions by direct genomic sequencing will allow cost-effective screening of any person's retinoblastoma gene to determine whether that person is genetically predisposed to developing the tumor. Currently such screening is expensive and time consuming.

The retinoblastoma gene has been shown to be lost or inactivated in many human tumors, even where it has no obvious role in the etiology of that tumor. These tumors include, among others, small-cell carcinoma of the lung, bladder cancer, breast cancer, and melanoma.

The retinoblastoma gene also plays a role in the etiology of both the sporadic and the hereditary forms of osteosarcoma. In human breast cancer the loss of the retinoblastoma gene seems to correlate with progression of malignancy.

Choroidal Melanoma

COMS is under way in evaluating the relative efficacy of enucleation versus radioactive plaque for the treatment of medium-to-large melanomas. This randomized clinical study holds promise of providing an answer to the following question: Which of these treatment modalities is most effective? If it is determined that there is no difference between the two treatment modalities, that result would be equally important since a nondisfiguring treatment such as local brachytherapy could be safely recommended in preference to enucleation in the treatment of these tumors.

Progress has been made in the development of alternate treatment modalities and approaches for choroidal melanoma. Low-energy isotopes that can be shielded from exposing the orbit and bone to radiation are available for use in brachytherapy. Adjuvant hyperthermia has been shown to be effective when combined with radiotherapy in the treatment of choroidal melanomas. Unfortunately relatively little progress has been made in understanding the etiology of choroidal melanoma.

Important Research Questions to Be Addressed

Dramatic, rapid advances in molecular biology and immunology as well as the success of multimodality therapy in other areas of oncology will have a major impact on priorities for basic and clinical research in oncology. The following set of questions may serve to stimulate new investigations in area of ocular tumors:

What is the function of the retinoblastoma gene product at both the cellular and the molecular level in the etiology of retinoblastoma and in the embryological development of the retina?

The key to treatment and prevention of retinoblastoma may well lie in our complete understanding of the function of the retinoblastoma gene. Specifically at the cellular level, more information is needed about the effect of transfection on the retinoblastoma gene into tumor cells both *in vitro* and *in vivo.*

Additional pertinent questions are as follows: Does the retinoblastoma protein play a role in the process of mitotic spindle formation? At the molecular level, does the Rb-1 gene product have an effect on replication and/or transcription? Precisely how does phosphorylation regulate the retinoblastoma gene? Is there gene regulation at the transcription level?

Are genetic changes other than those at the Rb-1 locus required for tumorigenicity of retinoblastoma?

Other chromosome-specific changes (e.g., the presence of four copies of the short arm of chromosome 6 and changes in chromosome 1) are associated with retinoblastoma. The 6p changes are specific for retinoblastoma. The genes present in this extrachromosomal material and the role they may play in the etiology or progression of retinoblastoma are unknown. The definition of the genetic events that prevent retinoblastoma formation after terminal differentiation may provide clues to the role that the retinoblastoma protein may play in terminal differentiation. Also needed to be determined is whether the domains of the retinoblastoma protein are shared by other proteins that play a role in terminal differentiation.

How will understanding of the retinoblastoma gene, its genetic changes, and its function affect the prevention and treatment of retinoblastoma?

The enlarging body of information about the nature of the genetic changes predisposing to retinoblastoma makes it imperative that such information be factored into designing rational treatment and prevention protocols. Errors at mitosis including chromosomal breaks play a major role in the etiology of retinoblastoma, osteosarcoma, and other solid malignancies to which individuals with the retinoblastoma susceptibility gene are predisposed. It becomes increasingly important to design rational treatment protocols that minimize the use of modalities known to cause chromosomal damage, particularly if normal tissue is included in the radiation field as is the case with externalbeam radiotherapy (EBR). Perhaps enucleation should be used more frequently, especially in group V disease. The development of a multimodality treatment regimen for primary groups I-IV retinoblastoma that minimizes EBR should be developed. This might provide the best hope for not only improving morbidity and mortality but for reducing the unwanted genetic damage and side effects.

In summary, knowledge of the retinoblastoma gene sequence and gene product should allow early identification of individuals who are genetically predisposed to retinoblastoma. However, technology for accurate and cost-effective molecular diagnosis of the genetic predisposition to retinoblastoma needs to be improved.

Do oncogenes or antioncogenes play a role in the etiology of choroidal melanoma?

Tantalizing suggestions have been made that genetic predisposition to choroidal melanoma does exist. There are a number of rare families with a genetic predisposition to both cutaneous and ocular melanomas (the B-K mole syndrome). A study of these families for clues to chromosomal localization for the predisposing gene for choroidal melanoma may be useful. An obvious starting point would be the investigation of the status at the loci known to be associated with the development of the cutaneous melanomas. A study of these genes and these families may be to melanoma what the 13 deletion syndrome was to retinoblastoma.

In the classic experiments of Stanbridge and colleagues, suppressor chromosomes were identified in human ß human hybrids. Because this fused cell nucleus is unstable, chromosomes are lost randomly. If the tumor phenotype is suppressed by the hybrid, it should be possible to determine its reappearance associated with the loss of a particular human chromosome. This might give a clue to the relevant genes and their chromosomal localization in choroidal melanoma.

How can both morbidity and mortality be improved in the treatment of retinoblastoma and choroidal melanoma?

It is clear from other branches of oncology that the steady progress in improving mortality from cancer has for the most part been a result of the introduction and refining of multimodality treatment protocols. In ophthalmology it has been the accepted procedure to treat these tumors with a single modality such as radiation and wait for a response before considering a second treatment with that or another modality. We should encourage and rapidly explore protocols for multimodality treatment of both retinoblastoma and ocular melanoma from the time of initial diagnosis. The use of adjuvant modalities such as hyperthermia in both retinoblastoma and melanoma as well as immunotherapy in choroidal melanoma should be strongly encouraged.

Can new approaches to the treatment of choroidal melanomas and retinoblastoma be developed?

In addition to the multimodality approach mentioned above, and because choroidal melanomas share cell origin similar to that of cutaneous melanomas, it would be appropriate to consider treatment of primary and metastatic choroidal melanoma with regimens known to be useful against cutaneous melanoma. Examples are interferon a (IFN-), IL-2, and other vaccines currently under development.

Other questions that need to be addressed include the following: Is there a role for immunotherapy or immunoaugmentation? Is this role preferentially in small melanomas where the tumor load is relatively minimal? Hyperthermia has been shown in pilot studies to be an effective adjuvant modality to use with choroidal melanoma and its investigation should be encouraged. When this treatment is combined with radiotherapy, the reduction of the overall dose of radiation to achieve tumorcurative regimens would be a goal. Laserthermia or through-the-pupil radiant hyperthermia using the 1064-nm Nd YAG laser may be useful in combination with chemotherapeutic agents such as carboplatin. Ultrasound, microwave, high-frequency radio waves, and laser hyperthermia modalities should all be compared for efficacy, safety, and side effects as sources for clinical hyperthermia. New and improved photosensitive dyes that produce fewer side effects than the porphyrins used in the experimental studies in the past should be sought.

Can noninvasive diagnostic or treatment methods with acceptable side effects be developed for use in diagnosing and treating small malignant melanomas?

The COMS currently calls for the enrollment of only those choroidal melanomas greater than 10 mm in largest diameter. For smaller, pigmented lesions there is no generally acceptable method of treatment. Over the years a "watch and wait" approach has developed. However, if more sensitive diagnostic methods for differentiating small melanomas from choroidal nevi as well as treatment modalities that would not threaten loss of macular function as a side effect were available, this "watch and wait" approach would be outdated. Dermatologists routinely remove suspicious lesions because the removal process is rarely associated with significant morbidity. A goal for the management of these small, intraocular lesions should be the development of treatment modalities with relatively few side effects. Then treatment of a choroidal nevus would be no worse than excising a benign but suspicious nevus from the skin.

Part Four

Corneal and Retinal Disorders

Chapter 27

The Cornea and Corneal Disease

What is the cornea?

The cornea is the transparent tissue that covers the front of the eye (see diagram). An easy way to locate the cornea is simply to look at your eye in the mirror. You will notice a clear surface covering the iris (the colored part of the eye) and pupil. This is the cornea.

What is the function of the cornea?

Because the cornea is as smooth and clear as glass but as strong and durable as plastic, it helps the eye in two ways:

- The cornea provides a physical barrier that shields the inside of the eye from germs, dust, and other harmful matter. It shares this protective task with the sclera (the white of the eye).

- It acts as the eye's outermost lens. When light strikes the cornea, it bends—or refracts—the incoming light onto the crystalline lens. The lens then focuses the light onto the retina, the paper-thin tissue at the back of the eye that starts the translation of light into vision.

NIH unnumbered document, May 1994.

Although much thinner than the lens, the cornea provides about 65 percent of the eye's power to bend light. Most of this power resides in the center of the cornea, which is rounder and thinner than the outer part of the tissue and is thus better suited to bend lightwaves.

How important is the cornea to good vision?

The cornea is essential to good vision. As the eye's outermost tissue, the cornea functions like a window that controls the entry of light into the eye. For example, the cornea filters out some of the most damaging ultraviolet (UV) wavelengths in sunlight. Without this protection, the crystalline lens and the retina would be highly susceptible to injury from UV radiation.

If this "window" is curved too much, as is the case in some nearsighted people, faraway objects will appear blurry because distant light waves will refract imperfectly on the retina. If this "window" has imperfections or irregularities, as is the case in people with an astigmatism, light will refract unequally, causing a slight distortion of the visual image. But, if this "window" is of normal shape and curvature, light will refract with exquisite precision to the crystalline lens.

What problems may affect the cornea?

The cornea copes very well with minor injuries or abrasions. If dirt scratches the highly sensitive cornea, epithelial cells slide over quickly and patch the injury before infection occurs and vision is affected.

But if the scratch penetrates the cornea more deeply, the healing process will take longer, resulting in greater pain, blurred vision, tearing, redness, and extreme sensitivity to light. These symptoms require professional treatment. Some of the more serious problems that affect the cornea are:

Microbial Infections (keratitis)

When the cornea is damaged, such as after a foreign object has penetrated the tissue, bacteria or fungi can pass into the cornea, causing a deep infection and inflammation. This condition may cause severe pain, reduce visual clarity, produce a corneal discharge, and perhaps erode the cornea.

As a general rule, the deeper the corneal infection, the more severe the symptoms and complications. It should be noted that microbial infections, although relatively infrequent, are the most serious complication of contact lens wear.

Minor corneal infections are commonly treated with anti-bacterial or anti-fungal eye drops. If the problem is more severe, a person may receive more intensive antibiotic treatment to eliminate the infection and may need to take steroid eye drops to reduce inflammation. Frequent visits to an eye care professional may be necessary for several months to eliminate the problem.

Conjunctivitis ("pink eye")

This term describes a group of inflammatory and often contagious diseases of the conjunctiva (the protective membrane that lines the eyelids and covers exposed areas of the sclera, or white of the eye). These diseases can be caused by a bacterial or viral infection, drug allergy, environmental irritants, or a contact lens product.

At its onset, pink eye is usually painless and does not adversely affect vision. The infection will come and go in most cases without requiring medical care. But for some forms of pink eye, such as epidemic keratoconjunctivitis, treatment will be needed. If treatment is delayed, the infection may worsen and cause corneal inflammation and a loss of vision. Depending on the type of pink eye that a person develops, treatment often consists of antibiotics and steroids.

Ocular Herpes

Herpes of the eye is a recurrent viral infection that affects an estimated 400,000 Americans with herpes. Although ocular herpes can result from the sexually transmitted herpes simplex 11 virus, it is usually caused by herpes simplex virus I (HSV I), the virus responsible for cold sores. In about 12 percent of those with ocular herpes, both eyes are involved.

Ocular herpes produces a relatively painful sore on the surface of the cornea. Prompt treatment with antiviral drugs helps to stop the herpes virus from multiplying and destroying epithelial cells. In time, the infection may also spread into the stroma, causing the body's immune system to attack and destroy stromal cells. This more severe infection, called herpes simplex stromal keratitis, is harder to treat and can scar the cornea, causing vision loss. It may also produce an infection of the inside of the eye. Like other herpetic infections, herpes of the eye remains a controllable, but incurable, problem. For those who lose vision to ocular herpes, it usually results from recurrent attacks that lead to severe stromal keratitis. Studies indicate that after a person has had an initial outbreak of ocular herpes, he or she has better than a 50 percent chance of having a recurrence of the disease. This second outbreak could come weeks or decades after the initial attack. In one large study, researchers found that recurrence rates were 10 percent after one year, 23 percent at two years, and 63 percent at 20 years. Some factors associated with recurrence include fever, stress, sunlight, and trauma.

Anyone with ocular herpes should avoid using over-the-counter steroid eye drops. Steroids cause the virus to multiply and the infection to worsen.

Herpes Zoster (shingles)

This infection is produced by the varicella-zoster virus, the same virus that causes chicken pox. After an initial outbreak of chicken pox (often during childhood), the virus remains dormant within the nerve cells of the central nervous system. But in some people, the varicella-zoster virus will reactivate at some time during their lives. When this occurs, the virus travels down long nerve fibers and infects some part of the body, producing a blistering rash (shingles), fever, painful inflammations of the affected nerve fibers, and a general feeling of malaise.

Varicella-zoster virus may travel to the head and neck, perhaps involving an eye, part of the nose, mouth, cheek, and forehead. In about 40 percent of those with shingles in this area, the virus infects the cornea. These zoster-related corneal lesions will usually clear up on their own. But without early anti-viral treatment, a person runs the risk of the virus infecting cells deep within the tissue, causing inflammation and scarring of the cornea. The disease may also cause decreased corneal sensitivity. For many, this decreased sensitivity will be permanent.

Although shingles can occur in anyone exposed to the varicella-zoster virus, several studies have established two general risk factors for the disease: (1) advanced age and (2) a weakened immune system. Studies show that people over age 80 have a five times greater chance of having shingles than adults between the ages of 20 and 40. Unlike herpes simplex I, the varicella-zoster virus does not usually flare up more than once in adults with normally functioning immune systems.

Be aware that corneal complications may arise months after the shingles are gone. For this reason, it is important that patients schedule follow up eye examinations.

Corneal Dystrophies

There are over 20 corneal dystrophies that affect all parts of the cornea. Some of the most common are:

Keratoconus. The disorder arises when the middle of the cornea thins and gradually bulges outward, forming a rounded cone shape. This abnormal curvature changes the cornea's refractive power, producing moderate to severe distortion (astigmatism) and blurriness (near- and farsightedness) of vision. These changes may also disrupt the normal, light-conducting arrangement of corneal protein, causing swelling and a sight-impairing scarring of the tissue.

Studies indicate that keratoconus stems from one of several causes: (1) an inherited corneal abnormality. About 7 percent of those with the condition have a family history of keratoconus; (2) an eye injury, i.e., excessive eye rubbing or wearing hard contact lenses for many years; (3) certain eye diseases, such as retinitis pigmentosa, retinopathy of prematurity, vernal keratoconjunctivitis; or (4) systemic diseases, such as Leber's congenital amaurosis, Ehlers-Danlos Syndrome, Down's syndrome, osteogenesis imperfecta, and Addison's disease.

Keratoconus usually occurs during puberty, or shortly thereafter. At first, people can correct their vision with eyeglasses. But as the astigmatism worsens, they must rely on specially fitted contact lenses to reduce the distortion and provide better vision. Finding a comfortable contact lens can be an extremely frustrating and difficult process. However, it is crucial because a poorly fitting lens could further damage the cornea and make wearing a contact lens intolerable.

In most cases, the cornea will stabilize after a few years without ever causing severe vision problems. But in about 10 to 20 percent of people with keratoconus, the cornea will eventually become too scarred or will not tolerate a contact lens. If either of these problems occur, a person will probably need to replace the diseased tissue with a donor cornea, called a corneal transplant.

This operation is successful in about 9 out of 10 people with advanced keratoconus. Several studies have also reported that about 80 percent of these patients have 20/40 vision or better with contact lenses after the operation. In fact, about 60 percent of transplant recipients will need to wear contact lenses after the surgery to correct astigmatism and nearsightedness.

For those with no scarring near the center of the cornea and 20/40 vision or better with contact lenses, another option is surgically grafting a layer of epithelial cells to flatten the cone-shaped cornea. This process is called epikeratophakia. It has comparable results to corneal transplantation and, if unsuccessful, it can be followed with corneal transplantation.

Map-Dot-Fingerprint Dystrophy. The epithelium is separated from the stroma, in part, by a membrane. It serves as the foundation on which the epithelial cells anchor and organize themselves. In map-dot-fingerprint dystrophy, the membrane develops abnormally. Like building a house on a damaged foundation, the epithelial cells anchor to a irregular membrane that, in turn, may make the epithelium slightly irregular.

The condition, which tends to occur in both eyes, usually affects adults between the ages of 40 and 70. It is also occasionally inherited—in which case it arises at about age 6. Map-dot-fingerprint dystrophy gets its name from the unusual appearance of the cornea during an eye examination. Most often, the epithelium will have a map-like appearance, i.e., large, slightly cloudy bodies that look like a continent on a map. This configuration is actually the irregular pattern of the membrane extending into the epithelium. There may also be a sequence of opaque dots—formed from cellular debris—underneath or close to the map-like patches. Less frequently, the irregular membrane will form concentric lines in the central cornea that resemble small fingerprints.

Most people will never know that they have this corneal dystrophy, since they will never have any pain and vision loss.

But for others, the disease will cause recurrent epithelial erosions—possibly from poor epithelial adhesion to the membrane. These erosions can be a chronic problem. They alter the cornea's normal curvature, causing periodic blurred vision. They may also expose the nerve endings that line the tissue, causing moderate to severe pain for several days. Generally, the pain will be worse in the morning. Other symptoms include: sensitivity to light, excessive tearing, and foreign body sensation in the eye.

Typically, the problem will flair up occasionally for a few years in adults and then go away on its own, with no lasting loss of vision.

However, if treatment is needed, the doctor will try to control the pain associated with the corneal erosion. He or she may do this by patching the eye to immobilize it or by prescribing lubricating eye drops and ointments. With effective care, the pain will subside in about 10 days, although periodic flashes of pain may occur for several weeks thereafter.

Fuch's Dystrophy. Fuch's dystrophy is a slowly progressing disease that usually affects both eyes and is slightly more common in women than in men. Although doctors can often see early signs of Fuch's dystrophy in people in their 30s and 40s, the disease rarely affects vision until a person reaches their 50s and 60s.

Fuch's dystrophy occurs when endothelial cells gradually deteriorate without any apparent reason, such as trauma or inflammation. As more endothelial cells are lost over the years, the cornea becomes less efficient at pumping water out of the stroma. This causes the cornea to swell and to distort vision. Eventually, the epithelium also takes on water, resulting in great pain and severe visual impairment.

Epithelial swelling damages vision in two ways: (1) changing the cornea's normal curvature, and (2) causing a sight-impairing haze to appear in the tissue. Epithelial swelling will also produce tiny blisters, called guttata, on the corneal surface. When the blisters burst, they are extremely painful.

At first, a person with Fuch's dystrophy will awaken with blurred vision that will gradually clear during the day. This occurs because the cornea is normally thicker in the morning, and it retains fluids during sleep that evaporate in the tear film while we are awake. But as the disease worsens, this swelling will remain constant and reduce vision throughout the day.

When treating the disease, doctors will try first to reduce the swelling with ointments or soft contact lenses. They may also instruct a person to use a hair dryer, held at arm's length or directed across the face, to dry out the epithelial blisters. This can be done two or three times per day.

But when the disease makes even the most simple tasks hard to complete, a person may need to consider having a corneal transplant to restore sight. The short-term success rate of corneal transplantation is quite good for people with Fuch's dystrophy. But, some studies do suggest that the long-term survival of the donor cornea can be a problem.

Lattice Dystrophy. Although lattice dystrophy can occur at any time in life, the condition usually arises in children between the ages of 2 and 7. It is characterized by an accumulation of abnormal protein fibers (amyloid) throughout the middle and anterior stroma. However, the disease is NOT related to amyloidosis, a serious systemic disease.

Lattice dystrophy gets its name from the amyloid deposits, which during an eye examination can appear as clear, comma-shaped dots and branching filaments that overlap each other in the stroma, creating a lattice effect. Over time, the lattice lines will grow opaque and involve more of the stroma. They will also gradually coalesce, giving the cornea a slight cloudiness that may also reduce vision somewhat.

In some people, abnormal protein also accumulates under the epithelium. This may result in poor adhesion between the stroma and epithelium, causing periodic epithelial erosions. The erosion will: (1) alter the cornea's normal curvature, resulting in temporary vision problems such as astigmatism and nearsightedness, and (2) expose the nerves that line the cornea, causing severe pain. In fact, even the involuntary act of blinking can be painful.

To ease this pain, a doctor may prescribe eye drops and ointments to reduce the friction on the eroded cornea. In some cases, an eye patch may be used to immobilize the eye. With effective care, the pain will subside in about 10 days, although occasional sensations of pain may occur for about the next 6 to 8 weeks.

By about age 40, some people will have scarring under the epithelium. As a result, a haze will develop on the cornea that can greatly obscure a person's vision. In this case, a corneal transplant may be needed. Patients with lattice dystrophy have an excellent chance for a successful transplant with good vision. However, in as little as three years, lattice dystrophy may also arise in the donor cornea. In one study, in fact, about half of the transplant patients with lattice dystrophy had a recurrence of the disease from 2 to 26 years after the operation. Of these, 15 percent required a second corneal transplant.

Structure of the Cornea

Although the cornea is clear and seems to lack substance, it is actually a highly organized group of cells and protein. The cornea receives its nourishment from the tears and aqueous humor that fills the chamber behind it. Unlike most tissues in the body, the cornea contains no blood vessels to nourish or protect it against infection. It must remain transparent to refract light properly, and the presence of even the tiniest capillaries would interfere with this process.

The tissue is arranged in three main regions, or layers:

Epithelium. As the cornea's outermost region—comprising about 10 percent of the tissue's thickness—the epithelium functions primarily to: (1) block the passage of foreign material—such as dust or water—into the eye and other layers of the cornea, and (2) provide a smooth surface that absorbs oxygen and other needed cell nutrients that are contained in tears. This layer, which is about five cells deep, is filled with thousands of tiny nerve endings that make the cornea extremely sensitive to pain when rubbed or scratched.

Stroma. Located behind the epithelium, the stroma comprises about 90 percent of the cornea. It consists primarily of water (78 percent); layered protein fibers (16 percent) that give the cornea its strength, elasticity, and form; and cells that nourish it. The unique shape, arrangement, and spacing of the protein fibers are essential in producing the cornea's light-conducting transparency.

Endothelium. This single layer of cells is located between the stroma and the aqueous humor. Because the stroma tends to absorb water, the endothelium's primary task is to pump excess water out of the stroma. Without this pumping action, the stroma would Swell with water, become hazy, and ultimately opaque.

Current Corneal Research

Although vision researchers have learned much about the structure and function of the cornea in health and disease, many important scientific questions remain to be answered. For example, vision researchers supported by the National Eye Institute, one of the Federal government's National Institutes of Health, are beginning to identify the specific genes that are activated, or switched on, in corneal cells. By understanding more about these genes and how they produce and maintain a healthy cornea, it will help immensely in understanding and treating corneal disease.

Although about 90 percent of all corneal transplant operations are successful, it is preferable for people to retain their natural corneas. For this reason, vision researchers continue to investigate ways to enhance corneal healing and eliminate the sight-threatening scarring that can complicate this process. NEI-supported scientists took an important step forward in describing this process when they recently developed a method of culturing rabbit cornea tissue that allows the researchers to measure cell movement rapidly during healing. The culture is also being used to study drugs and biochemicals that may promote or slow corneal healing and identify those agents that promote better wound healing.

Another area of research interest is laser therapy. Several small-scale studies show that lasers may be effective in sculpting the cornea to improve its ability to refract light in people with myopia and astigmatism. While this news is hopeful, many questions need to be

211

answered about its short and long-term benefits before laser therapy can be recommended as a safe and effective treatment.

The NEI also supports the Herpetic Eye Disease Study (HEDS), a group of clinical trials that is designed to study various treatments for severe ocular herpes. Recently, HEDS researchers reported that orally administered acyclovir, a drug widely used for genital herpes, had no significant effect in treating herpes simplex stromal keratitis. The HEDS should provide eye care professionals with valuable information about when to use and not to use specific antiviral drugs for this condition. But, more importantly, these clinical trials will improve care for people with advanced ocular herpes.

Chapter 28

National Eye Institute Report on Inflammatory and Infectious Processes

Introduction

As a consequence of injuries and infection, the cornea often suffers a loss of tissue substance, stromal ulceration, and scarring that produce opacities and decreased vision. It has been estimated that approximately 100,000 cases of corneal opacity occur annually in the United States. Such conditions produce impaired vision and severe pain and result in decreased productivity and high medical costs for rehabilitation and therapy.

The growth of blood vessels into the normally avascular cornea may be a component of healing and may participate in arresting tissue destruction. However, inappropriate vascularization occurs in many blinding diseases, including trachoma and herpes simplex keratitis, causes decreased visual acuity, and exacerbates rejection of corneal transplants. Since the 1987 Evaluation and Update, there has been increased activity and interest in corneal inflammatory mediators and neovascularization. Attempts to better understand and control the sequelae of inflammation have met with some success.

The ocular surface, comprising cornea and conjunctiva, is highly specialized to carry out important physiologic functions. Consequently, immune responses initiated on or in these surfaces also are highly specialized. The tear film contains immunocompetent lymphocytes,

NIH Pub. No. 93–3186. Excerpt from *Vision Research: A National Plan*, pp. 131–37.

inflammatory cells, immunoglobulin molecules, and proteins such as complement and lactoferrin that contribute to specific and nonspecific host defense mechanisms. The conjunctival surface is protected immunologically by a special component of the immune apparatus called the mucosal immune system. The ocular components of this system include secretory IgA antibodies in tears, IgA-secreting plasma cells in the lacrimal glands, lymph follicles of the subconjunctiva, and a unique population of recirculating T- and B-lymphocytes with special affinity for mucosal surfaces. In addition to providing immune protection, the tears as well as the subconjunctiva contain and/or elaborate cells and molecules that are critical to nonspecific host defenses, such as complement and clotting proteins, acute phase reactive proteins, antibacterial proteins, arachidonic acid-derived mediators, and so on. By the interplay of specific immune effectors with nonspecific defense mechanisms, expression of immunity within the conjunctiva and adnexal structures is appropriate, protective, and similar to that expressed on other mucosal surfaces.

The conjunctiva and adnexal structures also are equipped with mast cells and IgE-secreting plasma cells, rendering these tissues susceptible to inflammation of the allergic type. In this regard, the connective tissues of the ocular surface resemble connective tissues elsewhere in the skin. Disorders of this system potentially include vernal conjunctivitis, giant papillary conjunctivitis in contact lens wearers, and phlyctenular keratoconjunctivitis. By contrast, the cornea is an immunologically privileged site, permitting it to accept foreign tissues and pathogenic materials without immune destruction; therefore, the cornea, as an allograft, is relatively invulnerable to immune rejection. The specialization of the immune system with respect to the cornea is unique and distinctly different from the type of immunity found in the conjunctiva.

The unique and distinctive specializations of the immune response observed within these two ocular surface tissues account, in part, for the vulnerability of the ocular surface to certain infectious processes and perhaps for its susceptibility to certain inflammatory diseases with immunopathogenic components. The ocular surface frequently is infected with herpes viruses, adenoviruses, certain bacteria (especially Pseudomonas aeruginosa and Staphylococcus aureus), fungi, and parasites, of which Acanthamoeba is particularly prominent. In addition, the immune system plays a pathologic role in certain blinding and disabling inflammatory diseases of the ocular surface, such as cicatricial pemphigoid; the peripheral keratitis of rheumatoid arthritis, Reiter's disease, and Mooren's ulcer; and Sjogren's syndrome. Moreover, the clinical success of orthotopic corneal allografts, in relation to all other types of solid tissue allografts in man, also is related to these unique immunologic features.

Subprogram Objectives

- To elucidate the molecular genetic basis for inflammatory reactions within the conjunctiva and cornea.
- To understand the function of conjunctival-associated lymphoid tissues.
- To determine the physiologic basis for immune privilege in the cornea.
- To characterize the nonspecific host defenses on the ocular surface.
- To delineate the basis for irreversible corneal allograft failure.

Current Level of National Eye Institute Support

In FY 1992 the NEI supported 29 research projects at a cost of $5,318,948. This total includes studies of ocular surface disorders, inflammation, and corneal transplantation.

Recent Accomplishments

The response of the cornea to inflammation involves the interplay of several mediators, some of which come from corneal cells and others from recruited inflammatory cells. It is well established that stimulated granulocytes can release free arachidonic acid from membrane phospholipids to form leukotrienes, prostaglandins, and thromboxanes. Prostaglandins participate in the inflammatory response by causing a breakdown of the blood aqueous barrier and changing the intraocular pressure. Leukotrienes C4 and D4 may cause capillary leakage and edema, while leukotriene B4 is a potent chemoattractant for cells such as the leukocytes. Within the cornea, precursor fatty acids are stored as a component of cell membrane phospholipids and are released enzymatically by phospholipase A2 in response to various stimuli. Arachidonic acid is oxygenated rapidly, either by cyclooxygenase to prostaglandins or by lipoxygenases to leukotrienes. Corneal cells have both muscarinic cholinergic receptors and the inositol phospholipid pathway. Further work suggests that muscarinic cholinergic receptors may be an important regulator of the phosphatidylinositol cycle.

Nonsteroidal anti-inflammatory drugs like suprofen have been shown to inhibit cyclooxygenase, preventing formation of prostaglandins. Noninfected, inflamed rabbit eyes treated with lipoxygenase inhibitors exhibited decreased leukocyte infiltration, neovascularization, and edema, whereas cyclooxygenase inhibitors had little effect on any of those parameters. Other studies examining the effects of lipoxygenase inhibitors on the arachidonic acid cascade in rabbit cornea after cryogenic injury showed that the inhibitors differentially affected products of the cascade. The effects of new selective lipoxygenase inhibitors on alterations in arachidonic acid metabolism and breakdown of the blood aqueous barrier during HSV infection of rabbit cornea also were examined. Topical application of the inhibitors reduced leakage of proteins into the blood aqueous barrier. These drugs may be of use in treatment of the inflammatory consequences of herpes keratitis with no exacerbation of the infectious process.

A stimulatory effect of leukotriene B4 on leukocyte infiltration of the cornea also has been observed. Topical conjunctival application of leukotriene B4 has been shown to induce the migration of polymorphonuclear lymphocytes (PMN) and eosinophils into the conjunctiva.

Therapy directed toward prevention of ulceration due to chemical injury and perforation has relied on inhibition of collagenases. Tetracycline compounds recently have been shown to inhibit alkali-induced corneal ulceration, presumably by inhibiting collagenases. A newly developed synthetic thiol peptide, B-mercaptomethyl tripeptide, also has been promising. Thiol-treated corneas that did not ulcerate contained relatively fewer PMNs, whereas untreated corneas demonstrated marked inflammation at the site of ulceration. The development of standardized animal models of corneal injury should allow more precise study of the individual events of inflammation, ulceration, and vascularization during corneal disease.

Studies continue on the localization and distribution of complement components in both cornea and sclera. The anterior sclera and the cornea have been shown to contain more complement component C1, the recognition unit of the classical pathway, than does the posterior sclera. Important inflammatory functions of activated complement are well known and include increased vascular permeability, chemotaxis, release of histamine from mast cells, immune adherence, and cytolysis.

New methods for examining corneal neovascularization involving computer image analysis have been developed. These allow rapid, quantitative analysis of neovascularization. Such techniques have been used to evaluate the effects of several inhibitors of arachidonic acid metabolism on corneal neovascularization in the rat. Corneal angiogenic responses could be reduced by inhibition of cyclooxygenase as well as by other mechanisms that are steroid dependent. The role of phorbol ester tumor promoters in corneal angiogenesis *in vivo* also was examined. Several active tumor promoters that activated protein kinase C were found to stimulate angiogenesis in a dose-dependent manner. The data suggest that phorbol esters may be indirect angiogenic factors, since no mitogenic effect on bovine capillary endothelial cells in culture was detected.

The external ocular surface is protected immunologically by mucosal lymphoid tissues. Located beneath the conjunctiva and within the lacrimal glands are collections of lymphoid cells capable of responding to ocular surface antigens, chiefly by production of IgA antibodies. In animal models, lymphocytes that specifically are home to conjunctival lymphoid nodules and to lacrimal glands have been demonstrated and found to be different from cells that migrate to nonmucosal sites. Tears contain IgA antibody as well as lactoferrin and inhibitors of activated complement components. Despite high levels of this antibody in tears, it has not been shown yet to confer protection in ocular bacterial infections.

The cornea is particularly and peculiarly vulnerable to certain types of infectious diseases, because it has a nonkeratinizing epithelium, relying primarily upon the tear film to provide a surface barrier. There are no blood or lymphatic vessels in the stroma, and the entire anterior chamber has an immune privileged status. Damaged or wounded corneas can lose these properties, transiently or permanently, at which times the spectrum of corneal disease vulnerability may be exaggerated or even changed.

During the past 5 years immunologists have directed considerable research attention to limbal Langerhans cells. This research has focused on defining factors that govern migration into the central corneal epithelium, interaction between Langerhans cells and viruses and other microbial agents, and relationships between Langerhans cells and corneal tissue as allogeneic transplants. Some pathogenic stimuli to the corneal surface induce Langerhans cell migration into the central epithelium. Altered corneas that contain Langerhans cells induce allograft immunity and corneal graft rejection, as well as

217

generate cytotoxic and delayed hypersensitivity T cells in allogeneic recipient mice. However, normal corneas, which are virtually devoid of Langerhans cells, fail to induce delayed hypersensitivity and are less able to induce allograft immunity. In addition, the incidence and severity of HSV-1 stromal keratitis is increased in corneas containing central Langerhans cells.

The immunologic status of the cornea has been shown to influence immune responses to antigens within the anterior chamber. Anterior chamber-associated immune deviation develops following inoculation of many different types of antigens into the anterior chamber of eyes with normal corneas. By contrast, conventional immunity, including delayed hypersensitivity, occurs if the same antigens are placed in the anterior chamber of eyes with corneas containing central Langerhans cells. Thus, the condition of the anterior surface of the cornea unexpectedly influences immune responses within the globe itself.

The most significant recent advances in our fundamental understanding of the basis of corneal allograft acceptance and rejection have come from creating rodent models of orthotopic cornea grafting. It has been clearly demonstrated that rejection of orthotopic grafts strongly correlates with the presence of Langerhans cells in the graft. It also has been demonstrated that Langerhans cells in corneal allografts promote the development of both delayed hypersensitivity and cytotoxic T cells against graft antigens. Thus, Langerhans cells, which may be silently present in a cornea that otherwise appears normal, are a significant risk factor for graft rejection.

It has been established that rejecting corneal allografts up-regulate expression of major histocompatibility complex (MHC) molecules on epithelial cells, keratocytes, and endothelium. Yet, it remains unclear which of these cell types is the "true" target of the rejection reaction. Moreover, it has yet to be determined which immune effector modalities play the most important roles in corneal allograft rejection. During and following rejection of corneal allografts, the serum of some individuals contains antibodies that react specifically with cornea tissue. A 54-kd molecule has been identified as a target antigen on corneal epithelial cells. The role of these "autoantibodies" in corneal allograft rejection has yet to be determined.

The immunosuppressive drug cyclosporin A (CsA) is being investigated as a possible treatment for corneal graft rejection, but it is not yet known whether CsA will offer a significant improvement over existing therapies. Evidence from clinical studies indicates that human lymphocyte antigen (HLA) matching of donor and host has little effect on outcome, while ABO blood group matching is both a less expensive and more effective strategy. For high-risk patients, postoperative steroids treatment increases graft survival.

There also have been advances in the area of corneal preservation for transplantation. Obviously, there is an unavoidable period of time between the death of a corneal donor and the opportunity to transplant the donated cornea into the eye of a recipient. The adequacy of corneal preservation during this period of storage determines the results of the transplantation. Improvements in corneal storage techniques have resulted from recent studies of the beneficial effects of chondroitin sulfate in the preservative solution for storage at both 4° C and 34° C. At both these temperatures, however, there is a time-dependent deterioration of the tissue; so early transplantation is preferable. In general, corneal storage is limited to 1 week at 4° C and 1 month at 34° C. Recent studies suggest that corneal preservation by vitrification could eliminate this deterioration and extend corneal preservation. Continued research in corneal preservation techniques is needed to assure improved corneal viability at the time of transplantation, optimum tissue distribution, and the opportunity for true banking of tissue-typed corneas for high-risk procedures.

Important Research Questions to Be Addressed

During the next 5 years emphasis should be placed on understanding the cellular and molecular basis for corneal inflammation. The following important questions need to be addressed:

What is the role of Langerhans cells in corneal physiology and immunology?

Although a role for Langerhans cells in the induction of immune reactions in skin and cornea has been elucidated, the influence of these cells on nonimmune properties of the cornea and limbus is virtually unexplored. Do these cells participate in maintaining the microanatomic and physiologic parameters of the normal cornea? Do Langerhans cells contribute to corneal abnormalities when they have been induced to penetrate into the central epithelium? It is not clear whether Langerhans cells abnormally present in the central cornea have a pathogenic role in this site, perhaps as antigen-presenting cells for the expression of immunity. Model systems in mice and other laboratory animals now exist for use in exploring these important issues.

What is the molecular basis for lymphocyte traffic into the conjunctival-associated lymphoid tissues?

It is likely that lymphocytes participate in the pathogenesis of dry eye disorders, but the precise mechanisms by which tear secretion is abnormal and impaired remain undetermined. Interactions between lymphocytes and endothelial cells of vessels supplying the eye-associated tissues need to be clarified, and strategies for influencing these processes need to be developed.

What are the roles of nonimmune defense molecules in the tear film?

The presence and even concentration of molecules such as cytokines, complement components, and lactoferrin in tears have been described. Now research should begin to analyze the mechanisms by which these various factors provide protection against ocular pathogens.

How do the cornea and anterior chamber of the eye function as immune-privileged sites?

It is apparent that immune privilege in the anterior chamber and in the cornea are not maintained independently and that abnormalities in one site can influence privilege in the other site. Studies are needed to determine to what extent perturbation of the cornea leads to alterations in the immune properties of the anterior chamber and vice versa.

What processes are involved in corneal graft rejection?

Studies are needed to determine whether stromal vascularization and/or Langerhans cells are primarily important during induction of immunity to transplantation antigens on the corneal grafts or, rather, are chiefly responsible for promoting immune effector mechanisms that produce graft failure.

What is the basis of corneal allograft failure?

Recent evidence indicates that autoimmune responses against cornea-specific antigens may be evoked by corneal allografts. To what extent does autoimmune reactivity contribute to corneal allograft failure? The development of orthotopic corneal grafting in laboratory rodents makes it possible for basic scientists to approach these critical questions directly with model systems that faithfully mimic the clinical situation. Not all corneal allograft failures can be ascribed to immunity directed at transplantation antigens on the graft. Among factors that could play an important role in graft failure is latent infection of corneal tissue with HSV. It is important to determine whether the act of corneal grafting can lead to activation of latent virus infection in either the donor corneal button or the recipient bed, thereby placing the graft at additional risk of failure from virus infection.

What immunosuppressive agents should be used to treat failing corneal grafts?

Cyclosporin and FK506 are merely the most prominent of recently developed drugs that are significantly more selective in their action on the immune system. These and other agents need to be examined for their potential therapeutic usefulness, especially in laboratory rodents. Results of these types of studies are critical to the ultimate development of better therapeutic agents for use in humans.

Chapter 29

National Eye Institute Report on Corneal Structure and Function

Tears and Octal Surface of the Epithelium

Introduction

Abnormalities of the ocular surface continue to represent a major portion of eye care problems. These problems result in pain, redness, photophobia, and reduced vision. If the problems are chronic, they can lead to ulceration and scarring of the cornea and thus permanent visual impairment. Therapy is inadequate for many of these diseases, not only because their causes often are unknown, but also because many therapeutic agents do not penetrate well.

The previous NEI National Plan and the NEI-sponsored Tear Film Symposium in 1986 have led to a heightened interest in the tear film and its disorders. A lacrimal gland study group now meets annually. There has been a surge of interest in the cell biology of the ocular surface epithelium and more researchers have recognized that the cornea is an excellent model for study of the mechanisms of wound healing. Basic scientists have applied contemporary techniques to the study of the ocular surface, and results of this new research should translate into better therapies for surface disorders such as persistent epithelial defects, corneal ulceration, and inflammation.

NIH Pub. No. 93–3186. Excerpt from *Vision Research: A National Plan*, pp. 114–31

Subprogram Objectives

- To elucidate the composition and function of the tear film and its changes with aging and disease.
- To investigate the molecular mechanisms of tear film formation.
- To evaluate and more accurately diagnose tear film abnormalities and to develop new therapeutic approaches.
- To define more completely the cell and molecular biology, biochemistry, and physiology of the ocular surface epithelium.

Current Level of National Eye Institute Support

In Fiscal Year (FY) 1992 the NEI supported 35 research projects at a cost of $5,989,777. These grants included studies of the normal composition, function, and control mechanisms of the tear film; treatment of dry eye patients; interrelationships between the tear film and the ocular surface; development of organ and cell culture of the lacrimal and meibomian glands; the roles of lacrimal gland and duct obstruction in the production of dry eye; epithelial healing; and evaluation of stimuli for conjunctival growth onto the ocular surface.

Recent Accomplishments

The external ocular surface is a wet, remarkably smooth, refractile surface. The apical epithelial cells are covered by a tear film secreted by the lacrimal gland. Lipid from the meibomian glands spreads over the tear film, and additional products are added by accessory lacrimal glands. The past 5 years have seen an increased level of understanding of the factors controlling lacrimal gland protein, electrolyte, and water secretion. This increase in knowledge has been facilitated by development of techniques for primary culture of lacrimal gland acinar cells. Accessory lacrimal gland secretion has been shown to be increased by increased levels of cellular cAMP. In an animal model of Sjogren's syndrome, it has been found that androgens suppress lymphocytic invasion of the lacrimal gland. Other studies suggest that a retrovirus antigenically related to HIV or to Epstein-Barr virus may trigger the lymphocytic abnormality and subsequent immunopathology seen in Sjogren's syndrome. Still others suggest a defect leading to aberrant auto-antigen presentation. These findings open research avenues for developing new treatments for the respective diseases in humans.

The past 5 years have seen improved classification and diagnosis of keratoconjunctivitis sicca (KCS). Clinical use of topical vitamin A has been found to be effective in treatment of cicatricial diseases of the conjunctiva. A number of discoveries of the cellular biologic aspects of normal and healing ocular surface epithelium has been made since the 1987 update. Data are accumulating to support the hypothesis that the stem cells of the corneal epithelium are the limbal basal cells. The cells of this region are mitotically slow-cycling cells that have keratin antibody-binding patterns different from those of corneal epithelium; moreover, these limbal region cells grow better in culture than do those of the peripheral or central corneal epithelium. Clinically, it has been demonstrated that limbal autograft transplants are effective in treatment of patients with widespread damage to the ocular surface.

There has been general recognition that the mitogenic effect of epithelial growth factor and fibroblast growth factor enhances epithelial wound healing. Despite much interest in the role of growth factors in epithelial wound healing, translation of this interest into a clinical treatment for persistent epithelial defects has not been forthcoming. Similarly, although there has been much interest in the effect of exogenously applied extracellular matrix components (especially fibronectin) on epithelial healing rates, the resulting studies have had variable results. This has sparked a search for extracellular matrix receptors in the corneal epithelium that parallels the search for and major discoveries of such receptors in nonocular systems. Identification of matrix receptors in corneal epithelium has begun and should yield more reliable data upon which to base new therapies.

A major finding in the corneal wound-healing response is that synthesis of the protein vinculin is dramatically enhanced during epithelial migration. Vinculin is known to be a component of the cell-substrate junction known as a focal contact. These junctions may be the provisional adhesion junctions that replace hemidesmosomes during the period of epithelial migration. It also has been found that neutral glycosphingolipids are synthesized to a greater degree in migrating epithelium than in stationary epithelium. Characterization of these glycosphingolipids may yield information on their function during migration.

Major understanding of how the epithelium adheres to the stroma has been realized. The linkage of hemidesmosomes through the basement membrane to the anchoring fibril network has been demonstrated. The pattern of reassembly of these structures after keratectomy or laser photoablation has been documented in species lacking a Bowman's layer, but more work needs to be done in the human.

Discovery of new members of the metalloprotease family of extracellular matrix-degrading enzymes has occurred during the past several years. Study of these enzymes as they relate to stromal ulceration is of obvious interest. That the epithelium plays a role in extracellular matrix maintenance and degradation is evidenced by the finding that the corneal epithelium can synthesize a 92-kd gelatinase (also known as type IV collagenase), a member of the metalloprotease family of extracellular matrix-degrading enzymes.

Important work is being done on ocular pharmacology for the treatment of disease. Resins have been found that will slowly release drugs into the precorneal tear film. A variety of gels have been developed that can be administered as a liquid and then gel in the eye. The most significant development has been the use of drug-containing collagen shields. These devices are changing the treatment of infected ulcers and permit the delivery of large molecules like heparin in a therapeutically effective way.

Important Research Questions to Be Addressed

The following questions need to be addressed:

What are the molecular biologic mechanisms that regulate ocular surface gland secretion?

This information should lead to development of specific treatments for tear insufficiency. It is also important to determine what controls normal lacrimal gland secretion and its changes during development and aging. This information could provide a scientific basis for the development of a cure for the lacrimal gland insufficiency that occurs in Sjogren's syndrome.

What diagnostic tests will distinguish among disorders of the lipid, aqueous, and mucin layers of the tear film?

Since there is little effective treatment for the many KCS diseases, continued research into the normal and pathological composition of tear fluid, the cellular control mechanisms of secretion by the individual orbital glands, and the role of the ocular surface on the function of the tear film is indicated. The physical chemistry and function of mucin need to be elucidated. In addition, there is the need for new diagnostic tests for tear film insufficiency that can be used widely.

What defines a stem cell and how does it function?

There is increasing evidence that limbal basal cells are stem cells of the corneal epithelium. We need to further understand stem cell differentiation and migration in normal epithelial maintenance. It will be important to determine what factors are involved in preventing reepithelialization, and strategies to enhance resurfacing need to be developed.

How are cell-cell and cell-matrix interactions regulated in the normal and healing ocular surface?

There are still no adequate treatments for the diseases that affect the ocular surface. A particularly urgent need exists for biologically based strategies to enhance permanent resurfacing of chronic, persistent epithelial defects and recurrent erosions. The cornea provides an excellent model for study of epithelial-mesenchymal interactions and the role of the epithelium in matrix synthesis and degradation. Despite much effort devoted to clinical trials of factors believed to affect epithelial wound healing (growth factors and fibronectin), adequate treatment for chronic, persistent epithelial defects is not available.

Transport

Introduction

The corneal endothelium is essential for maintaining corneal transparency, however, this is a delicate monolayer of cells with no natural regenerative and only limited reparative capabilities in man. If endothelial cells are diseased or absent, permanent corneal edema, loss of corneal transparency, and eventual blindness may occur. There are corneal dystrophies in which endothelial cells progressively lose their ability to maintain corneal transparency. Some ocular surgical procedures also lead to loss of endothelial function by mechanical trauma. Thus, in the future, the development of procedures to restore function or replace corneal endothelial cells can be expected to grow in importance.

For advanced endothelial dysfunction, the transplantation of a full-thickness donor cornea is the accepted therapeutic means for re-establishing normal vision. Replacement of the endothelial cell layer without corneal transplantation has been a long-term goal in ophthalmology, and some laboratories are evaluating such replacement by cultured cells. However, the problem of establishing a fluid pump system across a cultured endothelial cell layer remains unsolved. Even in isolated rabbit cornea, the endothelial pump fails within a few hours. Nevertheless, the use of cells from tissue cultures would have the advantage over the use of donor corneas by eliminating delays due to variation in availability of donor material, enabling selection of cultured cells with known transplantation antigens, and eliminating immune challenge currently arising from stromal antigens.

Current research in this area is largely directed toward clinical applications. A good deal of effort also is being spent in improving organ culture conditions to allow eye bank corneas to survive longer. Comparatively less emphasis has been placed on basic cellular biologic and genetic regulatory factors for endothelial cell growth and differentiation as well as the biology of corneal organ cultures.

Corneal transparency hinges on a precisely controlled degree of corneal hydration that is required to maintain corneal matrix structures correctly organized in space. Stromal proteoglycans are able to imbibe water beyond the point at which the cornea would lose its transparency. Hence, that tendency must be balanced by outward water movements across both limiting layers. There is continuous transport of fluid across the endothelium secondary to active electrolyte transport and there are diurnal osmotic water movements across the epithelium. The limiting cell layers thus mediate bulk fluid transfer, while at the same time keeping a constant internal milieu. Hence, studies of fluid transport mechanisms have focused on epithelial and endothelial ion pumps, electrolytes, solutes, and water membrane channels; mechanisms leading to the coupling of fluid flow to ion transport; roles of paracellular pathways; and links between cell metabolism and volume control. The epithelium functions as a high-resistance barrier against the penetration of fluid, microorganisms, and foreign matter. The endothelium continuously transports sizable amounts of fluid from the stroma to the aqueous humor while allowing small molecules to pass forward. The epithelium and endothelium appear to act in concert to prevent the corneal stroma from swelling.

Preservation of corneal transparency depends upon the structural and functional integrity of the epithelium and endothelium. Although most techniques for examining cell layer function have been designed for isolated tissues, some have been modified for use *in vivo*. Currently, no procedure is available to make early diagnosis of endothelial dystrophies or degenerations, although specular micrographs can document the presence of established disease. The development of the specular microscope and the confocal microscope has facilitated the morphological evaluation of the endothelial layer *in vivo*.

Subprogram Objectives

- To study the biology and function of endothelial cells.
- To determine the necessary conditions for a successful transplantation of cultured endothelial cells in humans.
- To identity the molecular components of the corneal transport systems and determine how they function in normal, injured, diseased, and aged eyes.
- To develop methods for assessing the relationships between images of corneal cells in vivo and their functional state.

Current Level of National Eye Institute Support

In FY 1992 the NEI supported 41 research grants at a cost of $7,333,545. Among the supported studies are those that seek to define *in vitro* needs of corneal endothelium in tissue culture, to develop techniques for transplanting tissue-cultured endothelium in man, to develop methods for in vivo assessment of epithelial and endothelial function, to compare membrane metabolic function of normal corneas and diseased corneas, and to evaluate neural and humoral factors that influence metabolism.

Recent Accomplishments

The ability to grow, maintain, and manipulate corneal cells in culture has continued to improve. The types of proteins expressed, their localization, and the regulation of their synthesis have begun to be scrutinized, and a variety of receptors and binding sites are being found. It is now clear that adrenergic receptors are present on epithelial membranes. This finding may facilitate research on the modulation of epithelial growth. Regulation of chloride transport by the epithelium has been found to depend on many factors, such as adrenoceptors and prostaglandins. The regulation of pH has been traced to an Na$^+$/H$^+$ exchange mechanism, and ATPase activity and stoichiometry have been investigated.

Cultured endothelial layers have been developed as key model systems. The question of Na$^+$ transport by the endothelium continues to receive attention and to merit investigation, and evidence has been presented that Na$^+$ enters the endothelium via apical channels inhibitable by amiloride. Work also continues on the function of the Na$^+$/K$^+$-ATPase, particularly its indirect role in junction maintenance. The characteristics of the bicarbonate transporting system continue to generate study and controversy. The effect of cell pH on endothelial sodium fluxes *in vitro* and the mechanism of its regulation in cultured cells also have received attention. Several ion channels have been found in endothelial cells in vitro by use of patch-clamp techniques. Finally, a second function of facilitative glucose transporters—to serve also as water channels—now is being explored.

Since the last survey, new noninvasive observation procedures have been developed. Microprocessors and acoustic microscope and ultrasonic techniques are being developed to read corneal thickness *in vivo*. Noninvasive metabolic analysis continues to be developed. Confocal microscopes can now perform optical dissections of circumscribed tissue layers in cloudy and diseased corneas. In addition, the emergence of new surgical procedures, such as radial keratotomy and laser ablation, make it imperative to monitor the functional state of the keratocytes and their effects on matrix structure for safety considerations. Developing such procedures will have diagnostic and therapeutic applications.

Important Research Questions to Be Addressed

On the basis of assessment of recent accomplishments, current activities, and important research questions to be addressed in this subprogram area, the Panel recommends increased support for this area. Advances in cell biology, molecular genetics, and biochemistry should provide the technology needed to allow tremendous advances in the areas of electrolyte and fluid transport, metabolism, proteins acting as carriers, channels, transporters, and receptor sites in the epithelium and the endothelium. Questions that need to be addressed include the following:

Which proteins confer the endothelium's characteristic functions?

Knowledge of the sequence, structure, and dynamic behavior of the fluid pump proteins would enhance understanding of the disease processes involved in endothelial dystrophies and could lead to more effective treatments.

What determines and regulates the repair and mitotic ability of corneal endothelium?

Corneal tissues, like others of embryonic neural crest origin, have a very limited mitotic activity. Many laboratories are attempting to determine why endothelial function deteriorates following cell loss, age, or trauma. Delineating the optimal conditions for the tissue culture of corneal endothelium will help evaluate the problems involved in transplanting these cultured cells and assuring their survival. With further refinement of endothelial culture techniques, it will be possible to determine whether cell-cycle stimulatory and inhibitory factors arise from other cells and whether the endothelium can be induced to repair itself *in vivo.*

How are corneal cells polarized for transport?

The roles of the endothelium and epithelium in controlling hydration have been studied most extensively in the amphibian and the rabbit. These studies have focused on the mechanisms of epithelial and endothelial water and solute permeability and transport. Since transport processes are a major factor in the preservation of corneal transparency, a thorough examination of these processes is necessary to explain the causes of corneal disease and dysfunction that result in stromal and epithelial edema and in subsequent blindness. With recent advances in cell biology, biochemistry, and molecular biology techniques, many possibilities exist for finding ways to modulate the permeability and transport properties of the corneal limiting layers. This could lead to forms of therapy other than corneal transplant surgery for these conditions.

What hormonal, neural, and pharmacologic modulators act on epithelial and endothelial transport processes?

It is important to identify physiologically active substances, determine which receptors are present on the cell membrane, and learn how these receptors function in signal transduction. A full understanding of these transport phenomena will require fundamental information regarding the sequences, structures, and dynamic mode of operation of transport-related membrane proteins; their genetic regulation; and how these molecules are transported to their proper cellular destination.

Stroma

Introduction

The human cornea contains extracellular matrices with distinct structures, macromolecular compositions, and functions. These matrices are arranged in clearly defined layers and are synthesized by and interact with distinct cell types. The stroma forms the bulk of the cornea and is unique among connective tissues in being transparent while retaining the requisite mechanical properties to ensure the integrity of the eyeball. The collagen fibrils in the stroma form lamellae, which run parallel to the corneal surface without interruption from limbus to limbus. The fibrils have small, uniform diameters and are spaced equidistantly. The interfibrillar matrix contains nonfibrillar collagen, proteoglycans, and other poorly characterized components.

Understanding corneal hydration, transparency, and development as well as such disorders as corneal edema, wound healing, and dystrophies requires a basic knowledge of corneal extracellular matrices. The corneal extracellular matrices are known to contain a large number of the known collagen types, three proteoglycan (PG) classes, and at least three glycoproteins. The composition of the different corneal matrices is distinct and changes during normal development and pathological disorders. Fundamental to the understanding of corneal function and its pathobiology are the elucidation of the biochemical composition, macromolecular interactions, matrix turnover, cell-matrix interactions, and the regulation of corneal matrix gene expression.

Subprogram Objectives

- To determine the molecular basis of corneal transparency.
- To determine the cellular, molecular, and biochemical bases of normal corneal development.
- To identify the factors controlling corneal matrix assembly, turnover, and remodeling.

Current Level of National Eye Institute Support

In FY 1992 the NEI supported 17 research grants at a cost of $3,428,571. This total included studies of edema and transparency, normal corneal development, corneal dystrophies, inherited disorders, and developmental anomalies.

Recent Accomplishments

Corneal development involves a series of regulated spatial and temporal events involving cell differentiation, migration, and extra-cellular matrix synthesis and assembly. An approach that has con-tributed to our understanding of corneal development has been the use of cornea-specific monoclonal antibodies. These reagents have been characterized for epithelial, basement membrane, and stromal epitopes and have been used to study cell-cell and cell-matrix inter-actions involved in corneal differentiation. Another approach that will contribute to the elucidation of the function of a particular component is the study of systems deficient in a particular macromolecule. For example, corneal development proceeds relatively normally in the MOV13 mouse, which is deficient in its expression of type I collagen; however, there are some abnormalities in other aspects of matrix or-ganization.

Our knowledge of the corneal collagenous matrix has increased rapidly during the past 5 years. Nine different collagen types have been characterized in different corneal systems and in different stages of corneal development. Considerable effort has gone into character-izing these different corneal collagens and determining their distri-bution and cell origin. In the corneal stroma, the collagen fibrils are heterotypic, containing two or more distinct types of collagen. Such interaction of different collagen types provides a mechanism whereby fibril architecture can be regulated. The human corneal stroma is relatively enriched for type V collagen, and the interaction of type V with type I is at least partially responsible for regulation of collagen fibril diameter. It is likely that heterotypic fibrils are the rule rather than the exception. Changes in the proportion of types I and V have been observed in scar tissue and may be related to the opacity of the scar. In the primary stroma of the chick, heterotypic types I and II containing fibrils are present, whereas in the human cornea types I and III collagen fibrils are present. It is possible that this difference in type of heterotypic fibrils is developmentally significant.

Cell-matrix interactions are important determinants of cell behavior. Corneal epithelial cell interactions with either the intact basal lamina or individual matrix components produce changes in cell shape and organization as well as synthetic rates. Specific receptors have been shown to mediate these interactions, and this is a rapidly expanding area in corneal cell biology. A variety of nonfibrillar collagens have been studied in the cornea. Type IV collagen, which is present in the basal lamina, has important structural properties as well as the ability to mediate specific cell-matrix interactions. Type VII collagen, which makes up the anchoring fibrils or filaments that attach the basal lamina to the underlying stroma, also has been studied in the cornea during development and wound repair. Type VI collagen is a filamentous collagen that forms networks in most soft connective tissues. Type VI collagen is very abundant in the corneal stroma, located between individual collagen fibrils and between fibrils and cells, and may play a role in the distribution and organization of connective tissue. The alteration in the proportions of type VI to other collagens in corneal scar tissue suggests a function in transparency. Type VIII collagen is a major component of Descemet's membrane. Its localization as well as its protein and genomic structure have been partially characterized. Corneal type IX collagen is fibril-associated and contains a chondroitin sulfate side chain. The type IX species located in the primary corneal stroma is missing a large terminal domain present in the cartilage form. This corneal form results from alternative splicing and the use of a distinct promoter. This collagen is present in a very narrow developmental window and thus may have an important regulatory function.

The gene for type XII collagen recently has been cloned and localized in mammalian and chick corneas. The predicted structure of type XII collagen suggests the presence of three 60 nm fingers and a 75 nm collagen tail extending from a central globular region. It is possible that the type XII molecule collagen tail binds to the surface of type I-containing collagen fibrils while the fingers project into the perifibrillar matrix.

Another recent advance has been the availability of collagen type-specific monoclonal antibodies which have made localization studies possible. Unfortunately, a large number of these probes do not cross-react with human corneal components, thus limiting the information gained in this system. A solution to this problem would be the production of human reagents, including cDNAs and genomic probes.

Corneal transparency appears to require a uniform spacing of stromal collagen fibrils. Since the space between collagen fibrils is occupied by PGs, their physical and chemical properties may play an important role in determining corneal transparency. PGs are highly anionic macromolecules that possess at least one sulfated glycosaminoglycan (GAG) chain covalently bound to a peptide core. The two major types of GAGs in the corneal stroma are keratan sulfate (KS) and dermatan sulfate (DS). Each GAG is a disaccharide polymer, which in KS consists of N-acetylglucosamine and galactose and in DS consists of N-acetylgalactosamine and glucuronic or iduronic acid. GAG sugars are sulfated to varying degrees. The large hydrodynamic volume of GAGs, their tendency to bind to other macromolecules through ionic interactions, and their location within the corneal stroma suggest an important role in the development and maintenance of corneal transparency. The structural relationships and functional properties of these PGs are poorly understood, although comparative analyses of PGs from rabbit, bovine, cat, and human indicate marked similarities among species.

PGs interact with collagens through their core protein as well as GAG chains; thus, detailed knowledge of the PG core proteins is central to understanding the function of these macromolecules. In this regard, the core protein for chick corneal keratan sulfate PG recently has been cloned and sequenced. It has been given the name "lumican" to indicate its important role in maintaining corneal transparency. PGs also play an important role in corneal hydration. The water content of the cornea and the water absorption capacity increase across the cornea from anterior to posterior stroma. This water gradient correlates with the distribution of stromal PGs.

Recent cloning and sequencing studies have demonstrated that the corneal PGs are part of a family of small PGs with similar core protein composition and sequence. Although the core proteins may be derived from different gene products, they all appear to be closely related to the core proteins of decorin, fibromodulin, and byglycan. The high degree of homology between bovine bone, human fibroblast, and chick cornea core proteins strongly supports the concept of an evolutionarily conserved single-copy gene for the decorin core protein.

Comparative analyses of proteoglycans from rabbit, bovine, cat, and human corneas indicate marked similarities among species.

The mechanism by which PGs are differentially attributed in the cornea is unknown, but oxygen is suspected of affecting GAG synthesis. Since the corneal epithelium is designated to break down glucose and glycogen to lactate by the Embden-Meyerhof pathway, restrictions in oxygen quickly accelerate anaerobic glycolysis, release lactate to the stroma, and precipitate a cascade of metabolic events that may lead to alterations in PG precursors and arachidonic acid metabolites. Thus, moderate restrictions in the availability of oxygen to the cornea, such as those produced by extended wear contact lenses, may result in profound alterations in PG synthesis.

The strength of GAG interactions with other matrix proteins can be related to GAG charge density, and these interactions generally lack specificity. The core proteins also have been shown to bind to collagen and other matrix components. The fibroblast PG "decorin" (also known as PG40 or PGII) binds to collagen and fibronectin through its core protein. The high degree of homology between bovine bone and human fibroblast core proteins strongly supports the idea of an evolutionarily conserved single-copy gene for the decorin core protein. Cytochemical and physical evidence indicate that the keratin sulfate proteoglycine recently named "lumican" and decorin interact with corneal collagen fibrils at specific sites. The rapid turnover of the corneal PGs suggests potentially important roles in extracellular matrix organization and in mediating interactions between stromal cells and their environment.

Pathologic conditions affecting the corneal stroma result in edema and reduction of corneal transparency. The normal endothelium maintains a constant stromal water content through the action of a pump mechanism, which counteracts the osmotic properties of the hydrophilic stromal PGs. In rabbit cornea, transient stromal edema due to surgical damage to the endothelium is accompanied by changes in corneal PGs. Perfusion of rabbit cornea with calcium-free medium damages junctions between endothelial cells, swells the tissue, and causes ultrastructural changes consistent with the loss of PGs. Marked loss of PGs is paralleled by alterations in the collagen fibrils, suggesting a role for PGs in maintaining the structure of the stroma. Thus, the ultrastructural association and hydrophilic properties of corneal PGs are factors in stromal hydration as well as in the regular arrangement of collagen fibrils.

A new treatment has been developed for removal of corneal crystals by topical cysteamine in nephropathic cystinosis. This autosomal recessively inherited disorder is characterized by impairment of normal carrier-mediated transport of cystine across the lysosomal membrane leading to an accumulation of cystine crystals. Clinically, the intralysosomal cystine interferes with the function of different organs at different rates, but cystine generally appear in the cornea by age 1 and are pathognomonic of cystinosis. Although corneal cystine crystals do not interfere with visual acuity, they do cause severe discomfort, photophobia, blepharospasm, and recurrent corneal erosions. Tissue culture studies have demonstrated that cystinotic corneal cells lose their cystine after exposure to cysteamine (ß-mercaptoethylamine, a free thiol which reacts with cystine to form a mixed disulfide which traverses the lysomal membrane in a normal fashion). Following this observation, randomized placebo-controlled clinical trials now have established topical cysteamine eye drops as a treatment of choice for this condition.

The corneal stroma contains a variety of collagen types that change during development and repair. This changing matrix composition with accompanying changes in matrix-degrading enzymes of differing specificities may be an important regulatory mechanism. The matrix metalloproteinases (MMPs) are important for this process. The MMPs can be grouped into three subfamilies on the basis of their substrate specificities. Collagenases degrade native types I, II, or III collagens; stromelysins specifically cleave PGs, fibronectin, and laminin; and gelatinases hydrolyze denatured collagen molecules (gelatin) as well as native types IV, V, and VII collagens. Although controlled expression or activation of gelatinases might facilitate homeostatic processes, overexpression or inappropriate activation of these enzymes could have detrimental effects. Corneal ulceration can be considered to be a disorder of tissue maintenance. Its physical manifestation, corneal "melting," results from an excess of matrix-degrading activities. Gelatinases may play an important role during the development of the epithelial defect that leads to corneal ulceration. It will be important to determine the factors that control expression as well as activation of the gelatinases by corneal epithelial cells and stromal fibroblasts.

Despite the relative infrequency of inherited corneal diseases, their study can lead to a better understanding of other corneal disorders. For example, determining the basis of abnormal stromal cell function might contribute to understanding the biochemical basis of corneal ulceration and scarring. The study of corneal dystrophies, a heterogeneous group of relatively uncommon but usually inherited disorders, also may contribute important information about modulators and stimulators of wound healing in general as well as the biochemistry of scarring and aging.

Keratoconus is a heterogeneous, progressive disease involving thinning and scarring of the central cornea. Characterization of keratoconus has been difficult because corneal tissues have been obtained from patients of different ages and with different stages of the disease, often with associated complications such as corneal scarring or edema. Recent studies have shown that although corneas obtained from patients with keratoconus contain significantly less protein per milligram of dry weight than corneas of normal controls, protein synthesis is normal in corneal stromal cultures derived from some keratoconus patients. These results have led to the hypothesis that degradation of macromolecules may be one of the mechanisms affected in keratoconus. In support of this hypothesis, keratoconus corneas have an increased collagenase activity and less KS than normal.

Important Research Questions to Be Addressed

Studies of stromal macromolecules have been restricted largely to characterization of the macromolecules and their interactions with one another. Although this structural cataloging is important, we need to know how the various components are synthesized and arranged in the tissue to produce a stroma; how their synthesis and turnover are regulated; and how they contribute to its mechanical strength, transparency, and proper refraction. The following questions need to be addressed:

What makes a cornea?

Although many macromolecules have been described in normal corneal stroma, new collagens and PGs have been discovered in fetal and healing corneas. Some of these macromolecules are unique to the cornea. Further studies are needed to complete the molecular inventory, determine the relevant physicochemical properties, and elucidate the molecular genetic mechanisms controlling expression of these macromolecules responsible for producing a functional stroma. It is particularly important to determine whether there are cornea-specific proteins, what genes are involved in their expression, and how these genes are regulated.

What events and interactions are involved in corneal cell differentiation?

Connective tissue cells associate intimately with their extracellular matrix environment, resulting in specific morphological and biochemical alterations in the cell. Very little is known of the mechanisms by which corneal cells use extracellular matrix information to undergo the differentiation necessary for construction of normal stroma or scar tissue. The importance of physical alterations in the environment and growth factor effects should be determined.

What mechanisms regulate the architecture of corneal extracellular matrices?

The morphogenesis of the corneal stroma requires mechanisms to control the synthesis, deposition, and breakdown of extracellular matrices at specific times and places. Scar formation and stromal ulceration are a result of the loss of this control. Future avenues of research should include an examination of the self-assembly mechanisms employed during the development of stromal architecture; the role of fibroblasts in matrix assembly; the existence of homeotic genes involved in coordinating expression of specific groups of genes responsible for normal morphogenesis; the role of specific subclasses of integrins, specific domains of adhesive glycoproteins, and other adhesion molecules; and the cellular, biochemical, and molecular genetic control mechanisms involved in the regulated synthesis and turnover of stromal matrix components.

What are the biochemical and biophysical properties of the cornea?

There is a dearth of detailed information on the microstructural organization and properties of the human cornea. Baseline work is needed to determine the material and elastic of the cornea, and we need to know how these vary with age and between individuals. New approaches must be developed to investigate the stress-strain parameters of living corneal tissue and to identify its load-bearing elements. Efforts should be targeted to develop and verify representative computer models of the fundamental elements of the cornea.

What are the cellular, biochemical, and genetic bases of corneal dystrophies?

Steps should be taken to identify appropriate kindreds carrying genes that encode corneal disorders. Pedigree analysis could then identify the chromosomal locus of any genes involved in these hereditary disorders. The identification of restriction fragment length polymorphisms associated with particular disorders could lead to fine mapping and eventual gene identification and cloning. Some work of this type has been done for macular corneal dystrophy and the keratomas. Existing genetic technology is ripe for pursuit of additional corneal disease genes.

Chapter 30

National Eye Institute Report on Infectious Diseases and the Cornea

Introduction

Approximately 500,000 cases of ocular herpetic keratitis caused by HSV are reported yearly in the United States. Stromal disease frequently produces irreversible structural alteration and corneal scarring, and once someone has had more than one attack of herpes, chances are high that the disease will recur. Since the *1987 Evaluation and Update,* increased research on the role of specific viral genes in the pathogenicity of HSV-1 and in establishment and reactivation of latency has proceeded by use of DNA technology. New and improved animal models have been developed, the role of the immune system in disease pathogenesis has been further elucidated, and new families of therapeutic drugs are being examined.

Common ocular complications caused by varicella zoster virus (VZV)—the agent that causes ophthalmic herpes zoster—include chronic corneal epithelial and stromal ulceration and excruciating neuralgic pain. Unlike those affected by HSV, zoster-scarred corneas are less amenable to successful transplantation surgery. Since the *1987 Evaluation and Update,* development of improved animal models of ocular disease continues, and early therapy with acyclovir has been shown to reduce the severity and complications of ocular disease.

Adenovlrus is the most frequent cause of epidemic ocular disease. The ocular route of adenoviral infection may lead to disseminated

NIH Pub. No. 93–3186. Excerpt from *Vision Research: A National Plan*, pp. 138–46.

disease, which can be fatal in children. Recently, an animal model for adenovirus infection has been developed and can now be used to study the pathogenesis of disease and potential therapeutic regimens. Since the *1987 Evaluation and Update,* there have been no significant research developments regarding anterior segment involvement or transmissibility of HIV, the causative agent of AIDS, by rears or donor corneal tissue from which the virus has been isolated.

The corneal surface normally is protected against bacterial and fungal infection by an intact epithelium and its associated tear film. Disruption of this mechanical and physiologic barrier by trauma such as contact lens abrasion predisposes the eye to pathogen adherence, proliferation, release of virulence factors, and invasion. Infectious disease is enhanced by bacterial factors as well as a myriad of host factors, including advanced age or immunocompromise. *Pseudomonas aeruginosa* is the most virulent of several bacterial corneal pathogens, producing stromal suppuration and corneal perforation. Since the *1987 Evaluation and Update,* increased research activity has occurred in the areas of bacterial adherence to cornea and contact lenses, and delineation of the significant host and bacterial pathogenetic factors continues. Development of organ and tissue-culture models has facilitated these studies.

Several infectious ocular diseases have emerged since the 1987 update. Lyme disease, caused by the spirochete *Borrelia burgdorferi* (transmitted by ixodes ticks), like syphilis may involve almost all ocular and periocular tissues. It has a relatively slow onset and tends to recur following antibiotic therapy. More than 6,000 cases were reported in 1987. The tick vector is widely distributed throughout America, Europe, and Asia, and the spirochete can be found in both mosquitoes and deer flies. *Acanthamoeba* keratitis, caused by several species of free-living amoebae, also is diagnosed more frequently. There has been an increased scientific interest in this area. Risk factors that have been identified with transmission of this disease include corneal surface trauma, use of contact lenses, poor lens hygiene, and contact with contaminated water.

Progress continues in research on onchocerciasis, a major health problem in many parts of Africa and Central and South America. The causative agent is *Onchocerca volvulus,* a filarial worm that lives in the subcutaneous tissues of the body. Approximately 2 million people worldwide are blind from this disease. In heavily infected individuals microfilariae larvae may invade the eye where they can be seen in copious numbers in the aqueous humor. The microfilariae can be

242

killed effectively, but once they are dead, the host mounts a pathologic immune response against the parasite. Without an acceptable animal model of the disease, it is essential to elaborate the immunopathologic mechanisms observed in this infection.

Chlamydia trachomatis causes both acute and chronic conjunctivitis and produces hyperendemic or blinding trachoma. In the United States, active trachoma exists in scattered areas in the Southwest. In developing nations, where good personal hygiene is not always practiced, chronic and recurrent infections lead to scarring of the conjunctiva, lids, and cornea. Since the update, there has been progress in the development of improved methods for diagnosing chlamydia conjunctivitis, and some progress has been made in elucidating the role of the immune system in this disease. Studies using oral immunization against trachoma have focused on a 40-kd major outer membrane protein as the vaccine candidate. Although specific therapy is available to shorten the course of the disease, little progress has been achieved in preventing neonatal chlamydial infections.

Subprogram Objectives

- To characterize the pathogenetic roles of virus and host factors in order to design strategies to prevent or lessen infectious ocular disease.

- To determine the mechanism of herpetic latency in order to prevent recurrent infection.

- To elucidate the effects of the host inflammatory response to microbial pathogens and develop methods to prevent or to control its destructive components.

Current Level of National Eye Institute Support

In FY 1992 the NEI supported 49 research projects in the areas covered in this subprogram at a cost of $7,639,109. Among ongoing studies are those that seek to define the roles of live herpes simplex, herpetic antigen, and antigenically altered corneal cell membranes in disease; isolate genes involved in the pathogenesis of ocular HSV-1 infection; develop and test new treatments in animal models of herpes zoster; establish diagnostic techniques and therapy for amoebic keratitis;

investigate the host immune system response in onchocerciasis; and define immune mechanisms in chlamydial disease.

Recent Accomplishments

The role of specific viral genes in the pathogenicity of ocular HSV infection has been explored by use of recombinant DNA technology. The immediate-early gene alpha 0 codes for the ICP0 protein. Although nonessential for productive HSV-1 infection *in vitro*, ICP0 is important in producing ocular infections and latent infections in mice and rabbits. The importance of the gene product alpha *trans*-inducing factor, a structural component of the virion, in *trans*-activating and promoting the expression of alpha genes has been demonstrated *in vitro*, and its role in acute ocular infections and latency is currently under active investigation. Additional studies with recombinant mutants further identified other regions of the HSV-1 genome that are important in neurovirulence and neuroinvasiveness.

The demonstration that at least one HSV-1 gene, latency-associated transcript (LAT), undergoes extensive transcription during latency has stimulated great interest. LAT was first demonstrated in latently infected trigeminal ganglia in rabbits and in dorsal root ganglia in mice. In three independent autopsy series, LAT was detected in 54 to 67 percent of unselected seropositive individuals. The LAT gene has been mapped and its transcripts characterized, but no LAT gene protein has been found. Animal studies suggest that LAT transcription is important for efficient reactivation from the latent state.

Although the primary site of HSV-1 latency generally is accepted to be sensory neuronal ganglia, the possibility of additional ocular latency sites has been suggested by clinical and experimental studies. However unequivocal proof of such additional latency sites has not yet been obtained.

Immune responses to HSV-1 antigens are thought to protect the corneal epithelium and curtail disease confined to this region. In contrast, the immune system is thought to play a pathogenic role in stromal, endothelial, and anterior chamber involvement during HSV-1 infection. Which immune effectors are responsible for clearance of the virus in epithelial disease versus which effectors participate in the pathogenesis of stromal keratitis and endothelitis is unresolved. Serum antibodies to the HSV-1 glycoprotein D appear to protect against primary infection. Other evidence suggests that polymorphism at the IgH-1 locus in the mouse (which encodes all the heavy chains of immunoglobulins) governs susceptibility to stromal keratitis. Despite evidence that delayed hypersensitivity is an important mechanism for viral clearance, the interplay of antibody and delayed hypersensitivity in protection/pathogenesis still needs to be described.

Immunologic communication between the cornea and anterior chamber has been revealed by experiments in which HSV-1 glycoprotein B was first injected into the anterior chamber. This induced HSV-specific anterior chamber immune deviation is characterized by impaired delayed hypersensitivity and reduced cytotoxic T cells. The experimental animals failed to develop stromal keratitis when their corneas were infected with HSV-1 by means of scarification. This suggests that T-cell-mediated immunity is an important factor in promoting stromal disease. Similarly, corneas with resident Langerhans cells in the central epithelium (induced via cauterization or spontaneously associated with corneal dystrophy) are particularly susceptible to development of stromal keratitis. The keratitis is correlated with early onset of systemic, virus-specific, delayed hypersensitivity.

New, improved animal models have been developed for the study of HSV-1 latency, reactivation, and recurrent ocular disease. The use of immunosuppression alone in rabbits and in combination with ultraviolet light in mice has proven to be effective. Intrastromal inoculation of sterile deionized water also has been shown to reactivate and induce ocular shedding of HSV-1 in rabbits.

An important epidemiologic study documents the incidence (20.7 episodes/100,000 person-years) and prevalence (149 cases/100,000 person-years) of ocular herpes simplex between 1950 and 1982 in Rochester, Minnesota. The efficacy of new immunologic tests for the rapid diagnosis of HSV in a clinical setting has been reviewed, and a multicenter, controlled-clinical trial Herpetic Eye Diseases Study to determine the efficacy of systemic acyclovir in the treatment of herpetic stromal keratitis and herpetic uveitis has been organized and currently is enrolling patients. Clinical interest continues in the development of an effective, attenuated livevirus vaccine or subunit vaccine for the prevention of ocular disease.

Important progress has been made in the understanding and treatment of VZV infections. The molecular characterization of the VZV genome continues, and similarities to and differences from HSV-1 have been reported for different genes. The question of whether VZV latency mimics HSV-1 latency remains unresolved, and the ganglion cell that hosts the latent VZV genome is disputed.

The development of an animal ocular model of VZV infection is ongoing. Acute infection of the cornea and the trigeminal ganglion and latent trigeminal ganglion infection have been achieved. Snout infection

245

of mice produces an ipsilateral disease that resembles herpes zoster infection in certain immunocompetent human beings. A small percentage of animals not only develops zosteriform skin lesions in the ophthalmic distribution of the fifth cranial nerve but also develops mild stromal keratitis and anterior uveitis. These latter manifestations are greatly exaggerated in mice whose corneas contain Langerhans cells at the time of infection. Many of these mice die of encephalitis. The circumstantial evidence implies that T-cell-mediated immunity, promoted by Langerhans cells in the cornea, is responsible for the increased morbidity and mortality. Thus, this particular strain of virus may serve as a model for herpes zoster infections that involve the eye and brain in man. Reactivation of VZV and clinical disease resembling herpes zoster ophthalmicus have not been achieved in any animal model to date.

The early initiation of therapy with acyclovir in patients with acute herpes zoster has had a major impact in reducing the severity of the ocular disease and the long-term ocular complications. However, the sequelae of visual loss from progressive corneal opacification, recurrent iridocyclitis, cataract, and secondary glaucoma have not been eliminated.

The binding of a pathogen to host tissue is requisite for subsequent infectious disease production. The host/pathogen interactions that facilitate this first step are of extreme importance, and this area of investigation has received considerable recent attention. In *P. aeruginosa* infections, cell-surface carbohydrates such as sialic acid have been shown to play a significant role in different *in vivo* disease models. *In vitro* models also have been developed in both the rat and the mouse. In the rat, mannose is involved in bacterial adherence to the trephine-wounded eye, and bacteria adhere to the denuded basal lamina just in front of the leading edge of the wound. This important finding may indicate that cells of the leading edge are synthesizing a product(s) that facilitates bacterial recognition and binding. In the mouse scarified cornea model, the ocular receptor for *P. aeruginosa* has been shown to be lipase sensitive; corneal binding could be blocked by pretreatment with the sialylated glycoprotein fibronectin or by the monosialoganglioside GM1. Transient blockage of the bacterial ligand was shown by its putative receptor gangliotetraosylceramide (asialo-GM1). In addition, tissue culture of rabbit corneal epithelial cells provided the important information that *Pseudomonas* bound to neutral glycosphingolipids but failed to bind to sialylated gangliosides. Bacterial adherence to inert materials, particularly contact lenses, is also an active area of research. Contact lens coatings, especially mucin, facilitate the adherence of *Pseudomonas* to soft contact lenses, and mucin-coated lenses induce pseudomonal corneal ulcers in a higher proportion of animals than do uncoated lenses.

The host response to bacterial pathogens such as *Pseudomonas* is also of prime importance. Host inflammatory processes mediated by the PMN have been implicated in augmenting the rapid and devastating destruction seen in *Pseudomonas* infection. Yet, it has been demonstrated recently that in aged mice, the phagocytic capacity of PMN cells that infiltrate the cornea is markedly impaired and that this impairment also may contribute to subsequent ocular damage.

The role of antibody and complement responses in bacterial disease also continues to be addressed. It is of interest that despite the fact that IgA is the preponderant antibody isotype at the ocular surface, it provides little protection following experimental corneal infection with either *Pseudomonas* or *S. aureus.* In both of these studies, the protective antibody response appears to be of the IgG and IgM isotypes. Moreover, susceptibility and resistance to corneal clouding in response to infection with *Pseudomonas* correlate positively with the rapidity with which serum IgG antibodies develop.

Since the first case was diagnosed in 1973 *Acanthamoeba* keratitis has been identified with increased frequency as clinicians have become aware of the disease's manifestations, and diagnostic procedures have become standardized. In 1986 calcofluor white was introduced as a means of identifying amoebic cysts. This chemofluorescent dye has an affinity for the polysaccharide polymers of the parasite. Concomitant inoculation of corneal tissue on nonnutrient agar overlaid with heat-killed *Escherichia coli* also has become a standard diagnostic technique. Only about 50 percent of cases are diagnosed before performance of penetrating keratoplasty. Treatment for *Acanthamoeba* keratitis also remains disappointing. Antiamoebic agents, usually used in combination, are only moderately effective. Recently several animal models have been developed that may prove useful in examination of disease pathogenesis.

Important accomplishments in onchocerciasis-related research include introduction of the drug ivermectin, which has been shown to be effective and to produce little or no ocular or systemic toxicity. An animal model of sclerosing keratitis has been developed in guinea pigs, as has a promising animal model using cynomolgus monkeys injected with microfilariae. Immunologic events related to mononuclear cell activation may be associated with ocular disease, and a recent study suggests that immunoregulatory events may protect against the development of ocular disease in infected individuals. In the absence of an *in vitro* culture system, the production of defined antigens utilizing a recombinant DNA approach may offer new opportunities for exploring immunologic mechanisms of ocular disease.

Endemic trachoma usually is caused by *C. trachomatis* serotypes A, B, Ba, and C. In the United States, ocular disease usually is caused by serotypes D through K, which also are common causes of genital tract infections. The application of molecular biologic techniques to chlamydia research has provided the basis for significant advances in the identification and characterization of important antigens. The most significant accomplishment has been the molecular characterization of the major outer membrane protein. It binds protective antibodies to *C. trachomatis,* and the sites for antibody binding are sequence variant. These findings have implications for understanding variation in immune protection and for developing new seroepidemiologic and diagnostic assays. Another important finding is that immunopathologic responses can be mimicked by use of antigen fractions and that heat shock proteins may play important roles in the immunopathologic host response. Ocular animal models are under investigation because of the need to develop a trachoma vaccine. The development of a trachoma model that proceeds to conjunctival scarring in nonhuman primates has been useful but is severely limited because of the small number of animals available. Moreover, the primate model differs from human trachoma in that it lacks corneal vascularization or keratitis. The alternative animal model is guinea pig inclusion conjunctivitis. This naturally occurring infection of guinea pig herds, caused by *C. psittaci,* resembles human trachoma. A chlamydia-derived 57-kd antigen can induce delayed hypersensitivity in guinea pigs, and it is hypothesized that such delayed hypersensitivity plays a role in ocular surface disorders.

Rapid diagnostic tests for chlamydia are now available commercially. These tests should make it possible to refine the clinical circumstances under which chlamydial eye disease is diagnosed accurately.

Important Research Questions to Be Addressed

The recent burst of experimental studies on ocular surface infections has resulted in a much more sophisticated set of experimental questions to address during the next 5 years. Studies are needed to identify specific factors responsible for adhesion, penetration, and invasion of ocular surface cells and to understand the molecular basis for these phenomena. Only then will it be possible to design therapeutic strategies in which agents can be targeted to interfere with one or another of these important steps in microbial pathogenesis. The following questions need to be addressed:

What specific host/pathogen interactions occur in ocular infectious disease?

Further studies of host/pathogen interactions are warranted. If the responsible molecules can be characterized, molecular biologic approaches could produce these molecules in sufficient quantities to determine their therapeutic potential. Application of cell and molecular biologic techniques to this research area should lead to development of effective vaccines.

What mediates the host destructive response to infection?

It is important to determine the host immune response to infection, including the role that antibody and cell-mediated immunity play in protection and/or pathologic responses. Questions concerning the roles of MHC and T-cell subsets and issues of local and systemic immune responses are now more amenable for study than in the past because of the development of molecular biologic approaches and the availability of new reagents for immunologic studies. It is possible that the inflammatory response in the eye may be modulated to produce less destruction of ocular tissues yet allow effective elimination of the invading pathogen. It is critical to understand which lymphoid populations affect such responses in the eye and to determine the exact mechanisms involved. The role of cytokines, complement, and other products of the immune system in infectious disease should continue to be investigated.

What is the pathogenesis of Acanthamoeba keratitis?

It is important to determine whether trauma is a prerequisite to the development of *Acanthamoeba* keratitis and to identify factors responsible for corneal epithelial adherence and stromal penetration. More effective chemotherapeutic agents must be developed.

What antigens produce onchocercal sclerosing keratitis?

Antigens produced by a recombinant DNA approach should be used to elucidate the immunologic mechanisms associated with ocular onchocerciasis. Several opportunities now exist for studies that could lead to a successful understanding of the pathogenesis of this disease.

How does the immune system regulate the host response to chlamydial infection?

Over the past few years, a wealth of information has been obtained on *C. trachomatis,* including structural information on the key surface determinants and the genes that code for these molecules. These investigations as well as comparative structural and genetic analysis of the serovars mediating ocular disease should be continued. It should be possible to apply molecular biologic approaches to develop effective vaccine candidates. Determining the precise roles that antibody and cell-mediated immune responses play in the development of protective and/or pathologic responses to infection and whether the ocular mucosal immune system is involved requires further efforts.

Chapter 31

National Eye Institute Report on Retinal Detachment and Vitreous Disorders

Introduction

Separation of the neural retina from the underlying RPE consti-
tutes a retinal detachment. Detachments can be divided into three
basic types: (1) rhegmatogenous retinal detachment (RRD), in which
a tear or hole in the retina allows fluid to enter the subretinal space
from the vitreous cavity; (2) exudative or serous retinal detachment
(SRD), in which there are no retinal tears and subretinal fluid collects as a result of leakage through intact but abnormal RPE or retina;
and (3) traction retinal detachment (TRD), in which the retina is
pulled away from the RPE by contractile tissue in the vitreous body
or on the surface of the retina. Of the three, RRDs constitute the most
common and generally greatest threat to vision. SRDs occur in association with a variety of disease processes and range from small focal detachments that often resolve spontaneously to highly elevated
extensive detachments. Management is directed at the underlying
disease process, but in some instances (e.g., central serous retinopathy),
the pathogenesis is poorly understood and specific treatment is not available. TRDs usually occur in association with proliferative
retinopathies, most commonly proliferative diabetic retinopathy or
proliferative vitreoretinopathy (PVR). These retinopathies are clinically significant when the macula is involved, in this case requiring

Excerpt from NIH Pub. No. 93–3186. *Vision Research: A National Plan*, pp.
65–73.

surgical intervention to relieve the traction and allow the retina to flatten. Some detachments involve more than one of the above mechanisms. Almost all RRDs involve an element of vitreous traction, which is the underlying cause of most retinal tears. In the setting of PVR, severe traction on the retina often causes retinal tears, converting a TRD into a combined traction-rhegmatogenous detachment.

Significant progress has been made in the management of retinal detachments, but they are still a major cause of visual morbidity and a significant drain on our health care resources. This will change only with fundamental advances in our understanding of the cellular and molecular events that lead to and accompany retinal detachment as well as a better grasp of the consequences of surgical interventions.

Subprogram Objectives

- To better understand the molecular basis of vitreous syneresis—the degeneration and collapse of the vitreous body that leads to posterior vitreous detachment, the leading cause of retinal tears and subsequent RRD.

- To better understand the factors responsible for normal and abnormal vitreoretinal adherence.

- To better understand the factors responsible for normal and abnormal retinal-RPE adherence.

- To better understand the factors responsible for fluid transport into and out of the subretinal space.

- To better understand the pathophysiology of PVR.

- To better understand cellular and molecular events associated with visual recovery after retinal detachment and reattachment.

Current Level of National Eye Institute Support

In FY 1992 the NEI supported 16 projects on retinal detachment and vitreous disorders through research grants at a cost of $2,939,630. These grants supported basic and applied research in areas relevant to retinal wound healing and PVR, including pathogenic mechanisms, pharmacologic management and drug delivery, and surgical techniques. Other areas of research supported included work on the interaction between the RPE and retina and the consequences of retinal detachment, as well as the biochemistry of the normal and the diseased vitreous body. A clinical trial investigating the role of silicone oil and long-acting gas bubbles in the management of PVR also was funded.

Recent Accomplishments

Over the past several years significant advances have been made in the surgical management of retinal detachment and the attainment of greater understanding of related cellular and molecular processes.

Surgical Management of Retinal Detachments

Pneumatic retinopexy, the intravitreous injection of a gas bubble combined with retinopexy surrounding all retinal breaks, provides a new management approach to uncomplicated retinal detachments as well as certain advantages. It eliminates the need for conjunctival incision and can be performed in an outpatient setting. As greater experience is gained with the technique, however, the list of potential complications is growing (e.g., new retinal tears, macular holes, and retinal folds through the macula). The gradual manner in which these complications have come to light illustrates our lack of understanding of how surgical interventions alter the physiology and cell biology of the retina and vitreous. At this time there is considerable controversy about when the benefits of pneumatic retinopexy outweigh the risks.

Scleral buckling remains the major primary procedure for the treatment of retinal detachment and has a success rate greater than 90 percent. The major cause of failure is PVR, but major advances have been made in its management. These include recognition of the importance of relieving all peripheral traction and the use of long-acting tamponades. The Silicone Oil Study is a national collaborative study designed to determine whether there are any advantages or disadvantages to the use of a long-acting gas bubble or silicone oil in the management of PVR. Although no results are available at this time, the study has provided some new approaches to standardization in PVR.

Liquid perfluorocarbons are denser than water; therefore, when infused during vitreous surgery, they flatten the posterior retina first and displace subretinal fluid through peripheral retinal breaks. They provide significant benefits in the management of giant retinal tears, and since they can help immobilize the posterior retina, they can be an aid in the dissection of peripheral epiretinal membranes. Because they rapidly undergo emulsification, they must be removed at the end of surgery.

Factors Responsible for Retinal Adhesion

Insight into potential mechanisms involved in retinal adhesion to the RPE has been gained. It is now apparent that interactions between aggregates or assemblies of interphotoreceptor matrix molecules and plasma membrane components of the cell types bordering the subretinal space may provide the molecular basis for retinal adhesion that has long been suspected but poorly defined. Aqueous insoluble domains, rod and cone matrix sheaths, have recently been demonstrated in the interphotoreceptor matrix and may play a critical role in adhesion.

Fluid transport across the RPE has also been implicated in retinal-RPE adhesion. The control of ion and water transport across the RPE is complex, since several transport systems across both the apical and basal surfaces contribute. A bicarbonate and chloride transport system appears to play an important role in controlling fluid transport across the RPE. There may be some relationship between this transport process and the observations that acetazolamide, a carbonic anhydrase inhibitor, increases water movement from retina to choroid across the RPE and increases retinal adhesion. In addition to providing basic information concerning retinal adhesion, this finding has provided an additional benefit in serving as the basis for a clinical trial in which acetazolamide was found to be helpful in the treatment of some types of macular edema. This is a clear example of how research related to retinal detachment has provided clinically useful information relevant to other retinal disorders.

Cellular and Molecular Events That Accompany Retinal Detachment

The cellular events that occur after retinal detachment have been described in several species of animals and include dedifferentiation, migration, and proliferation of all nonneuronal cell types. In addition, degeneration of photoreceptor outer segments and, later, inner segments, synaptic terminals, and cell bodies also occurs. Eventually photoreceptor cells die and are lost from the outer nuclear layer. Recently progress has been made in identifying some of the molecular changes that accompany these morphological changes. Within 3 days of detachment, there is a dramatic rise in the mRNA for glial fibrillary acidic protein (GFAP) in Muller cells followed by an equally dramatic rise in GFAP at a time when the cells undergo hypertrophy and proliferation. Another structural protein, vimentin, undergoes a similar increase in Muller cells after detachment, while the expression of two enzymes and two retinoid-binding proteins is decreased. Elucidation of alterations that occur in the expression of these and other proteins could shed light on functional changes that occur after retinal detachment and reattachment. In photoreceptors, some functions are maintained surprisingly well, whereas others decline rapidly after detachment. Studies in mammals have shown that transport of newly synthesized protein and, apparently, assembly of new opsin-containing disc membranes continue for at least 60 days after detachment even though the outer segments are severely disrupted and only a fraction of their normal length. Recent studies in amphibians, however, suggest that disk shedding in rods may be compromised even by detachment intervals of short duration. The effect of detachment on the many other processes involved in phototransduction has not been determined yet.

Retinal Wound Healing

Retinal wound healing shares important basic features with wound healing elsewhere in the body but also has some important differences due to the presence of the blood-retinal barrier (BRB) and other specialized features of the retina. The BRB is disrupted by a variety of insults to the retina, such as cryopexy or laser photocoagulation. Its rapid reestablishment may be one mechanism by which the retinal wound-healing process is limited, for the extent and duration of breakdown of the BRB correlates with extensiveness of traction retinal detachment in cell-injection models of PVR.

An important conceptual development during the past 5 years is the realization that, in addition to serum, inflammatory cells and cells of the retina may serve as sources of regulators of cellular migration and growth. Macrophages and RPE have been demonstrated to produce a number of biologic response modifiers (i.e., peptides and other substances that modulate the growth and differentiation of cells), including basic FGF, transforming growth factor beta, and platelet-derived growth-factor-like proteins. The exact role of these factors in normal and exaggerated retinal wound healing *in vivo* has not been determined, but studies using cultured RPE and retinal glia suggest that platelet-derived growth-factor-like proteins are the principal, known regulators of chemotaxis, while several growth factors act in synergy to stimulate cell proliferation. In addition to soluble factors, cell-cell and cell-matrix interactions modulate retinal cell growth in culture and may help to regulate growth and differentiation *in vivo*.

Visual Recovery After Retinal Reattachment

We do not understand why some patients rapidly recover visual function after retinal reattachment, whereas others do not. However, progress has been made in identifying some of the factors that play an important role in poor morphological recovery after retinal reattachment in cats and monkeys. In general, the degree of morphological recovery is inversely related to detachment duration and height (i.e., distance of the retina from the RPE). The molecular basis of this is unknown, but it is likely that several factors are operative. The choroid normally supplies oxygen and nutrients to the outer retina, and therefore a chronically detached, highly elevated retina may suffer greater permanent damage from lack of oxygen and nutrients. In addition, chronic detachment promotes Muller cell and RPE proliferation in the subretinal space, adversely affecting morphological recovery by creating a cellular barrier that prevents the photoreceptors from reestablishing their relationship with the apical processes of the RPE. A third possibility is that the detached retina may be deprived of critical trophic factors produced by the RPE and secreted into the interphotoreceptor matrix. This possibility is suggested by the recent demonstration that the interphotoreceptor matrix supports the survival of photoreceptors *in vitro*; this experiment was made possible by the recent development of cell-culture systems for the growth of isolated photoreceptor cells. The proposed trophic factor has been partially purified and is a heparin-binding protein that elutes from size-exclusion columns in two peaks corresponding to molecular weights of 33 and 400 to 450 kd, the latter apparently representing aggregates of the lower molecular weight form. Interestingly, basic FGF, which is also a heparin-binding protein, also supports the growth and maintenance of photoreceptors *in vitro* and is produced by RPE.

Retinoids play an important role in phototransduction and are also modulators of growth and differentiation of several cell types, including the photoreceptors and the RPE. Retinal detachment may prevent normal retinoid shuttling and therefore may result in retinoid depletion in both the photoreceptors and the RPE. The degenerative changes observed in the photoreceptors of vitamin-A-deficient animals are similar to those seen after retinal detachment. Therefore, disturbed retinoid metabolism could play a role in photoreceptor damage after retinal detachment and also could contribute to observed changes in the RPE.

Recent evidence suggests that ischemic damage to retinal cells may involve an initial insult followed by local chemical and cellular changes that may ultimately lead to cell death. Several agents, including dextromethorphan, calcium channel blockers, antioxidants, nerve growth factors, and steroids, have been demonstrated to decrease retinal cell death after ischemia or photocoagulation. This suggests the possibility of maximizing visual recovery after retinal reattachment by pharmacologically limiting photoreceptor cell damage while the retina is detached.

Important Research Questions to Be Addressed

The following important questions need to be addressed:

What is the molecular basis of vitreous syneresis?

As pointed out above, we have made significant progress in treating retinal detachments and understanding their sequelae. However, the ideal approach to limiting the significant expense and visual morbidity associated with retinal detachments would be in developing better preventive measures. It is known that the vast majority of retinal tears and subsequent detachments occur shortly after posterior vitreous detachments, but the major barrier in this area is our almost complete lack of understanding of vitreous syneresis, the degeneration and collapse of the vitreous that leads to posterior vitreous detachment. It will be important to determine the molecular basis of vitreous syneresis and how conditions such as high myopia and aphakia contribute to its occurrence.

Wagner's disease, Stickler's syndrome, and Goldmann-Favre's vitreotapetoretinal degeneration are hereditary conditions with prominent vitreous degeneration and liquefaction. Patients with Stickler's syndrome or Goldmann-Favre's vitreotapetoretinal degeneration are at high risk for retinal detachment, whereas those with

Wagner's disease are not despite vitreous degeneration of a similar appearance. What are the underlying genetic abnormalities in each of these entities that lead to premature vitreous degeneration, and why are the vitreous changes in Wagner's disease less prone to cause retinal detachment? Not only might answers to these questions provide information helpful to patients with one of these three disorders, but they also could provide new insights into the pathogenesis of vitreous syneresis and its relationship to retinal detachment.

What is the molecular basis of vitreoretinal adherence?

Retinal tears occur at sites of abnormal vitreoretinal adherence. A better understanding of the vitreoretinal interface and the factors responsible for normal and abnormal vitreoretinal adherence is needed. This would provide insight into retinal tear formation and how it might be prevented but might also be relevant to the pathogenesis of idiopathic macular holes.

What are the factors that contribute to retinal adherence?

A relatively small proportion of retinal holes and tears lead to retinal detachment, and although some detachments spread rapidly, others remain limited for years. This suggests that retinal adhesion may vary significantly among individuals. A greater understanding of the factors responsible for normal and abnormal retinal adhesion is needed. The structural and functional characteristics of the interphotoreceptor matrix and cone and rod matrix domains should be completely described. An important barrier in retinal adhesion research is the rapid decay in adhesion that occurs post mortem. This provides a formidable technical challenge to the design of experiments but also may provide an important research question whose answer may greatly advance our knowledge of the forces responsible for retinal adhesion.

What are the mechanisms by which fluid is transported into and out of the subretinal space?

Further elucidation of how the various RPE pumps contribute to fluid transport across the RPE and the mechanisms by which they are modulated should increase our understanding of retinal adhesion and might also provide critical information concerning macular edema and serous retinal detachments.

What are the pathogenic mechanisms involved in the formation of serous retinal detachments?

Management of nonrhegmatogenous detachments is hampered by a lack of understanding of the critical conditions that cause subretinal fluid to accumulate or be absorbed under pathologic conditions. The development of an animal model of serous retinal detachment would be a significant benefit for *in vivo* studies aimed at investigating the pathogenesis of these disorders and the clinical usefulness of pharmacologically modulating RPE pump function. If transport modifiers can be found, are there ways to deliver active agents to the retina and the RPE without systemic effects? Conversely, RPE transport is known to be modulated by certain systemic factors including adrenergic stimulation; therefore, it is possible that selected systemic therapies could play a role in the management of serous detachments.

How can we improve our surgical management of retinal detachment?

Several questions related to our current surgical management of retinal detachments need to be addressed. What is the appropriate role for pneumatic retinopexy, what is the basis for its complications, and how might they be prevented? One of the major barriers to advances in our knowledge about the best management of complicated retinal detachments is that assessment of any treatment modality must somehow account for variability from case to case in both critical prognostic features of the disease process (e.g., the amount of traction on the anterior retina and ciliary body or the amount of retinal foreshortening) and the ability of individual surgeons to deal with them. The Silicone Oil Study is attempting to control for this inherent variability and thereby determine whether there is a particular advantage to silicone oil or long-acting gas tamponade in the treatment of PVR. The results of this study should help to define the feasibility of future clinical studies in other important areas, such as the efficacy of adjuvant drug therapy or the role of liquid per fluorocarbons. Further work also is needed in animals to establish clearly the toxicity of long-acting tamponades such as silicone oil. The development of tamponading agents that are denser than water and can be left in the vitreous cavity for a prolonged period of time without significant toxic effects or emulsification would simplify the management of particularly difficult cases.

A new area of investigation that may be important in the future is diagnostic and therapeutic surgical manipulation of the retina and subretinal space. This includes chorioretinal biopsies, removal of blood and scar tissue from the subretinal space, and delivery of biologic response modifiers to the subretinal space.

What is the pathogenesis of PVR?

Research to optimize our management of PVR is important, but it should be noted that the success rate for reattaching the retina in eyes with PVR is already quite good (i.e., 80 to 85 percent). The vast majority of successfully treated eyes suffer from poor vision, however, and the cost of treatment is high, since multiple procedures are frequently needed and the convalescent period is usually several months, resulting in a patient's prolonged absence from work. Therefore, prophylaxis should be the major priority with respect to PVR. This can only be achieved through a better understanding of the pathogenesis of PVR.

Perhaps the greatest barrier to a greater understanding of the pathophysiology of PVR is the lack of an appropriate animal model. The animal models thus far developed have relied on the injection of cells or growth factors and do not provide a means of directly studying many of the early critical events involved. A physiologically relevant model would allow the retina of the experimental animal to be somehow stimulated to produce the regulators of scarring *in situ.* Such a model would allow investigators to ask realistic questions concerning the nature of these important macromolecules and the regulation of their production, and it would provide a means of evaluating new medical therapies for PVR.

Another barrier to understanding the pathophysiology of PVR is the lack of adequate analytic techniques for the study of proliferation *in vivo.* Examples of such techniques are nonradioactive methods for the study of gene expression by *in situ* hybridization and better means of detecting and purifying new gene products from small amounts of tissue.

There are several specific questions in the area of PVR and retinal wound healing that need to be addressed. What factors cause migration, proliferation, and phenotypic alteration of retinal cells? What is the role of macrophages and other blood-borne cells in PVR? Although it is now known that inflammatory cells may be present at various stages of PVR and that these cells are capable of influencing cellular proliferation, the role of macrophages in PVR has not been determined. What is the role of the BRB in PVR, and how can it be modulated? A better understanding of the BRB and how it is modulated might provide a substantial opportunity for medical intervention in PVR and several other disease processes.

How do RPE and Muller cells modulate their own growth and differentiation as well as that of other cells?

There is compelling evidence that the RPE is one of the principal cellular sources of regulatory factors that direct the overall course of PVR. Although some limited knowledge of the specific growth factors secreted by these cells exists, additional avenues of research should be pursued. First, it is important to determine which growth factors RPE and Muller cells are capable of producing and how the expression of these proteins is modulated. Second, it will be necessary to examine which of the factors expressed by RPE and Muller cells *in vitro* is actually expressed in these same cells *in vivo* and whether their production is under the same control mechanisms. Third, it will be important to determine the best mode of delivery of drugs and biologic response modifiers to the retina.

What are the factors responsible for return of visual function after retinal reattachment?

Gaining greater insight into the factors responsible for return of visual function after retinal reattachment should be emphasized over the next several years. As noted above, we have made substantial progress in determining the morphologic changes accompanying retinal detachment and reattachment, but our understanding of why they occur is incomplete. The exact role of the various contributing factors should be determined, and attempts should be made to modulate their effects. As noted above, it has been demonstrated that pharmacologic agents can decrease the degree of cell death after ischemic insult to retinal tissue. It will be important to determine whether these agents can lessen photoreceptor and RPE deterioration after retinal detachment. We are in the early stages of understanding how retinal detachment affects the expression of specific proteins. This line of investigation could provide the keys to understanding functional as well as morphological changes.

The process of photoreceptor outer segment regeneration should be studied in detail. Further characterization of agents responsible for photoreceptor maintenance and differentiation *in vivo* and *in vitro* is needed. Molecules such as the partially purified trophic factor in interphotoreceptor matrix can be isolated, and further, its corresponding gene can be identified and cloned. Once this is done, the factors that control the expression of this trophic agent can be determined. The effect on photoreceptors of other growth factors produced by the RPE also should be determined. These investigations are relevant to retinal degenerations as well as photoreceptor regeneration after retinal reattachment and could greatly enhance our understanding of the interdependence of photoreceptors and RPE.

Chapter 32

Floaters and Flashes

What are floaters?

You may sometimes see small specks or clouds moving in your field of vision. They are called floaters. You can often see them when looking at a plain background, like a blank wall or blue sky.

Floaters are actually tiny clumps of gel or cells inside the vitreous, the clear jelly-like fluid that fills the inside of your eye.

Anatomy of the eye

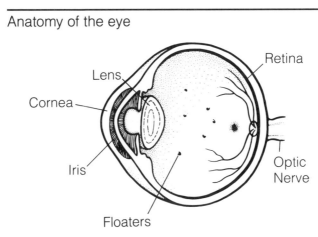

Figure 32.1. Although the floaters appear to be in front of the eye, they are actually floating in the vitreous fluid inside the eye.

American Academy of Ophthalmology, ©1985. Revised 1993. Used by permission.

While these objects look like they are in front of your eye, they are actually floating inside. What you see are the shadows they cast on the retina, the nerve layer at the back of the eye that senses light and allows you to see.

Floaters can have different shapes: little dots, circles, lines, clouds or cobwebs.

What causes floaters?

When people reach middle age, the vitreous gel may start to thicken or shrink, forming clumps or strands inside the eye. The vitreous gel pulls away from the back wall of the eye, causing a posterior vitreous detachment. It is a common cause of floaters.

Posterior vitreous detachment is more common for people who:

- Are nearsighted;
- Have undergone cataract operations;
- Have had YAG laser surgery of the eye;
- Have had inflammation inside the eye.

The appearance of floaters may be alarming, especially if they develop suddenly. You should see an ophthalmologist (a medical eye physician) right away if you suddenly develop new floaters, especially if you are over 45 years of age.

Are floaters ever serious?

The retina can tear if the shrinking vitreous gel pulls away from the wall of the eye. This sometimes causes a small amount of bleeding in the eye that may appear as new floaters. A torn retina is always a serious problem, since it can lead to a retinal detachment. You should see your ophthalmologist as soon as possible if:

- Even one new floater appears suddenly;
- You see sudden flashes of light.

If you notice other symptoms, like the loss of side vision, you should return to your ophthalmologist.

What can be done about floaters?

Because you need to know if your retina is torn, call your ophthalmologist if a new floater appears suddenly.

Floaters can get in the way of clear vision, which may be quite annoying, especially if you are trying to read. You can try moving your eyes, looking up and then down to move the floaters out of the way.

While some floaters may remain in your vision, many of them will fade over time and become less bothersome. Even if you have had some floaters for years, you should have an eye examination immediately if you notice new ones.

What causes flashing lights?

When the vitreous gel rubs or pulls on the retina, you may see what look like flashing lights or lightning streaks. You may have experienced this same sensation if you have ever been hit in the eye and seen "stars." [See Figure 32.2 on page 266.]

The flashes of light can appear off and on for several weeks or months. As we grow older, it is more common to experience flashes. If you notice the sudden appearance of light flashes, you should visit your ophthalmologist immediately to see if the retina has been torn.

Migraine

Some people experience flashes of light that appear as jagged lines or "heat waves" in both eyes, often lasting 10-20 minutes. These types of flashes are usually caused by a spasm of blood vessels in the brain, which is called migraine.

If a headache follows the flashes, it is called a migraine headache. However, jagged lines or "heat waves" can occur without a headache. In this case, the light flashes are called ophthalmic migraine, or migraine without headache.

How are your eyes examined?

When an ophthalmologist examines your eyes, your pupils will be dilated with eye drops. During this painless examination, your ophthalmologist will carefully observe your retina and vitreous. Because your eyes have been dilated, you may need to make arrangements for someone to drive you home afterwards.

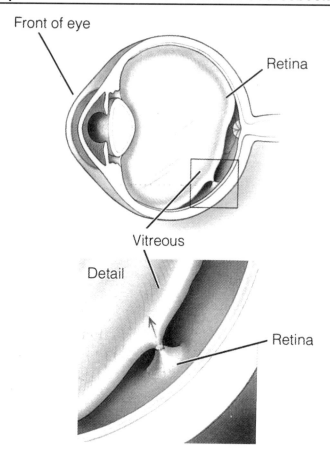

Figure 32.2. *When the vitreous rubs or pulls on the retina, it creates a sensation of flashing lights.*

Floaters and flashes of light become more common as we grow older. While not all floaters and flashes are serious, you should always have a medical eye examination by an ophthalmologist to make sure there has been no damage to your retina.

Chapter 33

DHHS Statement on Retinitis Pigmintosa

Most adults with blinding retinitis pigmentosa (RP) should take a daily, 15,000 IU vitamin A supplement, based on results from a large, randomized clinical trial published today in the Archives of Ophthalmology.

This recommendation is the first from a well-designed clinical trial indicating that people can be treated for this retinal disease. "This is exciting news," said Carl Kupfer, M.D., director of the National Eye Institute, which supported the six-year study. "While vitamin A supplementation certainly does not represent a cure, it does signify a first step in managing these diseases."

Eliot L. Berson, M.D., the study's principal investigator and Professor of Ophthalmology at Harvard Medical School, said that adults who supplemented their diets with 15,000 IU of vitamin A daily had on average about a 20 percent slower annual decline of remaining retinal function than those not taking this dose.

Based on this finding, Dr. Berson and his colleagues estimated that an average patient in the study who started taking a 15,000 IU vitamin A capsule at age 32 would retain some useful vision until age 70, whereas a patient not on this dose would lose useful vision at age 63.

The investigators also recommended that adults with RP should avoid taking high-dose vitamin E supplements. In the study, the disease appeared to progress faster on average in patients on a daily, 400 IU vitamin E supplement than in those taking a trace amount of the

---

DHHS unnumbered document.

vitamin. Dr. Berson said that the study showed no evidence that normal dietary or small supplemental amounts of vitamin E have an adverse effect on the disease.

Retinitis pigmentosa is a group of inherited retinal diseases that affects about 100,000 Americans and 1.5 million people worldwide. It causes the progressive deterioration of specialized, light-absorbing cells in the retina, the paper-thin tissue that lines the back of the eye like film in a camera.

As these cells slowly degenerate, people with RP develop night blindness and a gradual loss of peripheral vision. By about age 40, most have tunnel vision, although many may retain good central vision. Between the ages of 50 and 80, however, they typically lose their remaining sight. The extent of vision loss in people of the same age with RP may be different.

Dr. Berson stressed that adults considering vitamin A supplementation should first:

• Consult with their eye care professional about vitamin A supplementation.

• Have their blood level of vitamin A measured before starting treatment. If people have preexisting liver disease or abnormally high blood levels of vitamin A, they will need to adjust their vitamin A intake.

• Take vitamin A palmitate, as this was the form of the vitamin studied. Supplements of betacarotene, a natural precursor of vitamin A, are not a predictable source of the vitamin since each person breaks down beta-carotene differently.

• Make a point of eating a balanced diet, without selecting foods that are especially high in vitamin A.

• Avoid taking high-dose vitamin E supplements.

"One of my biggest concerns is that people will make the mistake of thinking that vitamin A supplementation in excess of the 15,000 IU recommended will provide even greater benefit," said Dr. Berson. "We have evidence in fact that supplementation of a regular diet with greater than 15,000 IU of vitamin A does not provide greater benefit. Moreover, a daily vitamin A intake exceeding 25,000 IU over the long term can be toxic in adults and may cause side effects such as liver disease.

"Our interpretation of the study results is that the course of the common forms of retinitis pigmentosa is slower on average among adult patients on a regular diet who take a daily, 15,000 IU vitamin A supplement in the palmitate form compared with the course of those patients not on this supplement," he said.

Because the study involved adults between the ages of 18 and 49, no formal recommendations can be made for patients under the age of 18.

Dr. Berson warned that women with RP should not take 15,000 IU vitamin A supplements during pregnancy because high doses of vitamin A have been linked to birth defects.

A single capsule containing 15,000 IU of vitamin A in the palmitate form will soon be available commercially. For further information on its availability, contact the RP Foundation Fighting Blindness toll-free at 1-800-683-5555.

Background Information on the Study

This study was a prospective, double-masked clinical trial (neither the patient nor the clinician knew to which treatment group the patient had been assigned). It was designed to assess the effectiveness of vitamin A and/or E supplements in halting or slowing the progression of RP. An independent Data Safety and Monitoring Committee provided advice to the investigators and monitored the accumulating data on a regular basis for evidence of harm or benefit to study participants.

A total of 601 RP patients from across the United States and Canada were enrolled in the study. All were in good general health, between the ages of 18 and 49, and entered the study with different initial levels of retinal function. Following an examination, participants were assigned randomly to one of four treatment groups:

- 15,000 IU vitamin A + 3 IU vitamin E
- 75 IU vitamin A + 3 IU vitamin E
- 15,000 IU vitamin A + 400 IU vitamin E
- 75 IU vitamin A + 400 IU vitamin E

Thereafter, the researchers examined each patient annually, with a mean follow-up time of 5.2 years. The electroretinogram (ERG) was used as the study's primary outcome measure. The ERG is a light-evoked electrical response from the retina that can be accurately measured using a special contact lens, much like an electrocardiogram measures coronary function. An ERG provides an objective measure of a person's retinal function. The scientists also used visual fields and visual acuity as additional measures of visual function.

This clinical trial was conducted at the Berman-Gund Laboratory for the Study of Retinal Degenerations at the Massachusetts Eye and Ear Infirmary in Boston, Massachusetts. It was supported by the National Eye Institute and, in part, by the RP Foundation Fighting Blindness in Baltimore, Maryland. The National Eye Institute, a part of the National Institutes of Health, is the Federal government's lead agency for the conduct and support of research on the human visual system in health and disease.

Chapter 34

National Eye Institute Report on Retinitis Pigmentosa and Other Inherited Disorders

Introduction

RP is the most common cause of inherited blindness. RP and other inherited disorders of the retina result in the degeneration of retinal photoreceptors, the RPE, or the choroid, which nourishes the retina. These debilitating and blinding disorders affect approximately 100,000 people in the United States and countless others around the world. The incidence has been estimated to be approximately 1 in 3,500 births, and all social, ethnic, and racial groups are affected. Approximately one-half of the patients with these conditions are born to parents with normal vision who nevertheless carry an abnormal gene for these disorders. The frequency with which an abnormal RP gene is carried in the general population is estimated to be approximately 1 in 80. The emotional and economic costs of these diseases to our society are enormous, particularly in view of the fact that no effective treatments are known for practically all types and that many patients become legally blind by the age of 40 or earlier.

In the recent past, dramatic progress has been made in understanding many aspects of RP and other inherited retinal disorders. Knowledge gained from studies of the structure, function, and metabolism of the normal retina and adjacent RPE has been applied to the understanding of these disease processes. Indeed, much of the progress in dealing with this important clinical problem has been

NIH Pub. No. 93–3186. Excerpt from *Vision Research: A National Plan*, pp. 41–55.

dependent upon advances made in research included in the Photore-ceptors and Pigment Epithelium Program. Use of noninvasive mea-sures of retinal function has provided insight into the early stages of these conditions and how they change year to year. The advances in our understanding of the human genome and our capacity to analyze the DNA from peripheral white blood cells by molecular biologic tech-niques have opened a new dimension in our ability to determine the precise gene defects responsible for these conditions and from that information to infer the mechanisms involved that lead to blindness. Analyses of the peripheral blood samples also have revealed biochemi-cal changes that in some cases may ultimately provide the basis for rational treatment strategies. Autopsy eyes with hereditary disease have been donated for research with increasing frequency, and these tissues have provided an opportunity for elucidating the various con-ditions at the cellular level by means of biochemical, immunocyto-chemical, and tissue culture techniques. Studies of animal models of hereditary retinal disease also have been important in determining specific genetic and biochemical defects that are being used as a ba-sis for seeking similar abnormalities in human retinal diseases. Ani-mal models, which now include transgenic mice, may provide a framework for considering tissue transplantation as a possible thera-peutic alternative for some of these diseases.

Subprogram Objectives

- To establish the degree and basis of genetic and clinical hetero-geneity found in RP and related disorders.

- To ascertain the specific cell(s) in which the various mutant genes are expressed in the different forms of RP and related disorders.

- To define the chromosomal location and characterize at the mo-lecular level the genes responsible for RP and related disorders.

- To determine the cellular processes that result from mutant gene expression and that lead to photoreceptor degeneration.

- To clarify the role of trophic, growth, nutritional, toxic, and en-vironmental factors in the degenerative processes of RP and re-lated diseases.

- To explore new research strategies for determining the causes, treatment, and prevention of RP and other inherited retinal degenerations.

- To explore potential therapeutic measures for RP and related disorders, such as gene transfer, tissue or cell transplantation, and pharmacologic intervention.

- To use the diagnostic, genetic, cellular, and molecular research findings ultimately to prevent photoreceptor degeneration in the many forms of RP and other inherited retinal degenerations.

Current Level of National Eye Institute Support

During FY 1992 the NEI funded 70 research grants in this subprogram at a total cost of $11,571,880. These included studies in RP and related disorders, as well as in normal retinal function. Also included were a clinical trial for dietary modification of RP and four cooperative agreements to produce animal models of inherited retinal degenerations.

Recent Accomplishments

Mapping, Cloning, and Molecular Characterization of Retinal Degeneration Genes

The keys to treating as yet incurable diseases are (1) accurate diagnosis and (2) determination of the pathophysiology of the disorders so that rational therapeutic measures can be developed. Inherited diseases have the complication of genetic mechanisms that lead to physiologic disorders and specific cell death. In the past 5 to 8 years, however, the powerful new tools of molecular genetics have revolutionized the field of inherited diseases. Through rapid advances in DNA technology, it has been possible to use readily available peripheral white blood cells to map many disease loci to specific chromosomes, thereby immediately offering in many cases early diagnostic and genetic counseling opportunities that previously did not exist. The linkage data can also be used with further DNA technology to clone mutated and normal genes and to characterize the genetic defects in molecular terms. This information ultimately can be used to define specific phenotypes that result from the genetic alterations and to devise means of treating the inherited diseases.

Researchers studying inherited retinal degenerations have participated in a major way in the recent explosion of molecular genetics advances in medicine. One form of X-linked RP was among the first of several genes to be mapped to the X chromosome by molecular methods. It is now known that at least two genetic loci for X-linked RP are found on the short arm of the X chromosome and that separate loci are present on the long arm for choroideremia and color blindness. One type of autosomal dominant RP has been found to map to the long arm of chromosome 3, but another type of autosomal dominant RP does not. Similarly, Usher syndrome type II recently has been mapped to the long arm of chromosome 1, whereas Usher syndrome type I has been excluded from this region. Other remarkable examples include the recent mapping of choroideremia, Norrie's disease, and retinoschisis as well as the elucidation of at least 25-point mutations of the ornithine aminotransferase gene responsible for gyrate atrophy (GA) of the choroid and retina.

A number of RP-related genes have been cloned, most notably the *rd* and *rds* genes in the mouse. In addition, many of the genes that cause retinal degenerations in the fruit fly, Drosophila melanogaster, also have been cloned. Once genes have been cloned or localized with molecular methods, DNA technology has allowed rapid characterization of exact nucleotide (and therefore protein) changes. For example, the finding that the gene for autosomal dominant RP was localized to human chromosome 3, and a previous finding that visual pigment rhodopsin was localized to this same region prompted scientists to ask whether the rhodopsin gene was defective. Very quickly, through the use of the powerful technology of polymerase chain reaction (PCR), they discovered a specific mutation in the rhodopsin gene that correlated with the disease. These researchers and others subsequently found numerous additional mutations in the human rhodopsin gene. Similarly, soon after the *rd* and *rds* genes in mice were cloned, scientists were able to determine that the specific gene product of the *rd* gene is the beta subunit of the rod specific transduction enzyme cGMP-phosphodiesterase and that of the *rds* gene is the photoreceptor outer segment disc protein *rds*-peripherin. Most recently mutations of the human homologue of the *rds* gene have been identified that cosegregate with autosomal dominant RP in separate family studies. Other important genes and their gene products have been characterized molecularly, including the cone visual pigment defects that lead to color blindness, different genetic mutations responsible for the ornithine aminotransferase deficiency in GA, and mitochondrial DNA abnormalities that lead to Leber's optic atrophy and the Kearns-Sayre syndrome. Overall, these achievements in the molecular biology of retinal degenerations have been among the most exciting and important in the field of medical genetics in the past few years, and they portend major advances in the coming years.

Initial Success with Gene Therapy

The powerful tools of molecular biology offer the hope of gene therapy as a cure for inherited diseases. One of the first examples of molecular genetic therapy was to cure a visual defect in Drosophila. Scientists were able to insert normal, wild-type rhodopsin genes into the eggs of flies that had defects in their own rhodopsin genes. The transfected genes corrected the defect. Some more recent experiments have been very promising. In the production of transgenic mice, scientists have been able to insert a normal, wild-type gene of the *rds*-peripherin locus into the eggs of *rds* mice, and the wild-type gene of ß-subunit of phosphodiesterase into the eggs of *rd* mice. In both cases the resulting transgenic mice showed a full or partial rescue of the inherited retinal degenerations. These mice studies represent the first *in vivo* genetic corrections of inherited retinal degenerations in vertebrates.

The family of lysosomal storage diseases known as the mucopolysaccharidoses often have retinal degeneration as a component of the syndrome. Researchers have recently been successful in using retroviral vector-mediated gene transfer to restore the enzymatic deficiency and to correct the metabolic defect associated with RPE and other cells in mucopolysaccharidosis VII. By transferring a rat cDNA of the lysosomal enzyme beta-glucuronidase into deficient canine RPE cells in primary cultures, the vector correction restored normal processing of specific glycosaminoglycans in the lysosomal compartment of the cells.

Advances in Noninvasive Diagnostic Methods and Sub-classification

There is general agreement that RP and allied blinding disorders can be detected in early life, often years before patients develop symptoms or before changes are clearly visible on ophthalmoscopic examination. Affected patients show reductions in amplitudes and delays in the temporal aspects of their light-evoked electrical responses from the retina (i.e., electroretinograms). Two rare forms of RP that are associated with the Bassen-Kornzweig syndrome and Refsum's disease, respectively, have yielded to dietary treatment when the disorders have been detected in early stages. GA patients can have the severity of their disease ameliorated by putting them on a low arginine diet. These experiences point out the importance of careful clinical classification of retinal degenerations and determination of the biochemical abnormalities that, in turn, can lead to rational treatment.

A major advance in the field of noninvasive measurements of retinal function occurred with the recent publication of recommended standards and protocols in clinical electroretinography. Potential problems with reproducibility in clinical electroretinography were highlighted in studies that quantified the effect of light adaptation on the electroretinogram. Psychophysical methods to assess rodand cone-mediated function in a clinical setting and techniques for making noninvasive measurements of visual pigments (i.e., fundus reflectometry and retinal densitometry with a confocal scanning laser ophthalmoscope) have been refined.

Progress in the understanding of the abnormal retinal mechanisms in the hereditary retinopathies achieved by use of noninvasive tests of visual function has led to the realization that there are different functional phenotypes within the genetic types. In autosomal dominant RP, studies using dark-adapted perimetry, adaptometry, and fundus reflectometry have demonstrated at least three types of rod photoreceptor-mediated dysfunction. These techniques have been used to define the exact functional abnormalities in autosomal dominant cone dystrophy, and three different patterns of dysfunction have been found in autosomal recessive cone-rod dystrophy. The exact dysfunctional mechanisms in the stationary night-blinding disorders are also being clarified, and two retinopathies with unusual types of shortwavelength-sensitive cone system involvement have recently been identified.

Knowledge of the natural history of these conditions has provided a framework for considering factors that may modify the cause of degeneration in well-defined subsets of patients. Moreover, advancements in subclassification provide a more accurate means for counseling patients on their visual prognoses and providing homogeneous patient populations for biochemical and molecular genetics studies.

Treatment of Cystoid Macular Edema in Patients with Retinitis Pigmentosa

Although central vision is traditionally said to be maintained until advanced stages, a significant percentage of RP patients will manifest degenerative changes within the macula consisting of a lesion of either atrophic or cystic appearance. These changes often are associated with a notable decrease in central vision. Clinical scientists have recently demonstrated the efficacy of acetazolamide (Diamex), a carbonic anhydrase inhibitor, in the treatment of cystoid macula edema in some RP patients. An improvement in central visual acuity was noted in a significant proportion of such patients, and angiographic improvement was seen in the cystoid macular edema of many of them. Improvement was noted even when edema had been present for more than a decade. This finding is new and remains to be fully evaluated. Nevertheless, this important observation may offer the opportunity for improvement in central acuity in some patients with RP; therefore, it will be necessary to determine the mechanism by which this drug acts so that other drugs with fewer side effects may be developed.

Detection of Systemic Manifestations of Retinitis Pigmentosa

Scientists have long sought evidence of systemic manifestations of RP and related disorders since such effects might offer clues to defective metabolic processes and possibilities for drug or dietary therapy. For example, thin hair and partial alopecia occur in GA and may be related to abnormal amino acid metabolism. Recently there have been a number of research findings of blood lipid abnormalities in patients with RP. Hyperlipidemia and an increase in serum cholesterol have been reported in some RP patients as compared with controls; reduced levels of docosahexaenoic acid (a major fatty acid of photoreceptor lipids) has been observed in the plasma of many families with X-linked and autosomal dominant RP as well as Usher syndrome; and a high incidence of relatively rare apolipoprotein phenotypes also has been observed in some families. Moreover, recent studies have demonstrated similar deficiencies in blood lipids in the miniature poodle with a progressive rod-cone degeneration. Taken together, while not conclusive, these findings raise the possibility of abnormalities in lipid metabolism in some forms of RP, an important area that needs further clarification.

Another systemic manifestation of RP is related to possible common developmental progenitors of photoreceptors and other cells. Photoreceptors, auditory hair cells, vestibular hair cells, and nasal olfactory epithelial cells develop from ciliated progenitors, and axonemes are present in mature photoreceptors and vestibular hair cells. Axonemes are ciliary organelles composed of nine interconnected peripheral doublet microtubules with a complex assembly of associated proteins. Sperm cell tails also contain axonemes. Scientists examined the structure and function of sperm cells in male patients with Usher syndrome, a recessive form of RP combined with a congenital hearing impairment and a vestibular system defect. A significant decrease in sperm motility and velocity was found in those patients, as were increases in the incidence of abnormal sperm tail axonemes seen by light and electron microscopy. Abnormal axonemes also were found in remnant photoreceptors of a donor eye from a patient with Usher syndrome. Furthermore, similar abnormalities in sperm tail axonemes have recently been found in patients with X-linked RP. Thus, if the axoneme abnormalities in cells with similar progenitors are found to be common among several or all RP subtypes, then the sperm tail abnormalities may offer another approach to studying the pathogenesis of RP at various times in the life of male patients. The significance of sperm tail abnormalities in RP should be determined in further research studies.

Photoreceptor Rescue by Retinal Pigment Epithelium Cell Transplantation

A significant achievement in retinal degeneration research has been the rescue of photoreceptor cells in the rat of the Royal College of Surgeons (RCS) by transplanting normal RPE cells. In the RCS rat the mutant *rdy* gene is expressed in the RPE cells, and this secondarily leads to photoreceptor cell death. When vision scientists transplanted normal RPE cells into the subretinal space, the transplanted cells established proper relationships with the rods and cones. Those photoreceptors adjacent to the transplanted RPE cells survived, whereas those located far away degenerated and were lost. Although many questions remain, the successful rescue of photoreceptors by RPE cell transplantation represents the first time that any inherited or degenerative disorder has been arrested in the central nervous system of man or animal. Further research offers the possible application of this procedure to those forms of retinal degeneration that have a primary RPE cell defect. This underscores the need for defining the cellular site of mutant gene expression in all forms of RP and allied retinal disorders to determine those diseases that are candidates for such a procedure.

Transplantation of Neural Retina and Photoreceptor Cells

As an alternative to the transplantation of RPE cells, scientists have successfully transplanted portions of normal retina or isolated photoreceptors into the retinas of experimental animals that had lost their photoreceptors as a result of genetic mutations or light damage. The transplanted cells expressed photoreceptor-specific proteins and survived for several months. Many significant questions remain about the functional capacity of the transplanted cells and their integration into the neuronal circuitry of the retina. Nevertheless, these initial findings offer hope for a therapeutic approach to diseases in which the mutant genes are expressed in photoreceptor cells.

Delay of Retinal Degeneration by Growth Factors

Scientists have recently found that a photoreceptor survival-promoting factor is present in the interphotoreceptor matrix. In addition, it has been demonstrated that one of the almost ubiquitous growth factors, basic FGF also is present in the interphotoreceptor matrix and can dramatically delay the rate of photoreceptor degeneration in the retinas of RCS rats with inherited retinal dystrophy as well as in the retinas of light-damaged animals. These findings not only raise important questions about the role of growth factors in normal photoreceptor-RPE cell interactions but also suggest the possibility of the development of a therapeutic approach that uses a survival-promoting growth factor.

Cytopathologic Advances in Mechanisms of Retinal Degeneration

The analysis of retinas from various animal models and human donor eye tissues using structural, biochemical, and cell biologic methods has provided a much better understanding of the various forms of inherited retinal degeneration. Some of the areas that have been developed in the past 5 years in retinal degenerate tissues are the better characterization of retinal proteins, the finding of elevated or absent levels of cGMP correlating with the stage of photoreceptor degeneration, the localization of retinal- and photoreceptor-specific molecules intercellularly and extracellularly, the role in retinal degenerations of the interphotoreceptor matrix with its specialized cone- and rod-specific domains, the disturbance in opsin localization in the surface membrane of photoreceptors, and the localization and role of actin in the connecting cilium in abnormal outer segment disc morphogenesis.

Discovery and Production of Animal Models for Research in Retinitis Pigmentosa

The field of RP research is fortunate in having numerous forms of inherited retinal degenerations in mice, rats, dogs, cats, chicks, and other species with which to work. Approximately 5 years ago the NEI seized the opportunity afforded by these mutants and made eye tissues available to all qualified researchers through support of several colonies of mice, rats, and dogs, as noted above. Through the use of these animal models, accomplishments, including the cloning and molecular characterization of the *rd* and *rds* mutant genes, initial success in gene therapy, rescue of photoreceptors by RPE transplantation, use of retinal transplantation and growth factors, and discovery of the possible abnormalities of lipid metabolism in RP and related disorders have been achieved. Most recently the generation of a transgenic mouse model of autosomal dominant RP using the human mutant rhodopsin gene offers much promise. With these discoveries in hand, the immediate challenge for vision researchers is the application of this information to human-inherited retinal diseases.

Important Research Questions to Be Addressed

The field of RP and allied hereditary retinal degenerations is in a position dramatically different from that of 5 years ago. At that time relatively little was known about the molecular and cellular defects that lead to most of these diseases, and there were few clues about possible therapeutic or preventive measures. As described above, in the past 5 years there has been an explosion of new experimental approaches, improved diagnostic methods, new animal models, hints of systemic effects related to RP, and determination of mutant gene products for several of the disorders as well as some degree of success in therapeutic measures in experimental models of RP. Thus, the field of RP research is now at a point where many critical questions can be answered. Some of the key questions and the research opportunities for 1994-1998 are listed below:

What are the general approaches for molecular genetics research on RP?

The remarkable advances outlined above using molecular DNA technology call, quite simply, for the localization, cloning, and molecular characterization of all genes that cause RP and related disorders in human and animal retinas. Only when these data are available will the full range of retinal degeneration genetic mechanisms and possible avenues for therapy be understood. Particular emphasis should be placed on recessive diseases, which are intrinsically more difficult to resolve. Taking advantage of recent technological advances to develop new research strategies should be incorporated in all molecular and cellular approaches where applicable. The use of transgenic mice technology is strongly encouraged, as described below.

How do specific gene defects result in cytopathologic changes and death of photoreceptor cells?

Given the rapid pace of molecular biologic research, it is possible that a lack of knowledge of the biochemical defects, cell biology, and pathophysiology of inherited retinal degenerations may impede the application of findings of molecular biology to the problems of inherited retinal degenerations. This concern is illustrated by the first gene defect discovered for any form of RP. In a subset of autosomal dominant RP patients a point mutation in codon 23 of the rhodopsin gene located on the long arm of chromosome 3 results in a base transversion of C to A, causing the substitution of one amino acid for another: proline to histidine. The remarkable precision of this knowledge contrasts sharply with the equally remarkable lack of information on the role this or any change in opsin plays in photoreceptor degeneration. Little or nothing is known about how such a change affects opsin structure, activation capability, biosynthesis, or degradation. The questions to be answered are straightforward. How does the amino acid transversion in rhodopsin explain the discrepancy of a degenerative process that takes years to evolve despite the fact that the rhodopsin molecule has a total lifetime of only 10 days in mammalian photoreceptors? How does it explain the regional differences in rate of degeneration in rod photoreceptors within an affected eye? How does the genetic defect in rhodopsin, the visual pigment of rods, cause the death of cone photoreceptors and, for that matter, of rod photoreceptors? How does the genetic defect explain the clinical heterogeneity in visual function observed among some individuals with the same mutation?

Another important example is the *rd* mouse. The abnormality in the cyclic nucleotide cascade in this mutant is the most widely studied potential biochemical mechanism of cell death; yet the mechanism by which the phosphodiesterase defect results in rod cell death is unknown. Here, too, the cause of subsequent cone cell loss is unknown. All these questions point to how little is known about the cell biology and pathophysiology of the most extensively studied visual protein, rhodopsin, and of the widely studied transduction enzymes. When other genetic defects are identified in less well-defined proteins in photoreceptors and RPE cells there will certainly be even less known about their precise role(s) in retinal degenerations.

These examples point to the major concern that many of the advances in molecular biology will exist in a vacuum if the corresponding areas of retinal cell biology in both normal and mutant animals are not strengthened. The two are complementary. Thus, the danger of overemphasis of molecular biology at the expense of cell biology of retinal degenerations must be avoided if the goals of prevention and treatment of RP are to be achieved.

What models are needed to exploit rapid cell and molecular genetic advances?

Significantly more attention should be given to retinal degeneration mutants of Drosophila, where most of the genes for visual proteins have been cloned, where genetic manipulations are far easier to effect than in mammalian retinas, where selective photoreceptor cell death can readily be studied, and where pharmacologic treatments can be explored. In addition, gaining fundamental knowledge of two research areas in Drosophila, phototransduction and visual development, has the potential to provide a source of molecular probes. Research strategies should include using the human homologs of molecules identified in Drosophila as a source of candidate genes for investigating their role in genetic defects among humans with inherited retinal diseases.

One of the most promising techniques for studying inherited retinal degenerations is the use of transgenic mice as animal models. Their experimental application is several-fold. In defined retinal mutations, such as *rd* and *rds*, the transgenic introduction of functional genes paves the way for the use of these animal lines in the study of gene repair. It now appears possible to target genes to photoreceptors; consequently, the good copy of the gene should alleviate the defect or at least illuminate contributions of normal and defective alleles of the gene. One of the most attractive uses of transgenic mice is the introduction of human genes with specific defects into the mouse. Similarly, homologous recombination may be used to introduce the same defect in the mouse gene. Specific gene alteration through homologous recombination in embryonic stem cells makes it possible to create new retinal phenotypes after any specific gene is cloned and characterized, and the resulting mice should provide considerable insight into the effect of the point mutation. Once the transgenic mice are produced, they can be bred and widely distributed for study. The study of transgenics heralds possibilities for developing mechanisms for targeted gene repair and the introduction of factors for therapeutic treatment of inherited retinal disorders.

Other approaches for targeted gene repair and replacement should be applied to RP research as they are developed. Examples of these include the use of retroviruses and other viruses as vectors for inserting genes into genetically affected photoreceptors and RPE cells.

What is the degree of clinical and genetic heterogeneity in various forms of RP and other hereditary retinal degenerations?

It has repeatedly been shown that heterogeneity exists in the age of onset and rate of visual loss among individuals classified clinically with the same type of RP. This has sometimes been ascribed to inadequate diagnosis and classification. Recently clinical heterogeneity has been observed among RP patients defective in the rhodopsin gene where many different mutations result in the same gene causing the disease. Heterogeneity is also observed in RP patients with the same identical genetic mutation. Among patients with GA, which results from a defect in the gene for omithine aminotransferase and where there are multiple gene mutations, there is also considerable clinical heterogeneity. These observations point to the need for rigorous clinical classification of patients and close correlation with their genetic defects once these are defined. Only then will investigators be able to determine the true statistical correspondence between clinical and genetic subtypes and physicians be able to provide truly accurate patient counseling.

Are systemic, environmental, or toxic factors important in hereditary retinal degenerations?

The finding that patients with the same genetic defect in rhodopsin or in ornithine aminotransferase show clinical heterogeneity raises important questions about whether factors other than the mutant genes themselves affect the severity of these diseases. One of the more obvious factors is environmental lighting. Under certain conditions excessive lighting can destroy photoreceptors and RPE cells, and although those effects have been widely studied, the molecular mechanisms and means for preventing light damage to the retina still are not understood fully. Clearly, oxidative mechanisms are involved in some way, and antioxidants have been shown in some instances to ameliorate the damaging effects of light. These processes need to be better understood, as do their relationship to inherited retinal disorders. It is possible that photoreceptors undergoing an inherited degeneration may be more sensitive to the damaging effects of light than normal photoreceptors. Thus, variability of light exposure among individuals might contribute to the clinical heterogeneity found in RP and other retinal degenerations. An additional factor may be a gene or genes that regulate the susceptibility of the retina to light damage, as shown recently in mice. This significant problem is amenable to analysis in animal models and in careful epidemiologic studies of human RP patients. Such studies also should ask whether other environmental factors are correlated with the incidence of RP.

Another area that needs clarification is the role of polyunsaturated lipids in hereditary retinal degenerations. As already noted, abnormalities in blood lipids have been found in selected patients with RP and in miniature poodles with hereditary retinal degeneration. In addition, several studies have shown that rats, primates, and human infants suffering from omega-3 fatty acid deficiencies can achieve improved visual function when the omega-3 fatty acids are restored in the diet. Evidence to date supports an important role of the key omega-3 fatty acid 22:6 3 in retinal function. It is possible that deprivation of a dietary source of 22:6 3 or its precursor or impairment of its transport from the blood to the retina could result in alteration

284

in retinal function. Since aberrations in 22:6 3 metabolism have been suggested in some humans and animals with inherited retinal degenerations, it is important to search for biochemical mechanisms that may serve as markers or be causal in the disease process.

Which cell(s) expresses the mutant gene(s) in various forms of RP?

Although photoreceptor cells degenerate in most forms of RP, the complex interactions between photoreceptors and RPE cells, choroidal vascular elements, and Muller cells make it impossible to say which cell type(s) expresses the mutant gene in any form of RP until this is shown experimentally. A clear example is the RCS rat, in which the RPE expression of the *rdy* gene results secondarily in photoreceptor cell death. Answering the question is crucial, however, if rational therapeutic and preventive measures are to be developed. For example, it makes no sense to transplant RPE cells into a degenerating retina if the genetic defect is the photoreceptor cell. Unfortunately, we know the cellular site of action of only a few forms of RP and related disorders: the autosomal dominant forms of human RP with the recently defined rhodopsin and *rds*-peripherin defects, the RCS rat, and mice carrying the *rd* and *rds* mutations.

In the past the only approaches to defining the cellular site of gene action were the use of experimental chimeras, which was limited to testing the role of RPE, and the isolation of specific cell types in culture, which has intrinsic limitations for studying this issue. More recently diagnostic advances in molecular and cell biologic technology have allowed the identification of many rod-, cone-, RPE-, and Muller cell-specific proteins and the development of antibodies or oligonucleotide probes to each of them. These antibodies and probes should now be used with immunocytochemical and *in situ* hybridization methods on all of the available animal models and human donor eye tissues to determine which, if any, forms of RP show deficits or developmental abnormalities in these cell-specific proteins. Most critical, presumably, are the various photoreceptor-specific proteins, since in all forms of inherited retinal degeneration in which the gene product has recently been identified the defect has been in the photoreceptor transduction pathway or in a photoreceptor structural gene.

Can transplantation of retinal tissues or growth factors be used therapeutically?

Numerous questions must be answered before the transplantation of RPE or photoreceptors can be attempted in human retinas. For example, are the restored retinas functional? What are the short- and long-term immunologic consequences of transplantation into this region of the eye? What are the optimal source and age of donor tissue? Does the method work experimentally in the rat because of developmental peculiarities (e.g., RPE cell proliferation) at the time of transplantation in this species? Are there ways to increase the area of the transplant in the host eye? What are the best surgical procedures? Can missing factors be used to rescue photoreceptors instead of, or in addition to, RPE cells? And most significantly, which diseases are candidates for transplantation of which cells, tissues, or missing factors (i.e., what is the cellular site of mutant gene expression)? Because of the potential importance of transplantation and survival promoting growth factors as potential therapeutic procedure, research in this area is needed to answer these and other questions.

Chapter 35

Cryotherapy for Retinopathy of Prematurity

Purpose

- To determine the safety and efficacy of trans-scleral cryotherapy of the peripheral retina in certain low birth weight infants with retinopathy of prematurity (ROP) in reducing the number of infants who become blind from ROP.

- To study the natural history of retinal vascular development and ROP in children born with a very low birth weight.

Background

Until recently, more than 500 infants annually were blinded by ROP in the United States alone. ROP is a disease in which the retinal blood vessels increase in number and branch excessively, sometimes leading to hemorrhage or scarring. The number of babies at risk is increasing as survival rates for smaller premature infants improve. The lower the birth weight, the higher the incidence of ROP.

Over 30 years ago, the National Institutes of Health sponsored a clinical trial which showed that if premature babies are given oxygen only as needed, the number of infants who develop ROP drops dramatically. Subsequently, hospitals cut back on giving excessive oxygen routinely to premature babies. But, with improvements in

Clinical Trials Supported by the National Eye Institute, pp. 21–26.

neonatal care over the last two decades, more premature infants with very low birth weights are surviving, and the incidence of ROP has increased. In a recent NEI-supported study, very low-birth-weight infants' blood oxygen levels were monitored continuously by use of transcutaneous measurements as long as they needed oxygen therapy. The study showed that there is no statistically significant difference between the rates of ROP in infants monitored on continuous oxygen therapy and in those monitored only when they were receiving oxygen in excess of 40 percent. This and previous studies have led to the conclusion that factors other than oxygen must be involved in ROP.

Description In some infants who develop ROP, the disease spontaneously subsides, permitting development of normal vision. But others who progress to a severe form of ROP are in danger of becoming permanently blind. Although the cause of ROP is not fully explained, scientists sought ways in which ROP can be successfully treated, and to find the right time in the progression of the disease to use treatment. Cryotherapy, which destroys the edge of the retina through freezing, is the only treatment so far that has demonstrated substantial benefit to these eyes. The multicenter trial of cryotherapy for ROP enrolled almost 5,000 premature infants who weighed no more than 1,250 grams at birth. These infants were at risk of developing ROP. While still in the intensive care nursery, infants enrolled in the study had their eyes examined at intervals. The pupils were dilated with eye drops, and the eyes were examined by an ophthalmologist using a binocular indirect ophthalmoscope to visualize the developing retina. The natural history of the condition of each infant's retinas was thereby recorded. When examination disclosed the severe form of ROP (threshold ROP) in both eyes, and the parents gave informed consent, one of the infant's eyes was randomly selected to receive cryotherapy. In this technique, a cryoprobe was used to freeze and thus destroy the outer edge of the retina, thereby arresting the development of the blood vessels growing wildly toward it.

Outcome of the therapy was assessed at 3 months and 12 months following randomization by means of an extensive examination that included fundus photography of both the treated and the control eyes, as well as measurement of visual function using preferential-looking techniques. Such measurements allowed comparisons between fundus photographs and retinal function. The trained photograph readers who evaluated the pictures from both eyes were unaware of which eyes had received cryotherapy. Additional assessments of visual acuity and retinal status have been carried out at 2, 3 ½, 4 ½, and 5 ½ years following randomization.

Patient Eligibility

Premature infants of either sex eligible for the natural history study had weighed less than 1,251 grams at birth, survived the first 28 days of life, and had no major ocular or systemic congenital anomalies. Infants who met these criteria and also had a threshold level of ROP (stage 3+ of the International Classification of Retinopathy of Prematurity defined as five or more contiguous or eight cumulative 30* sectors [clock hours] of stage 3 ROP in zone 1 or 2 in the presence of plus disease) could be referred for examination to determine eligibility for entry to the cryotherapy portion of the trial.

Patient Recruitment Status

Recruitment began in January 1986 and was stopped January 22, 1988.

Current Status of Study

Ongoing.

Results

The Cryotherapy for Retinopathy of Prematurity Cooperative Group reported preliminary results in 1988. This study of the safety and efficacy of cryotherapy in treating severe retinopathy of prematurity (ROP) registered 9,751 infants with birth weights less than 1,251 grams at 23 study centers. Through a randomization protocol, 291 infants developed a defined threshold ROP.

Cryotherapy was performed in half of the eyes. Twelve months after randomization, the results of masked grading of fundus photographs of the posterior pole indicated an unfavorable outcome in 25.7 percent of the eyes that had received cryotherapy and in 47.7 percent of the control eyes. Masked Teller acuity card assessment of grating acuity indicated an unfavorable functional outcome in 35 percent of the treated eyes, compared with 56.3 percent of the control eyes. These results indicate that cryotherapy reduces the risk of unfavorable retinal and functional outcome from threshold ROP.

Although the surgery was stressful, no major complications occurred during or following treatment. Physician diagnoses and the unbiased photograph grading were statistically similar. These data support the efficacy of cryotherapy in reducing by approximately one-half the risk of unfavorable retinal outcome from threshold ROP.

Cryotherapy is now recommended for both eyes whenever stage 3+ retinopathy of prematurity involves the posterior retina (zone 1) of both eyes, and for "at least one eye" in cases of threshold ROP in zone 2. There are, as yet, insufficient long-term data to permit a firm recommendation to apply cryotherapy routinely to both eyes of all patients with bilateral threshold ROP, to apply cryotherapy in any different pattern than that used in this trial, or to apply it to patients with less severe disease.

All study patients, including those not randomized into the cryotherapy trial, were followed through their 12-month examinations. (More than 4,000 of these "natural history" infants were studied.)

Long-term follow-up (Phase II) is under way. A selected cohort of patients is being examined annually to evaluate both retinal structure and visual function. This cohort includes all 257 surviving randomized patients and 1,192 "natural history" patients. The patients are being followed until they reach the age of 5 ½ years. At the 5 ½ year examination, a Snellen visual acuity test is assessed for all study patients. Follow-up information allows physicians to answer three specific questions:

1. Are there long-term structural or functional ocular sequelae in eyes treated with cryotherapy that would require reevaluation of the risk/benefit ratio of recommending cryotherapy?

2. Do long-term data on structural and functional sequelae in untreated eyes with ROP indicate that the threshold for treatment should be reconsidered?

3. Is the incidence of structural or functional ocular abnormalities any different in infants with mild ROP than in infants with no ROP?

Publications

Cryotherapy for Retinopathy of Prematurity Cooperative Group: Multicenter trial of cryotherapy for retinopathy of prematurity: Preliminary results. *Arch Ophthalmol* 106:471–479, 1988.

Cryotherapy for Retinopathy of Prematurity Cooperative Group: Multicenter trial of cryotherapy for retinopathy of prematurity: Preliminary results. *Pediatrics* 81:697–706, 1988.

Cryotherapy for Retinopathy of Prematurity Cooperative Group: Multicenter trial of cryotherapy for retinopathy of prematurity: Three–month outcome. *Arch Ophthalmol* 108:195–204, 1990.

Dobson V, Quinn GE, Biglan AW, Tung B, Flynn JT, Palmer EA, for the Cryotherapy for Retinopathy of Prematurity Cooperative Group: Acuity card assessment of visual function in the Cryotherapy for Retinopathy of Prematurity trial. *Invest Ophthalmol* vis Sci 31: 1702–1708, 1990.

Watzke RC, Robertson JE, Palmer EA, Wallace PR, Evan MS, Soldevilla JED, for the Cryotherapy for Retinopathy of Prematurity Cooperative Group: Photographic grading in the Retinopathy of Prematurity Cryotherapy trial. *Arch Ophthalmol* 108:950–955, 1990.

Phelps DL, Brown DR, Tung B, Cassady G, McClead RE, Purohit DM, Palmer EA, for the Cryotherapy for Retinopathy of Prematurity Cooperative Group: 28-day survival rates of 6676 neonates with birth weights of 1250 grams or less. *Pediatrics* 87:7–17, 1991.

Palmer EA, Flynn JT, Hardy RJ, Phelps DL, Phillips CL, Schaffer DB, Tung B, the Cryotherapy for Retinopathy of Prematurity Cooperative Group: Incidence and early course of retinopathy of prematurity. *Ophthalmology* 98:1628–1640, 1991.

Hardy RJ, Davis BR, Palmer EA, Tung B: Statistical considerations in the early termination of the multicenter trial of cryotherapy for retinopathy of prematurity. *Controlled Clin Trials* 12:293–303, 1991.

Palmer EA, Hardy RJ, Mowery R, Davis BR, Tung B, Phelps DL, Schaffer DB, Flynn JT: Operational aspects of early termination of the multicenter trial of cryotherapy for retinopathy of prematurity. *Controlled Clin Trials* 12:277–292, 1991.

Quinn GE, Dobson V, Barr CC, Davis BR, Flynn JT, Palmer EA, Robertson J, Trese MT: Visual acuity in infants after vitrectomy for severe retinopathy of prematurity. *Ophthalmology* 98:5–13, 1991.

Summers GC, Phelps DL, Tung B, Palmer EA: Ocular cosmesis in retinopathy of prematurity. *Arch Ophthalmol* 110:1092–1097, 1992.

Quinn GE, Dobson V, Repka MX, Reynolds J, Kivlin J, Davis B, Buckley E, Flynn JT, Palmer EA: Development of myopia in infants with birth weights less than 1251 grams. *Ophthalmology* 99:329–340, 1992.

Gilbert WS, Dobson V, Quinn GE, Reynolds J, Tung B, Flynn JT: The correlation of visual function with posterior retinal structure in severe retinopathy of prematurity. *Arch Ophthalmol* 110:625–631, 1992.

Trueb L, Evans J, Hammel A, Bartholomew P, Dobson D: Assessing visual acuity of visually impaired children using the Teller acuity cards. *Am Orthoptic J* 42:149–154, 1992.

Cryotherapy for Retinopathy of Prematurity Cooperative Group: Multicenter trial of cryotherapy for retinopathy of prematurity: 42-month outcome structure and function. *Arch Ophthalmol* (1993).

Schaffer DB, Palmer EA, Plotsky DF, Metz HS, Flynn JT, Tung B, Hardy RJ: Prognostic factors in the natural course of retinopathy of prematurity (ROP). *Ophthalmology* (1993).

Clinical Centers

Alabama

Frederick J. Elsas, M.D.
University of Alabama at Birmingham
(Office Address) The Children's Hospital
1600 7th Avenue South, Room 555
Birmingham, Alabama 35233
Telephone: (205) 939-9778

California

Alan M. Roth, M.D.
Department of Ophthalmology
University of California at Davis Medical Center
1603 Alhambra Boulevard
Sacramento, California 95816
Telephone: (916) 734-6078

District of Columbia

David Plotsky, M.D.
650 Pennsylvania Avenue, S.E.
Suite 270
Washington, D.C. 20003
Telephone: (202) 544-1900

William S. Gilbert, M.D.
Children's Hospital National Medical Center
Retinal Group of Washington
5454 Wisconsin Avenue, Suite 1540
Chevy Chase, Maryland 20815
Telephone: (301) 656-8100

Florida

John T. Flynn, M.D.
Bascom Palmer Eye Institute
University of Miami School of Medicine
900 N.W. 17th Street
P.O. Box 016880
Miami, Florida 33101
Telephone: (305) 326-4476

Illinois

Marilyn T. Miller, M.D.
University of Illinois Eye and Ear Infirmary
1855 West Taylor Street, Room 144
Chicago, Illinois 60612
Telephone: (312) 996-7445

Indiana

Forrest D. Ellis, M.D.
Department of Ophthalmology
Indiana University School of Medicine
(Office Address) 702 Rotary Circle
Indianapolis, Indiana 46223
Telephone: (317) 274-7919

Kentucky

Charles C. Barr, M.D.
Kentucky Lions Eye Research Institute
University of Louisville
301 East Muhammad Ali Boulevard
Louisville, Kentucky 40292
Telephone: (502) 588-5466

Louisiana

Robert A. Gordon, M.D.
Department of Ophthalmology
Tulane University
School of Medicine
1430 Tulane Avenue
New Orleans, Louisiana 70112
Telephone: (504) 588-5804

Maryland

Michael X. Repka, M.D.
Wilmer Ophthalmological Institute
The Johns Hopkins Medical Institutions
Wilmer Building, Room B1–35
600 North Wolfe Street
Baltimore, Maryland 21205
Telephone: (410) 955-8314

Michigan

John D. Baker, M.D.
2355 Monroe Boulevard
Dearborn, Michigan 48124
Telephone: (313) 561-1777

Michael T. Trese, M.D.
Associated Retinal Consultants, P.C.
3535 West Thirteen Mile Road, Room 632
Royal Oak, Michigan 48073
Telephone: (810) 288-2280

Minnesota

C. Gail Summers, M.D.
Department of Ophthalmology
University of Minnesota
516 Delaware Street, S.E.
P.O. Box 493, UMHC
Minneapolis, Minnesota 55455
Telephone: (612) 625-4400

New York

Dale L. Phelps, M.D.
University of Rochester
(Office Address) Strong Memorial Hospital
601 Elmwood Avenue
Box 651, Neonatology
Rochester, New York 14642
Telephone: (716) 275-5884

North Carolina

Edward G. Buckley, M.D.
Susie Wong, M.D.
Duke University Eye Center
Box 3802
Durham, North Carolina 27710
Telephone: (919) 684-6084

Ohio

Miles J. Burke, M.D.
Department of Ophthalmology
Children's Hospital Medical Center
Pavilion 1–80
3300 Elland Avenue
Cincinnati, Ohio 45229
Telephone: (513) 559-4751

Ohio, continued

Gary L. Rogers, M.D.
Don L. Bremer, M.D.
Columbus Children's Hospital
(Office Address) 545 South 18th Street
Columbus, Ohio 43205
Telephone: (614) 224-6222

Oregon

Earl A. Palmer, M.D.
Casey Eye Institute
3375 S.W. Terwilliger Boulevard
Portland, Oregon 97201-4197
Telephone: (503) 494-5945

Pennsylvania

Graham E. Quinn, M.D.
David B. Schaffer, M.D.
Children's Hospital of Philadelphia
One Children's Center
Philadelphia, Pennsylvania 19104
Telephone: (215) 590-2390

Albert W. Biglan, M.D.
Magee Women's Hospital
(Office Address) Oakland Pediatric
Ophthalmology, Inc.
3518 Fifth Avenue
Pittsburgh, Pennsylvania 15213
Telephone: (412) 682-6300

South Carolina

Richard A. Saunders, M.D.
Storm Eye Institute
Medical University of South Carolina
171 Ashley Avenue
Charleston, South Carolina 29425-2236
Telephone: (803) 792-2761

Tennessee

Stephen S. Feman, M.D.
Department of Ophthalmology
Vanderbilt University
Nashville, Tennessee 37232
Telephone: (615) 322-3484

Texas

Rand Spencer, M.D.
1055 Wadley Tower
3600 Gaston Avenue
Dallas, Texas 75246
Telephone: (214) 8214540

Wichard A. Van Heuven, M.D.
Department of Ophthalmology
University of Texas Health Science Center
7703 Floyd Curl Drive
San Antonio, Texas 78284
Telephone: (210) 567-8400

Johan Zwann, M.D., Ph.D.
Department of Ophthalmology
University of Texas Health Science Center
7703 Floyd Curl Drive
San Antonio, Texas 78284-6230
Telephone: (210) 567-8411

Utah

Robert O. Hoffman, M.D.
Department of Ophthalmology, 1C447
University of Utah School of Medicine
50 North Medical Drive
Salt Lake City, Utah 84132
Telephone: (801) 581-4955

Resource Centers

Chairman's Office

Earl A. Palmer, M.D.
Casey Eye Institute
3375 S.W. Terwilliger Boulevard
Portland, Oregon 97201-4197
Telephone: (503) 494-5945

Coordinating Center

Robert J. Hardy, Ph.D.
School of Public Health
University of Texas Health Science Center
Coordinating Center for Clinical Trials
1200 Herman Pressler, Suite 801
Houston, Texas 77030
Telephone: (713) 792-4480

Ocular Pathology Center

David J. Wilson, M.D.
Casey Eye Institute
3375 S.W. Terwilliger Boulevard
Portland, Oregon 97201-4197
Telephone: (503) 494-7881

Visual Acuity Center

Velma Dobson, Ph.D.
Department of Psychology
University of Pittsburgh
Langley Hall, Room 462
Pittsburgh, Pennsylvania 15260
Telephone: (412) 624-4525

NEI Representative

Richard L. Mowery, Ph.D.
National Eye Institute
Executive Plaza South, Suite 350
6120 Executive Boulevard
Rockville, Maryland 20892
Telephone: (301) 496-5983

Part Five

Glaucoma

Chapter 36

Some Answers about Glaucoma

Forward

Glaucoma has caused more blindness in America than any other disease. Many cases of glaucoma would have been prevented with regular testing and early treatment.

Much about glaucoma remains mysterious. Although we do not know what causes it, there is no cure, we do know how to control it if detected early. There have been great improvements in available treatments over the past ten years. Much more, however, remains to be done.

National Glaucoma Research, a program of the American Health Assistance Foundation, is searching for answers to many of these unanswered questions. The program has helped fund studies on promising new drugs and improved methods of glaucoma testing. While we are eager to discover new secrets that lead to the prevention and treatment of glaucoma, we also desire to serve the many people who suffer from glaucoma.

We have therefore prepared this booklet as a public education service. We sincerely hope it answers some of your questions. Please write to us if we can be of any further assistance.

Eugene H. Michaels, President National Glaucoma Research

Some Answers about Glaucoma

Why You Should Be Concerned about Glaucoma

Glaucoma has caused more blindness in the country today than any other disease. It is one of four major causes of new cases of blindness: glaucoma, diabetic retinopathy, age-related cataract, and age-related macular degeneration. It is responsible for more than 5,400 new cases of blindness every year, most of which could have been prevented.

Vision experts estimate over two million Americans have glaucoma. In its early stages, glaucoma usually has no symptoms. More than half of the people with glaucoma do not know they have the disease. Without proper testing, substantial loss in vision can occur before even realizing anything is wrong. Glaucoma can be detected during a comprehensive eye exam. Once diagnosed, eyedrops and pills can control the disease and in almost all cases prevent it from damaging the eyes.

What Is Glaucoma?

Glaucoma is a group of diseases in which the pressure inside the eye is too high.

To understand the nature of the disease, it is necessary to understand the structure of the eye. (See diagram.) The eyes see through delicate camera-like structures at the front of the eye. The cornea serves as a clear window at the front of the eye. The iris, the colored part of our eye, controls the amount of light entering the eye. The lens of the eye focuses light on the retina at the back of the eye.

These delicate structures are constantly bathed by a clear fluid called the aqueous humor. This aqueous humor provides nourishment for the tissues of the interior of the eye. Aqueous humor is produced inside the eye and then must drain out of the eye through a spongy network of tiny drainage canals called the trabecular meshwork. The trabecular meshwork is located near the front of the eye.

Glaucoma causes this drainage network to stop working properly. The aqueous humor continues to be produced but cannot drain away properly. As a result pressure in the eye rises, similar to the pressure buildup in a hose if you forgot to open the nozzle. This pressure of the fluid within the eye is called intraocular pressure, or IOP, and an elevated IOP can be damaging.

304

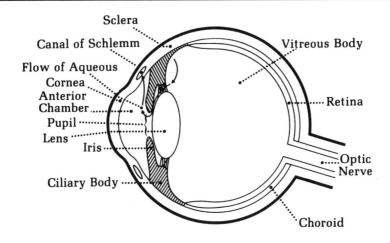

Figure 36.1. *The diagram of the anatomy of the eye.*

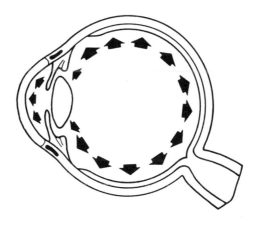

Figure 36.2. *Glaucoma—eye disease characterized by an increase in internal eye pressure leading to defects in vision.*

Messages from the eyes travel to the brain along the optic nerve. This nerve is damaged in glaucoma. When the eyes are affected by glaucoma, elevated pressure in the eye compresses the optic nerve. Nerve fibers are destroyed and vision is lost.

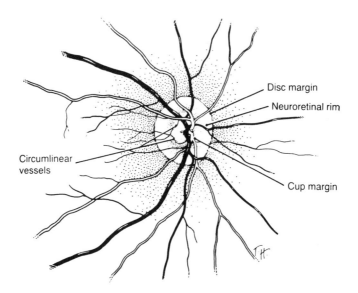

Figure 36.3. *Optic Nerve—nerve which carries the nerve signal to the brain enabling sight. This nerve is permanently damaged from the elevated pressure of the glaucoma.*

An individual with glaucoma may lose a portion of their sight and yet not notice it. This is because glaucoma generally attacks side or peripheral vision first. It is possible to have 20-20 eyesight and still have lost some peripheral vision because of glaucoma. During the course of the disease, if unchecked, the central vision, which is necessary for general vision such as reading or watching television, is adversely affected.

Once vision is lost due to glaucoma, it is gone forever. That is why glaucoma is such an insidious disease—it has been called the sneak-thief of sight.

Types of Glaucoma

Chronic Open-Angle Glaucoma. Accounting for about 80 percent of all cases, this is the most common type of glaucoma. It is generally painless and can be detected in its early stages only by an eye examination.

In this type of glaucoma, the rise in fluid pressure is so gradual the patient doesn't feel anything. But the elevated eye pressure does damage the optic nerve.

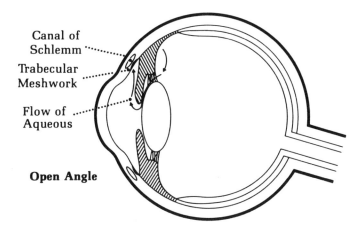

Canal of Schlemm
Trabecular Meshwork
Flow of Aqueous
Open Angle

Figure 36.4. *Open-Angle Glaucoma—the angle is not closed by the iris and the obstruction is caused by small invisible molecules within the drainage apparatus (trabeculum or canal of Schlemm).*

Acute or Closed-Angle Glaucoma. This is a sudden medical emergency. Eyes may become red and tear a lot. Vision may be blurred. There may be pain in or around the eye, nausea, and vomiting. If it is not treated, acute glaucoma can produce blindness in just a few days. Laser treatment and sometimes surgery are required.

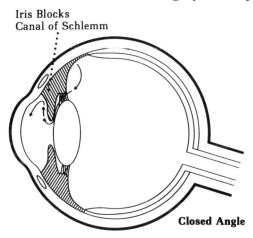

Iris Blocks
Canal of Schlemm
Closed Angle

Figure 36.5. *Closed-Angle Glaucoma*

Secondary Glaucoma. This is caused by an eye injury, inflammation, or tumor and includes Pigmentary, Traumatic and Neovascular Glaucoma. Advanced cases of cataracts or diabetes may also cause secondary glaucoma. Treatment is required for both the glaucoma and its underlying cause.

Normal or Low Tension Glaucoma. A few patients experience loss of vision when the intraocular pressure seems to be normal or low. The average intraocular pressure in the population is about 15 millimeters of mercury (15 mm Hg). Most healthy eyes have pressures below 21. In general as pressure increases above this level, the risk of damage to the vision increases though some patients with pressure above 21 never experience damage to their eyes. In low tension glaucoma, some patients with intraocular pressure below 21 experience glaucoma damage.

Infantile Glaucoma. This is a rare condition—an infant who has glaucoma. Symptoms include excessive sensitivity to light and unusual tearing of eyes. If present at birth, it may be called Congenital glaucoma.

What Are the Danger Signs?

Most of the time, a person with chronic glaucoma feels no symptoms at all. If there are any symptoms, they may include:

- Frequent changes of eyeglasses, which do not seem to help.
- Aching or discomfort around the eyes.
- Blurred vision or halos around lights.
- Difficulty in adjusting to darkened rooms.

Glaucoma usually affects both eyes. It is not an infection, and it is not contagious.

Who Is at Risk of Developing Glaucoma?

Few people under age 35 develop chronic glaucoma. But, starting at age 35, the likelihood of the disease steadily increases. Most cases of glaucoma strike people over 50.

One exam for glaucoma is not enough. It is possible to be free of glaucoma now, but develop the disease within the next year or two. Doctors recommend an exam every two years after age 35, with more frequent exams for those at higher risk.

People whose blood relatives have glaucoma are especially at risk. Someone with a parent, brother or sister with glaucoma, has a 1-in-10 chance of developing glaucoma themselves.

This means that if you have a relative who has glaucoma, you should have your eyes checked yearly by a competent vision specialist. If you have glaucoma yourself, urge your relatives to go in regularly for an eye exam to prevent possible loss of vision.

The risk of glaucoma is also greater among black people. The glaucoma rate among middle-aged blacks is 15 times the rate for whites. No one knows why. Experts are conducting special studies to determine the reasons. Meanwhile, The American Academy of Ophthalmology recommends regular eye exams for blacks, starting at age 30.

A person who is very nearsighted also has a higher risk of glaucoma. They are also likely to suffer greater damage from a pressure within the eye than someone with the same pressure who is not nearsighted. Other people at greater risk are those who have diabetes, people who take steroid medicines like cortisone, and someone who has had an eye injury or eye surgery.

Screening Exams

Regular screening examinations for glaucoma are conducted by ophthalmologists and optometrists. Optometrists, eye specialists, can screen for vision problems and refer suspected cases of glaucoma to an ophthalmologist, a medically trained eye doctor, for diagnosis and treatment.

These screening exams use a test device called a tonometer, which measures the pressure in the eyeball. Often a non-contact tonometer is used, this device uses a puff of air to measure pressure in the eyeball.

The test is quick and painless, and serves as a quick way to see if the pressure inside the eye is normal, borderline, or high. This simple test can save your sight.

If this test shows your eye pressure is borderline or high, you must get more sophisticated tests. Make an appointment with an ophthalmologist, who has years of specialized training in the care of the eyes. Keep that appointment.

How Can the Doctor Diagnose Glaucoma?

Glaucoma can be a difficult disease to diagnose. It is impossible to determine the exact amount of pressure that will do damage to someone's eyes. The eyes vary individually in the amount of pressure they can withstand without damage to the optic nerve. Furthermore, the amount of pressure in the eye changes as you go through the day, just as your temperature, blood pressure, and weight all vary during the day.

Your doctor may want to see you for several visits, and take measurements at different times of the day, before coming to a firm conclusion on whether you have glaucoma. The doctor will measure the pressure in your eyes carefully using a device called an applanation tonometer. Because this tonometer must touch the surface of the eye, a drop of local anaesthetic will he put in the eye before the exam. The exam itself is simple and painless.

Pressure inside the eye is measured in millimeters of mercury (mm Hg) and 12 to 21 mm Hg is considered normal. At 21 mm a doctor may start considering treatment. However, only 5 to 10 percent of people with pressures above 21 mm Hg actually develop signs of damage to the optic nerve.

In addition to checking the pressure, the doctor will also check the optic nerve carefully. Using an optic disc analyzer, a recently developed testing device, the ophthalmologist is able to analyze the optic nerve in far greater detail and with much more precision than ever before. A computerized image analysis of the optic nerve allows detection of the damage much earlier An ophthalmoscope is also used to check the optic nerve. Using the ophthalmoscope, which looks like a flashlight with a peep-hole to look through, the doctor can see through the pupil of your eye and look directly at your retina and optic nerve. Any unusual appearance offers valuable clues about possible damage to your optic nerve.

A new sophisticated form of ultrasound called Standardized Echography is used to determine the actual condition of the optic nerve. Sound waves are bounced off the ocular tissues to create an oscilloscope "picture" for examination. The procedure takes only a few minutes and causes no discomfort to the patient. Two types of ultrasound are used. A-scan produces a one-dimensional display and B-scan produces a two-dimensional "picture" of the eye.

The ophthalmologist will also use a variety of tests to see if you have lost any vision. The doctor will give you a visual field test. This test shows how much you can see to the right and left, above and below and directly ahead. This is your field of vision. If your field of vision is unusually narrow, it is a sign of damage to your optic nerve. These tests check carefully for damage to your side or peripheral vision.

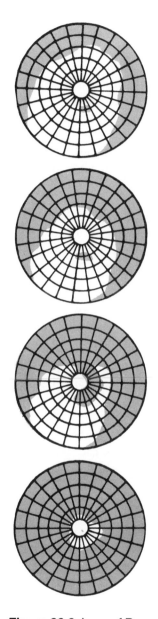

Figure 36.6. *Loss of Peripheral Vision—chronic glaucoma gradually destroys the side vision and then the central vision.*

The doctor may place a special contact lens on your eye which contains an angled mirror. The doctor is able to examine the structures inside the eye that can be problem spots in glaucoma through this gonioscopy test. Because the area between the iris and the cornea can be seen, this is especially helpful in detecting a narrowed angle which may suggest glaucoma.

An ophthalmologist will take all three measurements into account—the level of pressure within the eye, loss of visual field, and the appearance of the optic nerve and other structures within the eye—in deciding whether to start treatment for glaucoma.

Frequent examinations are necessary to determine if a patient has glaucoma and also to decide if the glaucoma is being adequately treated. The condition can get better or worse without the patient being aware of it. The sophisticated tests that only an ophthalmologist can do are essential for the proper care of the eyes.

If your doctor decides to treat you for glaucoma, you may wish to get a second opinion before starting treatment—that is a perfectly reasonable thing to do. You can ask your family doctor for a referral, or contact a local teaching hospital or university medical school and ask for the names of ophthalmologists with a special interest in glaucoma.

Adjusting to the Diagnosis

If your doctor diagnoses glaucoma and recommends treatment, allow some time to adjust to this new situation. Learning you have an illness is a surprise. Even if you have worried about a diagnosis ahead of time, it is still a shock when you actually receive the news. It can be hard to understand everything the doctor is saying. Fortunately there are support groups, literature and organizations available to help deal with this situation.

This chapter, and the other resource materials listed in the appendix, carefully answer many questions. Read more than one publication, as no one publication can cover the specific details of each individual situation. Make a list of questions you want to ask your doctor, and take the list with you on your next visit.

In addition, call a group like the National Society to Prevent Blindness. Their toll-free telephone hotline is listed in the appendix. They can put you in touch with experienced people in your area who have time to talk with you, possibly a self-help group. There are lots of ways to get the information you need.

Lifestyle Changes

The most important treatment for glaucoma is regular use of the medicines your doctor prescribes. In addition, there are a few simple things to keep in mind.

- A quiet life style and a calm disposition have beneficial effects on glaucoma. This does not mean that a hectic lifestyle causes glaucoma; no one knows why one person gets glaucoma and another does not. Some doctors believe a relaxed attitude toward daily problems can help reduce the pressure inside the eye associated with glaucoma.

- Drink any beverage you wish in moderation, but do not drink a large amount rapidly, the pressure inside your eyes may increase temporarily. A good rule of thumb is not to swallow more than two cups of water in five minutes.

- When you see a doctor or other health care professional, make sure they know you have glaucoma. List all the medicines you are using, including over-the-counter medications from the drugstore.

Medicines

A variety of eyedrops and pills are available to control glaucoma. An individual with glaucoma can expect to take them every day for the rest of their life.

Usually medicines for glaucoma are taken two to four times a day. Because the effect of each medicine only lasts a certain amount of time, it is important to follow the directions exactly. Develop a way to remember. Perhaps a beeper on your watch will work. Or if you are on a four-times-a-day schedule, you can schedule eyedrops or pills at breakfast, lunch, dinner and at bedtime.

When using eyedrops, you only need one drop at a time. Although more will do no harm, it is wasteful to use more. You want the drop to land in the space just inside your lower eye lid. This area can only hold one drop. If you miss the eye altogether try again. Do not blink, or you will squeeze the medicine out. Allow the medicine to sit on the eye for a few seconds so it can be absorbed.

Glaucoma medicines work in several different ways. Some improve drainage from the eye others reduce the production of fluid. Most medicines strong enough to produce the desired treatment can produce other undesired side effects as well.

You and your doctor must be a team, working together to find the best possible treatment program for your particular diagnosis. Your doctor cannot know how the medicine affects you unless you tell him.

There are so many medicines available to treat glaucoma that it would not be practical to list them all in this booklet. A brief description of those most commonly used follow:

Beta blockers decrease fluid production. At present they are the most widely used glaucoma medications. They include Timoptic, Betoptic, and Betagan. These drops are needed only once or twice a day. Side effects are rare. However aggravation of existing health problems, including asthma and congestive heart disease, may occur.

Adrenergic agents open the channels that allow fluid to leave the eye and they also decrease fluid production. Examples are Propine and several forms of Epinephrine. When the drops wear off, the eyes become somewhat red. Occasionally people develop allergies to these drops. Patients with heart disease or high blood pressure need to discuss possible side effects with the doctor before using these drops.

Miotics reduce the pressure in the eye by opening the drainage channels. One example is Pilocarpine, which has been in use for over a century and is one of the safest glaucoma drugs available. It comes

313

in eyedrops that range in strength from 1 to 4 percent. It is also available as a gel and as a tiny contact-lens-like insert that lasts for a week. Miotics constrict the pupil and may cause some dimming of vision.

Oral medications decrease fluid production. They include Diamox and Neptazane. Any medicine taken internally of course affects the whole body. These pills may have side effects that include tingling hands and feet, upset stomach, or a decrease in energy. Usually the side effects are mild.

A glaucoma patient usually does not take the same medicine on the same schedule for a lifetime. Some medicines may gradually lose their effectiveness over time. New medicines are always being developed to combat this problem. A change in medicines does not mean that glaucoma has gotten worse. It is part of the normal plan for treatment.

If you are having problems with eyedrops or pills, be sure to discuss them with your doctor. He or she needs to know. The doctor may want to change the dosage, prescribe a different medicine or ask you to continue for a few more weeks. Sometimes eyes are sensitive to a medicine at first, and then they adjust to it.

It is very important to continue with your prescribed glaucoma medication. It can be difficult to interrupt a daily schedule to take eyedrops. Experts estimate as many as 40 percent of those with glaucoma don't use their medicines as directed. Many will skip the eye drops a few times, then use them on the day they see the doctor.

This is a serious problem for several reasons. First, when you skip using the eyedrops, the pressure in your eyes increases. Second, when the doctor examines you and notices the increased pressure, his conclusion will be that your current prescription is not working well. The doctor will then probably recommend or change to a stronger medicine—one with perhaps more side effects.

It takes discipline and determination to take medicine for glaucoma regularly. But that is the only way to prevent blindness from this disease.

Laser Treatment

A recent development in glaucoma treatment is the use of lasers as an alternative to surgery in cases where eyedrops and pills are not enough to control the build up of pressure. Laser treatment has been so successful that researchers are now studying whether it may someday be an alternative to pills and eye drops.

A laser uses focused light energy to make tiny openings in the trabecular meshwork, where fluid drains from the eye. It is a noninvasive procedure, done in the doctor's office and taking only 20 minutes.

Laser treatment is used to control both open-angle and closed-angle glaucoma.

The term laser is an abbreviation for "Light Amplification by Stimulated Emission of Radiation." In the most commonly used ophthalmic lasers, a powerful electric current is passed through a tube containing one of several gases (Argon, Krypton or NeodymiumYAG). Energy is produced and the laser emits a narrow uniform light beam which, when focused through a microscope, produces either heat coagulation, cutting, or micro explosions in certain eye tissues.

Ophthalmic lasers are usually named according to the gas contained in the plasma tube. For example, the laser which uses the gas Argon, and emits a green or blue-green light beam, may be preferred to treat one eye disorder. The laser which uses Neodymium gas, called the YAG laser, which emits a near infrared light beam, may be preferred in treating another disorder.

Most of the time laser treatment is successful in substantially reducing the fluid pressure. The patient may still need to use eyedrops or pills after treatment. In some cases, however, laser treatment is not successful, and surgery is needed.

Surgery

Surgery always poses the risk of complications, so doctors avoid it as long as they have other options. Nevertheless, modern microsurgery is a relatively simple, low-risk procedure. A patient should not be excessively worried before an eye operation. It is somewhat natural to worry more about an operation on our eye than on another part of our body. This procedure is now done on a regular basis by qualified eye surgeons and can provide relief for many glaucoma sufferers. The operation takes only twenty to thirty minutes. Pain is minimal after the operation. The procedure is carried out with general anaesthetic, or with only a local anaesthetic with muscle relaxant drugs.

As a rule, only one eye is bandaged so that you can move around normally after the operation.

In closed-angle glaucoma, the excision of a tiny part of the iris, a procedure called an iridectomy, restores the connection between the posterior and anterior chambers which were blocked. This allows drainage to resume.

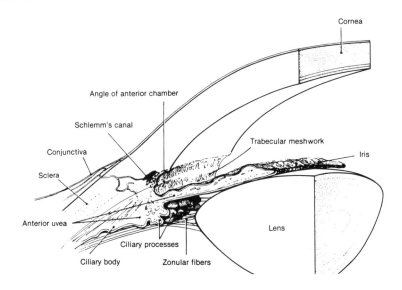

Figure 36.7. Cross Section of Eye—Aqueous is formed inside the eye behind the pupil. It flows into the anterior chamber and then into the canal of Schlemm in the area called the "anterior chamber angle" where the cornea and iris close together. Finally the aqueous leaves the eye through the veins on the outer surface of the eye and then passes into the body's blood circulation. The fluid inside the eye does not drain into the tears. This process maintains the eye at a certain intraocular pressure necessary for its health.

In primary open-angle glaucoma a new channel must be created through which the aqueous fluid can filter out and escape. At the same time, infection must be prevented from entering the eye. An opening must be made near the margin of the cornea and it must be covered over with a flap of eye tissue. Usually when the doctor speaks of surgery to provide a filter for the fluid, they will be speaking about creating a small opening as described.

A little bulge may be visible at the top of the edge of the cornea under the upper lid after the operation. This drainage bleb is the visible sign of the draining away of the aqueous fluid from the interior of the eye.

In some few cases, a surgeon will place a small plastic tube with a valve in the surgically made opening to assist the drainage of the aqueous fluid out of the eye.

It is particularly important to keep the eyes very clean after this operation. If you have to touch your eye, wash your hands first. You will need some time to recuperate. The exact amount of convalescence will depend on your age, physical condition, and lifestyle. Your eye will be protected by a patch for a week or so. You will need to avoid strenuous exercise for several weeks.

Finding Answers about Glaucoma Through Research

National Glaucoma Research, a program of the American Health Assistance Foundation, is supporting research to search for more complete knowledge of the disease and to develop more effective medical and surgical treatment.

Researchers are examining the trabecular meshwork, the network of drainage canals through which the fluid should drain, to find abnormalities which may be a cause of glaucoma. How the aqueous humor fluid is produced and ways to control the production and drainage of this fluid are being studied. Exactly what occurs in the aging eye and in eyes with glaucoma is being researched to provide clues to the causes and the potential cures for glaucoma.

Researchers are searching for new drugs and more effective drug therapies for treating glaucoma. Others are experimenting with new ways of delivering drugs to the eye, perhaps through an implant or slow release system. An artificial drainage system which would measure and control the rate of outflow of the aqueous humor is the subject of a study supported by National Glaucoma Research of the American Health Assistance Foundation.

Ways to improve conventional glaucoma surgery are being sought. The different forms of laser surgery are being carefully evaluated and improved laser treatments are being developed. The cellular and biochemical responses to laser trabeculoplasty are the focus of specific studies.

Self-Help Groups

Glaucoma can be controlled. Loss of vision can be prevented. The key factor is cooperation and determination to fight an illness that is an invisible enemy. It can be difficult to follow a lifelong medical regimen, especially one that results in unpleasant side effects.

An experimental program of self-help groups for glaucoma patients has been started in some areas. A self-help group is a small group of patients who meet regularly to learn more about their illness and share their own experiences and feelings. Patients can learn how others deal with problems, and offer each other emotional support as they make necessary adjustments in their lifestyles. Today there are groups in Florida, New York, Virginia, Ohio, Texas, Utah, Indiana, and Wisconsin. As the program grows, every glaucoma patient across the nation will be able to participate.

Most glaucoma self-help groups meet every month or so. Usually there is an information program featuring a local expert on glaucoma, followed by a discussion period. The facilitator, who recruits new members and coordinates the discussion period, is a glaucoma patient currently under treatment.

There may already be a self-help group in your area. If not, perhaps you can start one. The National Society to Prevent Blindness has a handbook and videotape available with information on how to start a self-help group.

A Few Tips to Remember—If You Have Glaucoma:

- Your blood relatives have an increased risk of glaucoma, so encourage them to have regular eye exams.

- When you see a doctor or other health care professional, make sure they know you have glaucoma.

- Carry an identification card in your wallet, listing all your medicines and your treatment schedule.

- Always keep an extra supply of medicine on hand in case it is lost.

- If you have any problems with your medicine, discuss them as soon as possible with your eye doctor.

Helpful Reading

Check your local library for useful material on glaucoma. Ask the reference librarian if there is a pamphlet file on the subject. You may also find useful material filed under "Eyes" or "Blindness."

If you live near a hospital, medical school, or medical library, you may be able to find more technical material available through these resources.

All About Glaucoma, Wolfgang Leydhecker and Ronald Pitts Crick. England: Faber and Faber, 1981. Paperback.

The only book on glaucoma currently in print that is written for the layperson. Your library may have a copy, or you can order it through your local bookstore.

This valuable book covers the various types of glaucoma, diagnostic procedures and treatments in great detail. It does not have the latest word on new treatments or current research in great detail. It contains basic information on glaucoma.

Understanding and Living with Glaucoma: A Reference Guide for Patients and Their Families. Foundation for Glaucoma Research, 490 Post Street, Suite 1042, San Francisco, California 94102.

A well-designed helpful booklet for glaucoma patients written by a patient. Many clear drawings, exceptionally useful patient tips Highly recommended.

Mutual Aid Glaucoma Groups—A Facilitator Handbook National Society to Prevent Blindness, 500 East Remington Road, Schaumberg, IL 60173.

A superb handbook that covers every aspect of starting a self-help group for glaucoma patients. Videotape and over-the-phone consultations on how to start a self-help group also available.

National Glaucoma Research Report (quarterly newsletter). National Glaucoma Research, American Health Assistance Foundation, 15825 Shady Grove Road, Suite 140, Rockville, MD 20850.

Information on current research funded by the organization and some patient-care information. Glaucoma patients can send in personal questions to a regular column, "Ask the Experts."

GLEAMS (quarterly newsletter). Foundation for Glaucoma Research, 490 Post Street, Suite 1042, San Francisco, California 94102.

Includes information on recent developments in glaucoma research and helpful hints for patients with glaucoma.

Glaucoma: It Can Take Your Sight Away. American Academy of Oph-thalmology, P. O. Box 7424, San Francisco, CA 94120-7424.

Brief, well-designed brochure.

Excess Risk of Glaucomatous Blindness in Blacks. American Academy of Ophthalmology, P. O. Box 7424, San Francisco, CA 94120-7424.

One-page fact sheet, technical and brief.

Glaucoma (NIH Publication No. 86–651). Public Information Office National Eye Institute, National Institutes of Health, Building 36 Room 6A32, Bethesda, MD 20892.

Clear, up-to-date brochure on glaucoma. Includes brief descriptions of current treatments and research programs.

Toll-Free Hotlines

The National Society to Prevent Blindness has a nationwide toll-free hotline. Call them at 1-800-221-3004 for information on available treatments, eye-care facilities, and publications.

The National Eye Care Project of the Foundation of the American Academy of Ophthalmology offers special services for people over age 65 who have not seen an ophthalmologist in the past three years be-cause of financial problems. Call 1-800-222-EYES for more informa-tion and a referral to an ophthalmologist who will do an eye exam and provide continuing care at no cost to the patient.

The American Foundation for the Blind has a toll-free hotline with information on visual impairment, employment of the visually im-paired, and a variety of services. Call 1-800-232-5463. New York resi-dents call (212) 620-2147.

National Glaucoma Research has a toll-free hotline offering cur-rent information on glaucoma research, treatments, and publications. Call 1-800-227-7998.

Organizations Concerned with Glaucoma

National Eye Institute
National Institutes of Health
Building 31 Room 6A32
Bethesda, MD 20892
(301) 496-5248

American Academy of Ophthalmology
655 Beach Street
P. O. Box 7424
San Francisco, CA 94120-7424
(415) 561-8500

American Optometric Association
243 Lindbergh Boulevard
St. Louis, MO 63141
(314) 991-4100

American Foundation for the Blind
15 West 16 Street
New York, NY 10011
(212) 620-2000

The Foundation for Glaucoma Research
490 Post Street, Suite 1042
San Francisco, CA 94102
(415) 986-3162

National Glaucoma Research
American Health Assistance Foundation
15825 Shady Grove Road, Suite 140
Rockville, MD 20850
1-800-227-7998

National Eye Care Project
Foundation of the American Academy of Ophthalmology
P. O. Box 6988
San Francisco, CA 94101-6988
1-800-222-EYES

National Society to Prevent Blindness
500 East Remington Road
Schaumberg, IL 60173
(312) 843-2020

Glaucoma screening, advisory and referral services, and educational programs are offered. Contact a local affiliate if one is near you. If not, call the national office for more information.

Local Affiliates

NSPB—Arkansas Division
400 West Capitol
Suite 2333
Little Rock, AR 72201
(501) 376-6217

Northern California Society to Prevent Blindness
4200 California Street
San Francisco, CA 94118
(415) 387-0934

Colorado Society to Prevent Blindness
3500 East 12th Avenue
Denver, CO 80206
(303) 399-8090

Connecticut Society to Prevent Blindness
1 Meriden Road
Middletown, CT 06457
(203) 347-6800

NSPB—Florida Affiliate
Main Office
4511 North Himes Avenue
Tampa, FL 33614
(813) 874-2020

Georgia Society to Prevent Blindness, Inc.
2025 Peachtree Road, NE
Atlanta, GA 30309
(404) 355-0182

Iowa Society to Prevent Blindness
309 Shops Building
8th and Walnut
Des Moines, IA 50309
(515) 244-4341

Indiana Society to Prevent Blindness
1425 East 86th Street
Indianapolis, IN 46204
(317) 259-8163

NSPB—Kentucky Affiliate
727 Starks Building
Louisville, KY 40202
(502) 584-6127

NSPB—Massachusetts Affiliate
375 Concord Avenue
Belmont, MA 02178
(617) 489-0007

NSPB—Mississippi Affiliate
115 Broadmoor Drive
Jackson, MS 39206
(601) 362-6985

NSPB—North Carolina Affiliate, Inc.
1033 Wade Avenue, Suite 126
Raleigh, NC 27605
(919) 832-2020

NSPB—Nebraska Affiliate
120 North 69th Street, Suite 203
Omaha, NE 68132
(402) 551-2198

NSPB—New Jersey, Inc.
303 George Street
New Brunswick, NJ 08901
(201) 545-2020

NSPB—New York Division
30 East 29th Street
New York, NY 10016
(212) 684-3222

NSPB—Ohio Affiliate
1500 West 3rd Avenue, Suite 200
Columbus, OH 43212
(614) 464-2020

Oklahoma Society to Prevent Blindness
6 Northeast 63rd Street, Suite 150
Oklahoma City, OK 73105
(405) 848-7123

NSPB—Pennsylvania Project
909 North 2nd Street
Harrisburg, PA 17102
(717) 234-2020

Puerto Rico Society for the Prevention of Blindness, Inc.
P.O. Box 3232
San Juan, PR 00904
(809) 722-3531

Rhode Island Society To Prevent Blindness
1800 17th Post Road (Airport Plaza)
Warwick, RI 02886
(401) 738-1150

NSPB—South Carolina Affiliate
5301 Trenholm Road, Suite C
Columbia, SC 29206
(803) 787-4040

Tennessee Society to Prevent Blindness
95 White Bridge Road, Suite 513
Nashville, TN 37205
(615) 352-0450

Texas Society to Prevent Blindness
Main Office
3211 West Dallas
Houston, TX 77019
(713) 526-2559

NSPB—Utah Affiliate
661 South 200 East
Salt Lake City, UT 84111
(801) 524-2020

NSPB—Virginia Affiliate
1004 North Thompson, Suite 100
Richmond, VA 23230
(804) 355-0773

Washington Society to Prevent Blindness
324 15th Avenue East
Seattle, WA 98112
(206) 324-9894

NSPB—Wisconsin, Inc.
759 North Milwaukee Street
Milwaukee, WI 53202
(414) 765-0505

Glossary

Acute-angle closure glaucoma. Sudden blockage of flow of aqueous humor resulting in severe pain, swelling of cornea, colored halos, iris fixed in mid-dilation and a red eye. Untreated it can lead to permanent loss of vision.

Angle-closure glaucoma. Blockage of flow of aqueous humor within the eye by closure of angle between the cornea and iris.

Adrenergic agents. A class of drugs used in the treatment of glaucoma to reduce pressure within the eye. Glaucon, Epitrin, and Propine are the most commonly used.

Aqueous humor. Fluid providing nourishment to the interior of the eye. Normal pressure within the eye depends upon the aqueous humor entering the eye at the same rate it leaves the eye.

Argon laser. One special type of laser used in glaucoma treatment. Lasers are extremely powerful focused light.

Ciliary processes. Site of production of aqueous humor.

Cornea. Tissue covering front of the eye.

Glaucoma. Eye diseases characterized by an increase in pressure within the eye leading to defects in vision and potential blindness.

Halo vision. Perception of a colored halo about a light source. Can be a symptom of glaucoma.

Infantile glaucoma. Glaucoma occurring early in life. Symptoms are tearing, blinking, and sensitivity to light. Requires prompt attention and usually surgery.

Iris. Colored portion of the eye with muscles that increase or decrease the diameter of the pupil to adjust the amount of light entering the eye.

Laser therapy. Light energy focused on the interior of the eye to alter the iris or trabecular meshwork, thus allowing drainage of the aqueous humor and lowering of the interior eye pressure.

Lens. A round tissue within the eye that actively focuses light on the retina by changing its shape to alter curvature of the light. With aging or disease the clear lens may become cloudy, a condition known as a cataract.

Miotics. A class of drug used to treat glaucoma by constricting the pupil Used in many forms of glaucoma.

Open-angle glaucoma. Occurs in eyes with open anterior chamber angles (between the cornea and iris). *Primary*—Not associated with other ocular disease. *Secondary*—Associated with other ocular disease.

Optic nerve. Structure that carries visual signals from the eye to the brain. Elevated pressure associated with glaucoma damages the optic nerve head, which can lead to blindness.

Ophthalmologist. A physician who specializes in the diagnosis and medical and surgical treatment of diseases and defects of the eye and related structures.

Ophthalmoscope. An instrument used to examine the interior of the eye through the pupil. Useful in detecting glaucoma damage to the optic nerve.

Retina. Light-sensitive part of the eye. Light is focused by the cornea and lens on photoreceptors in the retina.

Sclera. The white tissue making up the coat that surrounds the outside of the eye.

Steroids. A class of drugs used topically to reduce inflammation. Prolonged use of steroids can result in an elevation of pressure within the eye resembling open-angle glaucoma. Steroids are stopped when this occurs.

Tonometer. An instrument to measure pressure in the eye. There are two types of tonometers: *Non-contact*—deforms the eye with a puff of air and automatically records the pressure; *Applanation*—measures intraocular pressure by determination of the force necessary to flatten a cornea surface of constant size.

Trabecular meshwork. Sieve-like structure forming the canal leading to the channel between the cornea and sclera, the main route through which aqueous humor leaves the eye.

Tunnel vision. Vision in which the visual fields are severely constricted to about 10 degrees from the direction of the gaze. Common in retinitis pigmentosa and advanced chronic glaucoma.

Chapter 37

Take This Eye-Q Test on Glaucoma

Fifty million Americans are at risk for vision loss from glaucoma, a leading cause of blindness in the United States. Are you one of them? If you are, do you know how to reduce your risk of blindness? To determine how high your Eye-Q is, answer the following questions about glaucoma.

True or False?

1. Glaucoma is more common in Blacks than in Whites.

2. Glaucoma tends to run in families.

3. A person can have glaucoma and not know it.

4. People over age 60 are more likely to get glaucoma.

5. Eye pain is often a symptom of glaucoma.

6. Glaucoma can be controlled.

7. Glaucoma is caused by increased eye pressure.

8. Vision lost from glaucoma can be restored.

Unnumbered publication of the National Eye Health Education Program (a division of NIH).

9. A complete glaucoma exam consists only of measuring eye pressure.

10. People at risk for glaucoma should have an eye examination through dilated pupils.

To see if you have a perfect Eye-Q score, read the following answers. If you got 9 or 10 right, congratulations. You know a lot about glaucoma. If you missed some, review the answers so you can share your knowledge with your family and friends.

Answers

1. True. In a study funded by the National Eye Institute, researchers at The Johns Hopkins University reported that glaucoma is five times more likely to occur in Blacks than in Whites. In addition, glaucoma is four times more likely to cause blindness in Blacks than in Whites.

2. True. Although glaucoma tends to run in families, a hereditary basis has not been established. If someone in your immediate family has glaucoma, you should have your eyes examined through dilated pupils every two years.

3. True. The early stages of open-angle glaucoma, the most common form, usually have no warning signs. However, as the disease progresses, a person with glaucoma may notice his or her side vision gradually failing.

4. True. Everyone over age 60 has an increased risk for glaucoma. Other groups at increased risk include Blacks over age 40 and people with a family history of the disease.

5. False. People with glaucoma usually do not experience pain from the disease.

6. True. Although glaucoma cannot be cured, it usually can be controlled by eyedrops or pills, conventional surgery, or laser surgery. Sometimes eye care professionals will recommend a combination of surgery and medication.

7. True. In glaucoma, for reasons still not completely understood, fluid drains too slowly out of the eye. As the fluid builds up, the pressure inside the eye rises. Unless this pressure is controlled, it may cause damage to the optic nerve and other parts of the eye and loss of vision.

8. False. Vision loss from glaucoma is permanent. However, with early detection and treatment, the progression of visual loss can be slowed, or halted, and the risk of blindness reduced.

9. False. A measurement of eye pressure by tonometry, though an important part of a comprehensive eye exam, is by itself not sufficient for the detection of glaucoma. Glaucoma is detected most often during an eye examination through dilated pupils. This means drops are put into the eyes during the exam to enlarge the pupils, which allows the eye care professional to see more of the inside of the eye to check for signs of glaucoma. When indicated, a visual field test also should be performed.

10. True. An eye examination through dilated pupils is the best way to diagnose glaucoma. Individuals at increased risk for the disease should have their eyes examined through dilated pupils every two years by an eye care professional.

Get your eyes examined. Don't lose sight of glaucoma.

Chapter 38

National Eye Institute Report on Glaucoma

The word glaucoma is derived from the Greek and was used to describe blindness that occurred with age and that was associated with a bluish-green hue of the eye. The first association of disease with a rise in intraocular pressure (IOP) is found in 10th century Arabian writings. In the 19th century it was firmly established that glaucoma was separate from cataract and linked to elevated IOP.

Glaucoma is a heterogeneous group of disorders that share a distinct type of optic nerve damage which can lead to blindness. These diseases involve several individual tissues both at the front and the back of the eye and result in optic nerve damage, specifically the loss of retinal ganglion cells. Classically, it had been thought that IOP was the cause of glaucoma but it is now clear that IOP is only one of several risk factors. Indeed, there are some forms of glaucoma that seem to be independent of pressure within the eye. Recent advances in clinical and basic research have led to a greater understanding of the normal functions of the tissues usually involved in the disease. However, although this disease has been studied actively for over 100 years, we still lack understanding of the essential aspects of its molecular and cellular basis.

The heterogeneous nature of the disease is demonstrated by the variety of glaucoma syndromes that have been described. Primary open-angle glaucoma is the most prevalent form of the disease and generally is considered to be associated with a defect in the outflow

NIH Pub. No. 93–3196. Excerpt from *Vision Research: A National Plan*, pp.199–202.

drainage channel or trabecular meshwork (TM) in the front part of the eye. Angle-closure glaucoma is a mechanical form of the disease caused by contact of the iris with the TM, resulting in blockage of the drainage channels that allow fluid to escape from the eye. This form of glaucoma can be treated effectively in the early stages with a laser iridotomy procedure. More serious and harder to treat are congenital, developmental, and infantile glaucomas. Another group of glaucomas result from other ocular diseases that impair the outflow of aqueous humor from the eye and are called secondary glaucomas. Included in this category are glaucomas resulting from trauma and inflammatory diseases. Neovascular glaucoma can occur in people with retinal vascular disease, particularly diabetic retinopathy. Since people with diabetes now live longer, thanks to improved medical treatment, the incidence of this particular disease may increase.

Glaucoma is an insidious disease. Its most common form begins in midlife, progresses slowly, and robs functional vision until its progression is slowed by medical and/or surgical treatment. It progresses so slowly that some patients do not realize they have the disease until a large portion of their vision is irreversibly lost. One goal of research in early diagnosis of the disease is to recognize this early damage before it affects the patient's daily visual needs.

One major problem in glaucoma research continues to be the lack of an appropriate animal model system. Until one can be developed, the Glaucoma Program stresses the importance of clinical studies of human patients.

Program Description

Glaucoma is a major public health problem; approximately 80,000 Americans are blind from the most prevalent form of the disease, primary open-angle glaucoma. About 2 million people in the United States have the disease but, because of its insidious nature, a significant number of those afflicted are unaware of its presence. High IOP is the traditional indicator that one has the disease, and approximately 5 million Americans have elevated pressures. However, only a small percentage of these people actually will develop glaucoma. This subset of persons at risk for the disease but without actual visual field loss are called "ocular hypertensives." The dilemma for the clinician is whether or not to treat them as if they have overt glaucoma. Treatment trials designed to include a control arm of patients given no initial therapy have not been performed in the United States.

In the absence of better information, many clinicians treat these patients with medications—at considerable expense and attendant side effects.

The economic burden of glaucoma is difficult to estimate, but over 3 million annual office visits are needed in order to follow progression of the disease in the approximately 1 million patients under treatment. African-Americans have an age-adjusted risk for the disease about five times that of Caucasians. The rates for blindness due to primary open-angle glaucoma in African-Americans are six times higher than the rates in the rest of the population, reflecting not only an increased rate but more severe disease. Some patients, particularly those in socioeconomically disadvantaged minority groups, may have glaucoma but are slow to utilize health services to treat their disease. This is caused in part by the fact that they may not be able to afford treatment or may not have health insurance and in part by poor understanding of the disease.

Highlights of Recent Accomplishments

During the past 5 years there has been progress in both clinical and basic research in glaucoma. The techniques of molecular biology are being focused on the once intractable tissues involved in this disease. It has been known for some time that glaucoma patients are susceptible to steroid-induced increases in IOP. The use of cDNA cloning has made it possible to identify proteins induced in cultured human TM cells during exposure to steroids. A novel clone has been isolated that is expressed only in the presence of steroids. Thus, the linkage of a physiological event (i.e., response to steroids) with the induction of a specific protein may be an important clue in identifying the molecular mechanism of the pathogenesis of primary open-angle glaucoma. The presence of collagen has been studied in the optic nerve head. Cells of the lamina cribrosa, a meshwork of collagen and elastic tissue through which the individual nerves must pass on their way to the brain, have been found to produce increased type 1 collagen when exposed to increased pressure, as occurs in glaucoma. Since the optic nerve becomes damaged in glaucoma, any event that compromises the integrity of the nerve fibers, as might happen with increased buildup of collagen, could diminish optic nerve function and lead to vision loss.

Two clinical trials funded by the National Eye Institute (NEI) have yielded important information. Early results from the Glaucoma Laser

Trial (GLT) demonstrate that argon laser therapy may be a safe and effective alternative to medication as a first treatment for patients with newly diagnosed primary open-angle glaucoma. Traditionally medications are administered as the first therapeutic choice, but they are expensive and can have annoying and sometimes serious side effects. The Fluorouracil Filtering Surgery Study (FFSS) examined the effect of the drug 5-fluorouracil (5-FU) in slowing the growth of undesirable scar tissue, which may reverse the beneficial effects of surgery. This study showed an improvement in the surgical control of glaucoma in patients with certain poor-prognosis secondary glaucomas. Generally, patients receiving 5-FU were less likely to require further surgery and needed fewer or no daily medications.

An important diagnostic tool for detecting early disease is the noninvasive clinical assessment of the optic nerve head, which is the area in the back of the eye where all the retinal nerve fibers exit the globe to become the optic nerve. The earlier in the course of disease that loss of retinal nerve fibers can be detected, the earlier treatment can be instituted and vision spared. The development of computerized imaging techniques is in its initial stages and holds promise for early diagnosis of glaucoma and for following and comparing the effectiveness of treatment.

Recommended Program Structure

The Glaucoma Panel report is organized into the following two sections: (1) Epidemiology and Clinical Research and (2) Basic Science Research. The first section is divided into subprograms concerned with epidemiology, diagnosis, and treatment. The second section has been revised considerably from versions in previous NEI plans to reflect the growing opportunities and recent advances in such disciplines as molecular biology, cell biology, and physiology. This section reflects a philosophical shift in the program's description and direction away from the traditional anatomic sites of pathologic and structural change to the physiologic and biochemical mechanisms of disease. This has led to the new proposed Glaucoma Program structure listed below:

- Epidemiology and Clinical Research
  —Epidemiology
  —Diagnostic Modalities
  —Treatment.

- Basic Science Research
  - —Biochemistry
  - —Cell Biology
  - —Molecular Biology
  - —Pathobiology and Morphology
  - —Pharmacology
  - —Physiology.

Program Goals

The overall goal is to determine the pathogenesis of glaucoma in order to develop a better rationale for therapy. To achieve this, the following are important:

- To understand the cellular and molecular basis of ciliary body and TM function so that glaucomatous pathology can be understood better.

- To determine the physiologic mechanisms of optic nerve damage so that therapy can be designed to decrease the risk of vision loss from glaucoma.

- To determine the causes of glaucoma.

- To develop clinically relevant and reproducible diagnostic criteria for glaucoma and its progression.

- To identify risk factors for glaucoma.

- To develop more effective treatment of glaucoma.

- To determine the epidemiology of primary open-angle glaucoma in ethnically and geographically diverse subgroups.

Chapter 39

The Epidemiology of and Clinical Research on Glaucoma

Introduction

A description of the epidemiology of glaucoma requires definition of the disease itself. Traditionally, the glaucomas are defined as those diseases characterized by relative elevations in IOP with "pathologic" cupping of the optic disc. Cupping and visual field loss are considered to result from the elevation in pressure. The cause of this relative pressure elevation is often unknown.

In order to determine the public health burden of these diseases, their prevalence must be known. Prevalence refers to the number of cases existing in the population divided by the total number in the population, usually at a specific point in time. Prevalence data are important for planning economical health care delivery, and they provide clues to potential etiologic associations or risk factors. For example, an association between blood pressure and IOP was confirmed in the National Health and Nutrition Examination Survey prevalence data. If this association is found in subsequent incidence studies and if blood pressure influences the subsequent risk of developing open-angle glaucoma, appropriate treatment of blood pressure may alter disease progress and outcome.

Prevalence data also may provide clues about the existence of possible protective factors. For example, certain oxidative mechanisms

NIH Pub. No. 93–9186. Excerpt from *Vision Research: A National Plan*, pp. 202–14.

are related to aging in some body tissues. Antioxidants in the aqueous humor may play a role in delaying or preventing aging in the human trabeculum. Therefore, investigators are pursuing possible associations between oral intake of antioxidant nutrients and the prevalence of primary open-angle glaucoma. Finally, prevalence data provide important information for making policy decisions regarding payment for diagnostic procedures, therapy, and disability. Thus, accurate prevalence data are important for the allocation of scarce resources.

While prevalence data measure the magnitude of the problem, incidence data directly measure the risk of developing a disease. Incidence rates are computed on the basis of the subsequent development of a disease in a group of persons who are disease-free at a given time (usually determined during a prevalence survey). The defined group, or cohort, is then followed longitudinally for the development of new cases of the disease. In evaluating incidence data, comparisons are made between the rates of new disease in various defined subgroups to determine whether some have higher rates. Incidence data may give evidence of etiologic relationships. The incidence of primary open-angle glaucoma has been difficult to determine because of the large cohorts required in order to provide reliable estimates and the uncertainty surrounding the diagnosis of early disease. A consistent definition of disease would permit the computation and comparison of incidence rates.

African-Americans are at increased risk of primary open-angle glaucoma. An etiologic link between blood pressure and glaucoma should be investigated in African-Americans because they have a higher prevalence of high blood pressure, high IOP, and glaucoma. Potentially causal relationships such as these should be explored using incidence or longitudinal studies, because they allow evaluation of the antecedent-consequent relationships that are important in understanding the etiology of disease.

Epidemiology provides the tools necessary for developing etiologic insights and formulating hypotheses to develop meaningful, sight-saving interventions. Epidemiology is also the discipline that defines the frequency and scope of visual disabilities due to glaucoma that are an important public health problem in our community.

Subprogram Objectives

- To investigate differences in the distribution of primary open-angle glaucoma in communities of varying ethnic, social, and racial composition and to evaluate similarities and differences in risk factors between them.

- To use epidemiologic methods to develop reliable, valid criteria for the diagnosis and progression of primary open-angle glaucoma.

- To evaluate the distribution of diagnostic and therapeutic facilities and factors affecting patients' access to care, including cost barriers and geographic location, and how these influence disease outcome.

- To determine the public health burden of current visual impairment and blindness due to glaucoma and the cost-effectiveness of diagnostic and therapeutic regimens.

- To investigate the genetic components of primary open-angle glaucoma and determine whether there are specific inheritance patterns and genetic markers.

Current Level of National Eye Institute Support

The NEI supported seven grants for studies of the epidemiology of primary open-angle glaucoma in Fiscal Year (FY) 1992. Because this research area is of direct public health importance and is not significantly supported by other sources, expanded support through the NEI is needed. The total support for research in this subprogram area was $2,010,019.

Recent Accomplishments

Several large, population-based studies of prevalence and risk factors in primary open-angle glaucoma have been completed or are under way. They provide an opportunity for greater understanding of the relationship between IOP, other risk factors, and glaucomatous optic nerve damage.

Pilot data from the Barbados Eye Study, involving a predominantly African-American population, indicate that the prevalence of glaucoma in persons ages 54 or older is 13 percent. Preliminary data for the over 4,500 participants in this study confirm these findings and indicate a higher prevalence in males than females. Analyses are under way to determine factors that are associated with this high glaucoma risk. Additional information will be provided by the Barbados Incidence Study of Eye Diseases, which will follow up the Barbados Eye Study cohort, to measure incidence and further evaluate risk factors related to glaucoma development in the African-American population. Population-based studies, such as the Baltimore Eye Survey, the Barbados Eye Study, and the Saint Lucia Study, will provide additional information on the very high prevalence of glaucoma in African-Americans and the rates at which glaucomatous optic nerve damage increases with age. Data from the Baltimore Eye Survey suggest that glaucoma occurs four times more frequently in African-Americans than in Caucasians. The Baltimore Eye Survey documents that one-half of the individuals with primary open-angle glaucoma are unaware of it; one-half of the patients with glaucomatous optic nerve damage have IOPs less than or equal to 21 mm Hg at their baseline examination, again confirming the inadequacy of tonometry as a useful screening tool; and, very importantly from a health services standpoint, more than 90 percent of those who do not know they have glaucoma were seen by a primary care physician during the preceding 2 years.

The Beaver Dam (Wisconsin) Eye Study is a study—in a predominantly white population—of the most frequent causes of decreased vision in Americans. To date 3.1 percent report having glaucoma, 0.4 percent report having had glaucoma surgery, and 2.4 percent are taking drops for glaucoma. Of those with no history of glaucoma, 4.9 percent have IOPs greater than 21 mm Hg in at least one eye. Although preliminary, these data suggest that the frequency of glaucoma in the Caucasian population is also substantial. Prevalence data from the Beaver Dam Eye Study will provide some insight into questions regarding the effectiveness of care. Preliminary data indicate that about 40 percent of those with a history of glaucoma have IOPs higher than 21 mm Hg, and even among those who are taking medication, more than 40 percent have high pressures. Similar epidemiologic data are being accumulated in other countries.

Cohort studies indicate which of the factors measured in prevalence studies predict development or progression of glaucoma. Such research suggests that a glaucomatous eye with IOP within the "normal" range, but higher than in the fellow eye, may be predisposed to greater visual field loss than occurs in the fellow eye. In the current longitudinal studies, other prospective hypotheses will be investigated.

Important Research Questions to Be Addressed

The following research questions need to be addressed:

What are appropriate diagnostic criteria for primary open-angle glaucoma?

Comparative and collaborative efforts are needed to develop diagnostic criteria for primary open-angle glaucoma. Without development of uniform criteria, it is difficult to make comparisons between studies and even more difficult to define etiologic pathways.

Low-tension glaucoma by definition is not associated with relative elevations in IOP. There are many studies indicating that using an upper-bound IOP (e.g., >21 mm Hg) as the sole diagnostic criterion for glaucoma is not appropriate. Similarly, the optic nerve cup shows variable size within the normal population. Whether a "ratio" exists that is definitely abnormal is not clear. Additionally, most cups are not perfectly symmetric nor do their configurations always parallel the contours of the optic disc. Which geometric shapes are clearly pathologic needs to be defined. Hemorrhage on the optic disc needs further study to clarify its potential role in glaucoma pathogenesis.

To date, the visual field examination is the most important indicator of functional vision loss due to glaucoma. However, even its role as a definitive diagnostic test is being scrutinized. The frequency of true abnormalities of the visual field in populations free of glaucoma is not certain, and the importance of false-positive and false-negative responses is not known. Because it is a psychophysical test, perimetry requires some understanding, cooperation, and stamina on the part of the subject. Various investigators have suggested tests and parameters to be added to the list of criteria used to diagnose glaucoma.

What are appropriate criteria for diagnosing progression of open-angle glaucoma?

Agreement on these criteria would facilitate comparison of risk factors between studies and the effects of intervention on progression. Specification of these criteria for visual field endpoint criteria in glaucoma clinical studies was discussed at a workshop sponsored by the NEI in May 1990. No consensus could be reached, and it was clear from this meeting that the definition of clinically and statistically significant endpoints needs further refinement. It will be necessary to hold further dialogue on this subject.

What is the distribution of primary open-angle glaucoma in different racial and ethnic groups?

Important areas of further epidemiologic inquiry include descriptive studies of glaucoma in people of different ethnic and racial backgrounds. These groups include African-Americans, Native Americans, Hispanic Americans, Asian-Americans, and other ethnic groups in this country. Causal pathways of glaucoma-related optic nerve damage in those groups known to be at high risk need to be defined so that possibilities for prevention can be explored.

What are the risk factors for incidence and progression of primary open-angle glaucoma?

Longitudinal studies of patients whose disease spans the spectrum of severity and treatment are needed to determine the natural history of this disease. Then it will be possible to investigate some of the more difficult management questions.

How does glaucoma influence the quality of life?

There is a growing recognition of the importance of evaluating the health outcomes and quality-of-life changes imposed by glaucoma and its treatment. This is a relatively new area for disease-oriented epidemiology but is probably more important to the patient than change in IOP as a measure of successful glaucoma treatment.

Is there evidence of heritability of the types of open-angle glaucoma?

A positive family history has been noted in many cases of glaucoma. There are systemic and ocular developmental syndromes that appear to have clear genetic transmission patterns. For primary open-angle glaucoma, the relative influence of genetic and environmental characteristics is unknown. Some of the "family tendency" is speculated to be related to iris color or anatomy of the globe. Although some study designs and techniques are unique to population genetics, it may be for epidemiologists to estimate the heritable component for primary open-angle glaucoma.

Chapter 40

Basic Science Research on Glaucoma

Introduction

Biochemical approaches to study glaucoma focus on the characterization of extracellular matrix (ECM) components, cytoskeletal elements, and other proteins in the anterior chamber angle tissues and
in the optic nerve head. Hence, some subjects in this section overlap
with the Cell Biology, Molecular Biology, and other sections. However,
the Biochemistry subprogram distinguishes itself from others by placing emphasis on the identification, characterization, and enzymology
of specific biomolecules.

The ECM consists of various proteins that are linked together covalently or noncovalently to form an insoluble composite. Each of the
two major types of matrices, the interstitial matrix and the basal
lamina, contains collagens, cellbinding glycoproteins, and proteoglycans. These macromolecules, as well as cytoskeletal components and
other proteins, may be important in the regulation of outflow resistance through the TM in primary open-angle glaucoma. Cupping of
the optic nerve head, clinically associated with glaucoma, may result
from compression, stretching, and rearrangement of the connective
tissue of the lamina cribrosa. Although advances have been made and
valuable information has been acquired, the biochemical basis of outflow obstruction and the roles of aqueous humor constituents need to

NIH Pub. No. 93–3186. Excerpt from *Vision Research: A National Plan*, pp.
214–41.

be determined. A greater understanding of the basic biochemical alterations that occur in glaucoma is essential for improved treatment of the disease.

Subprogram Objectives

- To characterize specific macromolecules, such as ECM components and cytoskeletal elements in the TM, iris, ciliary process, sclera, and optic nerve head.

- To determine the roles played by specific macromolecules in outflow resistance and in maintenance of compliance and resilience of the optic nerve head.

- To evaluate changes in specific macromolecules as a function of age, race, and disease in order to determine the biologic significance of gene regulation by factors such as hormones and aqueous humor components.

- To investigate the influence of aqueous humor constituents in regulating levels of metabolic activity in the chamber angle tissue.

Current Level of National Eye Institute Support

In FY 1992 the NEI supported seven research grants at a total cost of $1,377,806 which included biochemical studies of the tissues and cells related to glaucoma. A majority of these grants supported research efforts dealing with the cellular and extracellular structure and materials in the TM, reflecting a traditional concentrated interest in this tissue.

Recent Accomplishments

The ECM components, especially proteoglycans, in TM tissues have been studied extensively. Three major types have been identified: (1) chondroitin, (2) dermatan, and (3) heparan sulfate proteoglycans. Hyaluronic acid also has been found. Enzymatic perfusion studies suggest that these molecules play a role in the maintenance of resistance to aqueous humor outflow. With aging there seems to be a loss of collagen-associated chondroitin and dermatan sulfate proteoglycans in both normal and glaucomatous tissues. A reduction in hyaluronic acid and an increase in an unidentified sulfated material also have been associated with glaucoma.

Interstitial collagen types I, III, and V; basement membrane collagen type IV; and collagen types VI and VIII have been identified in the TM. Many of these collagen types also have been found in such tissues as the conjunctiva, cornea, and the lung. Each tissue has its unique three-dimensional arrangement formed by the heterotypic mixture of collagen fibers. It is believed that the TM functions as a valve structure and its three-dimensional array is constructed to accommodate extensibility and resilience. The spatial organization of fibrils involves interactions between the collagens and such adhesion proteins as fibronectin and laminin. The presence of these proteins, as well as elastin, has been well demonstrated in the TM, although how the macromolecules are assembled and regulated remain unclear. The precise role of the ECM components in the outflow resistance also awaits clarification. Nevertheless it is significant that abnormal accumulation of extracellular plaque material containing type VI collagen and fibronectin has been found in the juxtacanalicular mesh work in glaucoma.

In the optic nerve head, interstitial collagen types I and III and elastin have been found in the core of the lamina cribrosa beams and optic nerve septa. Collagen type IV, laminin, and heparan sulfate proteoglycan are localized to the basement membranes of the vasculature and astrocytes. Type VI collagen is distributed under the basement membrane of the cribriform plates and blood vessel and throughout the core. Chondroitin/dermatan sulfate proteoglycans, heparan sulfate proteoglycan, and hyaluronic acid also are present. *In situ* hybridization has been used to identify specific cell types in the optic nerve head that synthesize types I and IV collagens. An increase in the level of these ECM proteins with aging has been observed. The age-related increase appears to be greater in blacks than in whites for collagen type I, but the pattern is reversed for type IV collagen. It also has been found that increased pressure causes lamina cribrosa cells to elongate and produce more collagen type I in tissue culture. In the lamina cribrosa of eyes with primary open-angle glaucoma, progressive changes in the distribution and amount of fibers of elastin have been described and correlated to the loss of optic nerve compliance.

The sclera contains mainly collagen types I, III, and V and two types of dermatan sulfate proteoglycans. Type IV collagen and laminin, which are found in the lamina cribrosa, have not been found in the sclera. Collagen type VI, fibronectin, and laminin have been demonstrated recently in the iris and the ciliary body.

The ECM may be remodeled in response to exogenous stimuli. The production of proteoglycans, collagens, fibronectin, laminin, and other glycoproteins by TM cells has been reported to be affected quantitatively and/or qualitatively by factors such as glucocorticoids, glycosaminoglycan-degrading enzymes, and ascorbic acid. The turnover of the protein components of ECM involves the following two main classes of enzymes: (1) the plasminogen activator/plasmin family and (2) the metalloproteinases. The former has been found in the TM, ciliary body, and optic nerve. Metalloproteinases also have been demonstrated in the TM. The transcription of the metalloproteinase genes is responsive to substances such as fibroblast growth factor and interleukin-1. Degradative enzymes also are implicated in the remodeling of connective tissues in the lamina cribrosa observed in glaucomatous conditions. Further studies, however, are necessary to discern the exact roles of the various enzymes and inhibitors.

TM cells contain three major types of cytoskeletal elements: actin filaments, microtubules, and intermediate filaments containing vimentin and desmin. Sulfhydryl agents, cytoskeleton-active drugs, and glucocorticoids cause marked alterations of these elements that correlate with changes in the overall cell shape and organization. However, it has yet to be established whether such changes have an impact on the function of TM cells *in vivo*. In the ciliary epithelium, coexpression of cytokeratin and vimentin has been detected. This pattern is similar to that found in other neuroepithelial cells with secretory function.

Analyses of protein profiles of the normal human TM suggest an age-related decrease in actin levels and an increase in type IV collagen. Comparison of proteins from calf and cow TM reveals that protein aggregation appears to occur with aging. The aggregation may result from oxidative stress and may relate to increased outflow resistance.

A series of recent studies has demonstrated that bovine aqueous humor obstructs flow through microporous filters. The aqueous humor contains many proteins; among them fibroblast growth factor, transferrin, and transforming growth factor B have been identified. The sources of these factors are as yet unclear. In glaucomatous eyes, the aqueous humor has a higher protein content than that of normal eyes, but there seems to be only minor changes in protein profiles.

Important Research Questions to Be Addressed

Research questions to be addressed include the following:

What is the molecular basis for conventional outflow resistance in normal and glaucomatous eyes?

Cytoskeletal elements, extracellular matrix, and hydrophobic proteins may be contributing factors, but it is still not clear what determines outflow resistance. Questions about the exact nature of these molecules and their assembly, regulation, and localization in the anterior chamber need to be addressed. As an aid to understanding how these molecules function in the tissues, antibody perturbation experiments may be used. Additionally, genes for a specific type of macromolecule may be deleted, altered, or expressed in transfected cells or transgenic animals in an effort to determine the full implication of a loss or gain of function phenotype.

What are the roles of ECM components in maintaining the compliance and resilience of the optic nerve head?

Characterization should be continued of both the ECM macromolecules in the optic nerve head and of the cells involved in the synthesis of ECM. The biomechanical properties need to be determined of the connective tissue and the structural and functional roles of ECM molecules.

What controls the production of ECM proteins, cytoskeletal elements, and other key proteins in the outflow pathway and in the optic nerve head?

Observations have been made of variation in expression of some proteins in the optic nerve head. Evaluation needs to be conducted on the basis of this variation and its relationship to glaucoma development and optic nerve cupping. Since the operative mechanisms may be different for each tissue, the processes controlling the gene expression of the various proteins need to be determined for all chamber angle tissues and for the optic nerve head. In addition, the following are of relevance and should be investigated further: gene regulation by hormones, growth factors, aqueous humor components, pressure elevation, mechanical force, and oxidative stress.

What regulates the metabolic activities of anterior segment tissues?

Cells communicate with various ECM components using surface receptors. Several classes of receptors, particularly one major gene superfamily called integrin receptors have been defined. The integrin receptors are transmembrane glycoproteins which bind to one or more ECM proteins, interact with cytoskeletal elements, and function as signaling molecules to initiate a cascade of intracellular events. In the anterior segment and the optic nerve head, work needs to be done to determine whether or which types of integrins and other classes of receptors are present. Are the receptors in the optic nerve head similar to those in the anterior segment? How do they regulate properties and functions of cells in the TM, ciliary body, and lamina cribrosa?

Changes in aqueous humor constituents have been noted in patients with glaucoma. Are such changes a result of the disease, or do they in fact cause glaucomatous conditions? How do these changes affect the cells in the anterior chamber? Cytokines and mediators secreted by immune cells and parenchymal cells of the eye have regulatory as well as immunosuppressive properties. Studies of such immunosuppressive factors may be relevant to wound healing and the growth of tissues and cells of the outflow track.

Chapter 41

National Eye Institute Fact Sheet on the Therapeutic Use of Marijuana for Glaucoma

Description of Glaucoma

In glaucoma, pressure within the eye is elevated to a level that leads to damage to the optic nerve and subsequent loss of visual function. The most common form of the disease, chronic, open-angle glaucoma, is a leading cause of blindness in the United States and the number one cause of blindness in Blacks.

In a normal eye, aqueous humor, a clear, nutrient-rich fluid secreted by the ciliary body passes continuously through the pupil and into a small space at the front of the eye, between the iris and the lens, called the anterior chamber. As it leaves this area, the aqueous humor flows to the periphery of the chamber, called the angle, where it exits through a complex channel system and drains into blood vessels in and near the sclera, the white outer coat of the eye.

In an eye with open-angle glaucoma, because of obstruction within this channel system that is not fully understood, the aqueous humor drains too slowly from the eye. This creates a chronic rise in intraocular pressure, resulting in progressive destruction of nerve fibers that are essential for vision.

At its onset, open-angle glaucoma usually has no symptoms. There is no pain, no blurring of vision, and no ocular inflammation to alert someone that he or she has the disease. But, as open-angle glaucoma progresses, it will slowly begin to destroy peripheral vision. It is at

NIH unnumbered publication dated June 1994.

this point that most people seek treatment. However, vision that has already been lost from glaucoma cannot be restored.

Effective Glaucoma Treatments

Although glaucoma cannot be cured, intraocular pressure can usually be effectively controlled with several existing medical and surgical treatments. These include:

Medications. Currently, 24 agents, all approved by the Food and Drug Administration, are incorporated into a variety of prescription drugs used for glaucoma treatment. These medications, in the form of eyedrops or pills, either enhance the drainage of fluid from the eye or decrease the production of aqueous humor. Unfortunately, because anti-glaucoma drugs enter the blood, they can cause various systemic side effects such as headaches and respiratory problems. In addition, a given drug may lose its effectiveness over time. However, because of the availability of so many different anti-glaucoma agents, when such problems occur eye care professionals can usually substitute alternative, effective treatment regimens.

Laser Surgery. Glaucoma treatment employing an argon laser has proved beneficial in NEI-sponsored clinical trials. In this form of treatment, a high-energy beam of light is directed onto the trabecular meshwork—part of the anterior chamber's drainage system—and approximately 100 tiny laser burns are made on its surface. The burns stretch the existing holes in the meshwork for better fluid drainage. Laser surgery, however, may be effective for only a short time and usually is used in conjunction with drops or pills.

Incisional Surgery. Several procedures may be performed to improve drainage flow, such as a trabeculotomy, trabeculectomy, and subscleral filtering surgery. All of these involve making a small hole in the anterior chamber through which fluid can leave the eye. Although these procedures have a fairly high success rate, they are generally reserved until medical therapy is no longer effective.

Marijuana as a Treatment for Glaucoma

Marijuana is a complex mixture of numerous chemical components, some of which have biological activity. Studies in the early 1970s showed that marijuana, when smoked, lowers the intraocular pressure in people with normal pressure and in those with glaucoma.

To follow up on these findings in an effort to determine whether marijuana and/or its derivatives might be effective as a glaucoma treatment, the National Eye Institute (NEI), one of the Federal government's National Institutes of Health, supported several research studies from 1978 to 1988. Studies using topical preparations containing marijuana derivatives did not demonstrate lowering of intraocular pressure in human subjects. Other studies demonstrated that one of marijuana's derivatives, delta-9-tetrahydrocannabinol (THC), as well as some other cannabinoids, lower intraocular pressure when administered by various routes: smoking, orally, or intravenously. However, none of these studies demonstrated that marijuana—or any of its components—could safely and effectively lower intraocular pressure enough to prevent optic nerve damage from glaucoma. Simply lowering intraocular pressure does not necessarily control the disease, as research with other potential glaucoma drugs has shown.

Furthermore, these studies have shown that smoking marijuana produces undesirable side effects for glaucoma patients, such as elevated blood pressure, dry eye, and euphoria in the majority of patients studied. Glaucoma patients who regularly and chronically smoke marijuana would also be at risk for respiratory system damage. In addition, the long-term ocular and systemic effects of marijuana use by glaucoma patients is unknown. There is considerable variability in the composition and quality of marijuana from supply to supply. In addition, smoking is a less than optimal drug delivery system. Without a standardized product and method of assuring the bioavailability of its active ingredients, marijuana is problematic as a therapy for glaucoma.

Conclusions

Presently, there is no scientifically verifiable evidence that marijuana or its derivatives are safe and effective in the treatment of glaucoma. The availability of a wide variety of alternative treatments that do not have marijuana's psychoactive and other specific side effects argues against the use of marijuana for treating glaucoma. Marijuana offers no advantage over currently available glaucoma drugs and indeed may be less effective than these agents.

Contacts

For general information on glaucoma treatments, individuals may contact:

Office of Health Education and Communication
National Eye Institute
Building 31, Room 6A32
Bethesda, MD 20892
(301) 496-5248

American Academy of Ophthalmology
P.O. Box 7424
San Francisco, CA 94109-7424
(415) 561-8500

For information on glaucoma treatment for specific patients, physicians may contact:

Wiley Chambers, M.D.
Supervising Medical Officer
Division of Topical Drugs
Food and Drug Administration
5600 Fishers Lane
Rockville, MD 20857
(301) 443-4310

Part Six

Cataracts

Chapter 42

Cataracts

What is a cataract?

A cataract is a cloudy or opaque area in the lens of the eye. The lens is located behind the pupil and iris. It helps focus light onto the retina, the light-sensitive tissue that lines the inside of the back of the eye. Usually, the lens is transparent. But if it becomes clouded, the passage of light is obstructed and vision may be impaired.

What causes a cataract?

When a cataract forms, there is a change in the chemical composition of the lens, but scientists do not know exactly what causes these chemical changes. The most common form of cataract is related to aging, although this type can occur at age 50 or even earlier. Cataracts also may be associated with diabetes, other systemic diseases, drugs, and eye injuries. Sometimes babies are born with congenital cataracts or develop them during the early years of life.

What are the symptoms of a cataract?

Cataracts usually develop gradually, without pain, redness, or tearing in the eye. Some cataracts never progress to the point where they seriously impair vision, whereas others eventually block most or all

NIH Pub. No. 93–201.

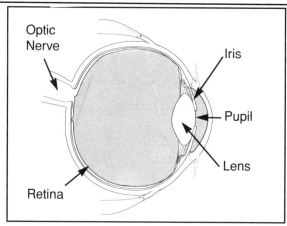

Figure 42.1.

vision in the affected eye. The effect of a cataract on vision depends on several things: 1) its size, 2) its density, 3) its location within the lens.

Among the signs that a cataract may be forming are:

• Hazy, fuzzy, or blurred vision. Double vision sometimes occurs, but this usually goes away as the cataract worsens.

• The need for frequent changes in eyeglass prescriptions. When the cataract progresses beyond a certain point, these changes no longer improve vision.

• A feeling of having a film over the eyes, or of looking through veils or a waterfall. The person with a cataract may blink a lot in an effort to see better.

• Changes in the color of the pupil, which is usually black. When the eye is examined, the pupil may look grey, yellow, or white, but color changes are not always noticeable.

• Problems with light. For example, night driving becomes harder because the cloudy part of the lens scatters the light from on-coming headlights, making these lights appear double or daz-zling. Also, the person with a cataract may have trouble finding the right amount of light for reading or close work.

- "Second sight"—a temporary improvement in reading vision experienced by some people when their cataract reaches a certain stage of development. As the cataract progresses, vision again worsens.

None of these symptoms necessarily means that a person has a cataract, or if a cataract is present that it must be removed. However, people who have any of these symptoms should see an eye doctor.

When should a cataract be removed?

A cataract should be removed surgically when it has progressed to the point where resulting vision problems interfere with one's daily activities. A second reason for cataract surgery, more urgent but less common than the first, is that the cataract has become completely opaque (mature). It is possible for a mature cataract to swell and even disintegrate inside the eye. Such changes can permanently endanger vision.

With congenital cataracts, it used to be standard practice to postpone surgery until the child was at least 6 months old. Recently, however, cataracts have been removed from the eyes of newborn infants with good results. Early removal of severe congenital cataract(s) is an important advance because it reduces the risk of visual loss resulting from the disuse of one or both eyes during childhood.

How are cataracts treated?

Treating cataracts really involves two steps. The first is removal of the clouded lens by an ophthalmologist. Surgery is the only method proven effective for removing cataracts. The second is finding an appropriate substitute for the natural lens. The decision about which substitute lens to use is usually made before surgery.

There are two general methods of removing a cataract: intracapsular and extracapsular extraction of the lens. Intracapsular extraction is sometimes used to remove senile cataracts. In this method, the entire lens, including its capsule, is removed.

Extracapsular extraction involves removal of most lens tissue but the back part of the lens capsule is left in place. In infants and young children, whose lenses are relatively soft, the lens tissue may be withdrawn through a hollow needle, a procedure called aspiration. A variety of extracapsular techniques are also used to remove the lens in adults.

One technique is called phacoemulsification. High-frequency sound vibrations (ultrasound) are used to soften and liquify the lens so it can be aspirated through the needle.

Phacoemulsification should not be confused with another form of eye surgery, photocoagulation, in which laser light—not ultrasound— is used to treat some eye disorders other than cataract. A laser cannot remove a cloudy lens or make it clear again. However, some doctors may use a laser to open the front part of the lens capsule before removing the lens or to help patients who develop "after-cataract." (See "What happens after surgery?")

How safe is cataract surgery?

Cataract surgery is one of the most successful operations done today—more than 90 percent of the people who have this surgery find that they can see better. Complications may occur, but most are treatable. Serious complications that threaten vision are rare.

Certain people may not benefit much from cataract surgery. They include people whose cataracts are not advanced enough to impair vision seriously and those whose vision is impaired by another eye disease as well.

In summary, each cataract patient should discuss the possibility of surgery with the doctor who examines his or her eyes to determine whether the potential benefits of cataract surgery outweigh the risks. It is also very important to decide in advance, with the help of the doctor, what form of substitute lens would be most suitable. Patients may want to get a second opinion on the advisability of surgery and on the most appropriate substitute lens to use after surgery.

What are the choices for a substitute lens?

There are three options for replacing the natural lens removed in cataract surgery: eyeglasses, contact lenses, or an intraocular lens implant. Each has advantages and drawbacks.

Eyeglasses. This is a safe and time-proven solution to the problem of seeing without a natural lens. But cataract eyeglasses can have some unpleasant effects. Patients may be bothered by the fact that these glasses magnify objects 20-35 percent, affect depth perception until the person relearns how to judge distances, and limit side vision.

If only one eye requires cataract surgery, eyeglasses may well cause problems because the person is unable to fuse the different-sized images

360

formed by the operated and unoperated eyes. Such patients are often advised before surgery that it would be best to use a contact lens, or have a lens implant.

Contact lenses. These usually provide better vision than eyeglasses and also are quite safe if handled and maintained properly. A contact lens may be especially helpful after cataract extraction in one eye. With a contact lens in the operated eye, the difference in the size of the images seen by the two eyes is much smaller. Soft contact lenses are commonly used for cataract patients.

Another option is the *extended-wear contact lens.* These lenses can be left in the eye for a longer period of time without being removed, even for sleep. They may be especially useful for people who have trouble inserting and removing a contact lens, because an eye care specialist can remove and clean them periodically. However, extended-wear lenses have some disadvantages: They are very fragile; some serious infections have been reported; their long-term safety is still being assessed; and they do require periodic removal, cleaning, and reinserting.

Intraocular lenses. These devices, sometimes called IOLs, are clear plastic lenses that are implanted in the eye during the cataract operation. Lens implants have certain advantages: They usually eliminate or minimize the problems with image size, side vision, and depth perception noted by people who wear cataract eyeglasses. Also, because lens implants remain in the eye and do not have to be removed, cleaned, and reinserted, they are more convenient than contact lenses. This is particularly true for people who have physical problems that would make it difficult for them to carry out the procedures involved in using contact lenses.

Because of these advantages, lens implants have been used with increasing frequency in recent years. About three-fourths of all people now undergoing cataract surgery have an IOL inserted at the same time, and the vast majority are very pleased with the results. Of course ophthalmologists will continue to study IOLs for many years in an effort to assess the long-term effects of implantation on the eye as well as the short-term complications.

What happens after surgery?

Most people who undergo cataract surgery are treated as outpatients and can go home the same day. For others, a stay in the hospital of 1 to 3 days may be required. In either case, during the early stages of recovery, patients need to take special care to avoid strenuous physical activity.

Sometimes people whose cataract surgery was performed by the extracapsular method develop a problem called "after-cataract." After the operation, the back part of the lens capsule left in the eye may become cloudy and interfere with passage of light to the retina.

The cloudy material must be cleared away, if possible, so that full vision can be restored. Ophthalmologists often treat after-cataract with an ophthalmic laser called the neodymium-YAG or "cold" laser. When this procedure is successful, the patient's vision is restored without additional eye surgery.

What research is being done on cataracts?

National Eye Institute supports and conducts research on the eye and its disorders, including cataracts. The major goals of this research are to learn more about how and why cataracts develop, to find ways of preventing cataracts or slowing their progress, to evaluate the safety and effectiveness of techniques for treating cataracts, and to devise better methods of correcting vision after cataract surgery.

Chapter 43

Lifting the Clouds of Cataracts

You're approaching retirement, feeling healthy and looking forward to many more active and productive years. But then your vision begins to grow cloudy. Everything you look at has a yellowish tint. Simple tasks like reading or driving a car become difficult. Street signs and faces aren't as sharp as they once were. Bright sun and auto headlights hurt your eyes. New eyeglass prescriptions improve vision for a while—but eventually they no longer help.

The culprit is cataracts, a condition that will beset most people if they live long enough. This disorder affects 60 percent of people older than 60 and occurs when the normally clear, aspirin-sized lens of the eye starts to become cloudy, impairing vision.

Experts estimate that 1.2 million Americans will be diagnosed in 1989 with cataracts that require treatment, compared with 123,000 in 1978. Most of the increase is due to the growing numbers of elderly in the United States, many of whom want to continue driving cars, reading and traveling—activities for which clear sight is vital.

Until recently, anyone who developed cataracts and needed surgery faced a procedure that involved pain and often less than satisfactory results. Until the late 1970s, doctors removed the cloudy lens in a surgical procedure that required a hospital stay of five to seven days. Afterward, the patient had to wear thick "Coke bottle" glasses or contact lenses—neither of which could completely restore vision to its previous level.

FDA Consumer Magazine. DHHS Pub. No. (FDA) 92–1183.

Today, there's little need for such complicated treatment. Advances in medicine have made cataracts much less worrisome. Now, the clouded lens is surgically removed and replaced with a plastic intraocular lens (IOL) in an hour-long operation that often requires no hospitalization.

"The intraocular lens has revolutionized the treatment of cataracts," says Carl Kupfer, M.D., director of the National Eye Institute in Bethesda, Md. "Implantation of the lens is one of the most successful operations in medicine."

How a Cataract Forms

A cataract forms in the eye's lens, the transparent structure behind the iris (the colored membrane surrounding the pupil). The lens focuses light on the retina, the light-sensitive membrane at the back of the eye which converts light impulses into nerve signals to produce clear visual images. Clouding of the lens—much like smearing grease over the lens of a camera—can develop at any age but most often appears in people older than 42.

Most cataracts are caused by a change in the chemical composition of the lens. In a small percentage of cases, the chemical changes are caused by a hereditary enzyme defect, trauma to the eye, diabetes, or use of certain drugs, such as the steroid prednisone.

Precisely why cataracts occur with age is unknown, but ultraviolet radiation, particularly from the sun, is thought to play a major role in creating the chemical change in the lens responsible for most cataracts. Experimental evidence suggests that UV radiation can cloud the lens by forming highly reactive chemical fragments called "free radicals." These, in turn, disrupt the delicate structure of the lens. The type of ultraviolet radiation from the sun called UVB—the kind that causes blistering sunburn and skin cancer—is thought to be a major factor because the lens absorbs these rays.

Indeed, in a recent study of 838 Chesapeake Bay professional fishermen, Hugh Taylor, M.D., of Johns Hopkins Hospital in Baltimore, Md., found a strong association between ultraviolet radiation and cataract formation. Fishermen with the highest levels of ultraviolet radiation exposure had three times the risk of contracting cataracts compared with those with the least exposure. Those with cataracts had 20 percent more exposure to sunlight in every year of life. Taylor's studies suggest that cataracts can be prevented by avoiding sun exposure between 10 a.m. and 4 p.m., when sunlight is strongest, and by wearing a wide-brimmed hat and sunglasses.

A cataract can develop so slowly that a person may not even know it's there. If the cataract is on the outer edge of the lens, no change in vision may be noticeable. Cloudiness near the center of the lens, however, usually interferes with clear sight.

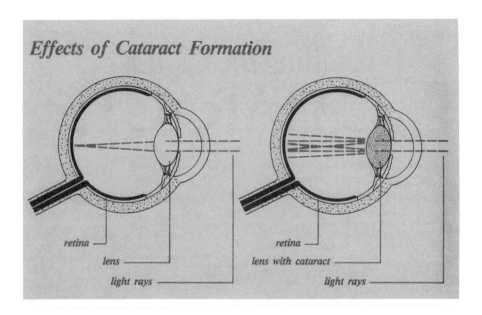

Effects of Cataract Formation

retina

lens

light rays

retina

lens with cataract

light rays

Figure 43.1. *In normal vision, the lens focuses light on the retina, producing clear visual images. When the lens is clouded by a cataract light cannot be properly transmitted to the retina, and vision problems occur.*

Symptoms

Symptoms of developing cataracts include double or blurred vision, sensitivity to light and glare (which may make driving difficult), less vivid perception of color, and frequent changes in eyeglass prescriptions. As the cataract grows worse, stronger glasses no longer improve sight, although holding objects nearer to the eye may help reading and close-up work. The pupil, which normally appears black, may undergo noticeable color changes and appear to be yellowish or white, says Peter Hersh, M.D., an assistant surgeon at Boston's Massachusetts Eye and Ear Infirmary.

Cataracts are typically detected through a medical eye examination. The usual test for visual acuity, the letter eye chart, may not, however, reflect the true nature of visual loss, says the American Academy of Ophthalmology. Other tests—which measure glare sensitivity, contrast sensitivity, night vision, color vision, and side or central vision—help nail down the diagnosis.

Because most cataracts associated with aging develop slowly, many patients may not notice their visual loss until it has become severe. Some cataracts remain small and never need treatment; others grow more quickly and progressively larger. Only when a cataract seriously interferes with normal activities is it time to consider surgery, doctors say. People who depend on their eyes for work, play and other activities may want their cataracts removed earlier than those whose needs are less demanding.

Some experts estimate that about 88 of every 100 persons receiving IOLs will achieve 20/40 vision or better. (An individual with 20/40 vision can read letters on an eye chart from 20 feet away, while a person with normal 20/20 vision can read the chart from 40 feet away; 20/40 vision is good enough to get a driver's license in most states.) Among those who do not have other eye diseases, about 94 of 100 will achieve 20/40 vision.

Treatment Options

During the diagnostic examination, an ophthalmologist will carefully measure the shape, size and general health of the eye to determine whether a lens implant will be effective. In the relatively small number of cases where it won't be, eyeglasses or contact lenses will improve vision after traditional cataract surgery. Glasses, while used for years, have drawbacks. Their extreme thickness makes them unattractive and heavy. Magnification and distortion of the visual image causes objects to appear closer and 25 percent larger than they are. Peripheral vision may be reduced. Contact lenses provide fairly good vision, but many elderly people have trouble inserting, removing and cleaning them.

An implanted IOL is usually the best replacement. Because the implant is placed in or near the original position of the removed natural lens, vision is restored with good peripheral vision and depth perception yet with minimal magnification and distortion.

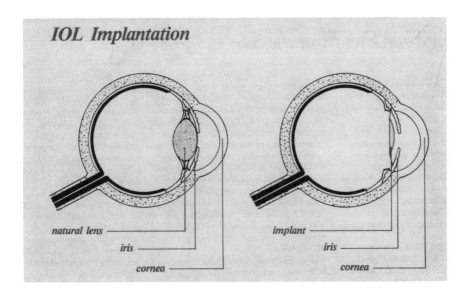

IOL Implantation

natural lens

iris

cornea

implant

iris

cornea

Figure 43.2. In IOL implantation, the clouded natural lens is removed and replaced by an implanted lens.

Getting an IOL

IOLs remain permanently in place, require no maintenance or handling, and are neither felt by the patient nor noticed by others. Eyeglasses with thin lenses for near or distant viewing may still be required, but thick glasses are not necessary. A doctor can determine the appropriate implant prescription with an ultrasound device that measures eye length and corneal curvature. These measurements are combined by computer to calculate the lens power required.

The standard surgical procedure, which ranges in cost from $3,000 to $5,000, is performed in a hospital or doctor's office. Peering through an operating microscope, the surgeon makes a minute, curved incision in the cornea—the surface of the eye. Then the clouded lens is cut loose with a thin needle and suctioned out, leaving intact the rear wall of the transparent capsule that encloses the lens.

The surgeon enlarges the original incision, and the new lens—a clear hard plastic disc—is then slipped in behind the iris and up against the back wall of the capsule. Two tiny "c" shaped arms attached to the lens eventually become scarred into the side of the eye and hold

367

the lens firmly in place. The incision is closed with 7 to 10 nearly invisible stitches of fine nylon or silk.

In a newer method, an ultrasonic probe enters the cut in the cornea and high-speed vibrations break the lens into microscopic flecks that are then removed by suction. A folded flexible plastic lens one-quarter of an inch in diameter can be inserted through the cut with a scissors-like device called an injector and positioned behind the pupil against the capsule wall. Once in place, the injector is removed and the lens opens.

The flexible lens is one of two advances already on the market in half a dozen European countries. This softer lens, designed to allow a smaller incision and thus less tissue damage than implantation of the standard hard lens, is now undergoing clinical trials in the United States and is expected to be available here in late 1990.

Some manufacturers are also developing bifocal IOLs, which may eliminate the need in some patients for prescription glasses after surgery. The bifocal IOLs could be on the market in the United States in 1991.

The procedure to remove the natural lens and replace it with a synthetic one is done under a general or local anesthesia with injections made in muscles around the eye. Recovery takes several hours in the hospital; in a few cases, it may require an overnight stay. The patient wears a metal shield over the eye at night; wraparound sunglasses are recommended during the day.

Within a few days of the operation, most people are back at work. In several office visits during the first six to eight weeks after surgery, the doctor will check for infections or other complications and fit the patient for reading glasses. Vision is significantly improved in 95 to 98 percent of cases.

However, results of the operation aren't always worry free. After the IOL implantation, a clouding of the lens capsule, known as a "secondary cataract," occurs in roughly 40 percent of cases. To restore vision, a pulsed yttrium aluminum garnet (YAG) laser is used to produce a hole non-thermally, by "optical breakdown," in the capsule to allow the normal passage of light rays back to the retina. This painless procedure takes a few minutes; improvement usually is immediate. Other problems that may occur in a small percentage of patients include swelling of the cornea, glaucoma, and swelling of the retina, which distorts vision. Overall, though, IOLs "have turned out to be much better than anyone ever expected," says Nancy Brogden, chief of the Food and Drug Administration's IOL branch.

At a time when more older Americans than ever before are looking forward to years of active life ahead of them, IOLs offer hope and a better life.

Shielding Your Eyes From the Sun

Headed for the ski slopes or beach? These pleasures can pose dangers to your eyes unless you take precautions against the sun's harmful rays.

Ultraviolet radiation is invisible and cannot be felt, yet long-term exposure to it may be associated with development of cataracts. Short-term exposure to very intense ultraviolet light—much as you get on a ski slope—can produce photokeratitis, also called actinic keratopathy or snow blindness. There is even some evidence ultraviolet radiation may damage the eye's retina.

By spring of 1990, a new voluntary labeling program developed by the Sunglass Association of America in cooperation with the Food and Drug Administration is expected to be in place to tell consumers how much UV protection they can expect from nonprescription sunglasses. (Prescription sunglasses already meet standards of protection against UV radiation and are not included in this labeling program.)

The voluntary labeling program calls for manufacturers to attach a tag to sunglasses that specifies the level of protection from the two types of ultraviolet rays: the longer wavelength ultraviolet A (UVA) radiation and the shorter wavelength ultraviolet B (UVB) rays. The standards were developed in 1986 by the American National Standards Institute in New York City through consultation with eye-care professionals and educators, research scientists, industry, and military and other government agencies. The labeling standards are the only recognized statement on the properties and performance of sunglasses.

The different categories describe minimum levels of protection and are designed to help consumers pick the best glasses for the types of activities they plan:

- Cosmetic: For non-harsh sunlight and around-town uses such as shopping. These will block at least 70 percent of UVB, 20 percent of UVA, and less than 60 percent of visible light.

- General Purpose: For most outdoor activities such as boating, flying, hiking, picnicking, and beach outings. They also can be used for snow settings. They will block at least 95 percent of UVB, at least 60 percent of UVA, and from 60 to 92 percent of visible light.

• Special Purpose: For very bright environments such as tropical beaches and ski slopes and for activities like mountain climbing. They will block at least 99 percent of UVB and 60 percent of UVA, in addition to from 20 to 97 percent of visible light.

The amount of visible light—glare—blocked by sunglasses depends on the darkness of the lenses. The darker shades of special-purpose sunglasses are intended for a high level of brightness, while the lighter shades can be used for less bright situations like skiing on a cloudy day.

In addition, within the categories, look for the actual percentage of the sun's UV radiation that each particular model of glasses claims to block. The greater the blockage, the lower the risk of UV damage to the eye.

Thomas Loomis, technical director of the Sunglass Association of America, offers this advice when buying nonprescription sunglasses:

First, decide on the purpose, color and fashion you want. Once you've made a selection, hold the sunglasses up at arm's length and look through them at an object with a straight border, such as a window or door frame. Move the glasses slowly across the line. If it seems to wiggle, sway or curve, the lenses contain an optical defect and should be replaced with another pair.

Since 8 percent of males and 3 percent of females have a vision color defect, be sure the glasses don't distort the colors of a traffic signal. Pay for the glasses, says Loomis, walk outside the store and conduct your own test. If they distort the colors, exchange them for another pair.

—by Ellen Hale

Chapter 44

Overview: Cataract in Adults

Background

A cataract is an opacity, or cloudiness, in the lens of the eye. Because a cataract blocks the passage of light through the lens to the back of the eye, it becomes difficult to see clearly. However, the amount of vision loss varies from person to person. Moreover, people vary in the amount of functional impairment caused by a cataract.

The development of cataract is a normal part of aging. More than half of Americans 65 years of age and over have cataracts, but opacities can occur in people of any age. However, most of them have little or no functional impairment.

Cataracts are so common among older people that cataract surgery is the therapeutic surgical procedure most often performed on Americans 65 years of age and over. No medical treatment can prevent cataract development or progression in adult eyes that are healthy in other respects. Although lens opacities are associated with various risk factors, not enough is known to provide guidelines on reducing the risk of cataract.

Addressing the Problem

Vision is directly linked to independence and quality of life. Decisions regarding the diagnosis, treatment, and followup care of patients

AHCPR *Guideline Overview*, February 1993, No. 4.

whose cataracts have caused functional impairment are critical to the well-being of many Americans. In 1990, the Agency for Health Care Policy and Research (AHCPR), an arm of the Federal Government's Public Health Service, Department of Health and Human Services, convened a panel of private-sector experts to review cataract literature and develop a clinical practice guideline.

AHCPR had several reasons for studying cataract in adults:

- The high prevalence of cataract in the elderly U.S. population.

- Decreased independence and quality of life for people whose cataracts cause functional impairment. Functional impairment is defined as difficulty in performing normal everyday activities, such as: personal care, taking medicine, cooking and homemaking, using the telephone, driving, shopping, working in one's occupation, enjoying leisure activities/hobbies, reading, watching television, and so on.

- The high volume of cataract surgery. About 1.35 million cataract surgeries and 640,000 laser procedures to treat posterior capsular opacification (a consequence of modem cataract surgery) were performed in the United States in 1991, at a cost of approximately $3.4 billion.

- Wide variation in cataract care practice.

- Lack of information on diagnosis and treatment of cataract for both health care professionals and the public.

Toward the goal of ensuring quality care for patients with cataract, the panel had these objectives:

- Aid decision making in the diagnosis and treatment of cataract.
- Reduce wide variations in clinical practice.
- Educate health professionals and consumers about cataract.
- Encourage further biomedical, clinical, and cost research on cataract.

The panel published the results in a clinical practice guideline, *Cataract in Adults: Management of Functional Impairment.*

Findings and Recommendations

Learning about cataract, exploring treatment alternatives. and weighing the benefits and risks of cataract surgery are responsibilities shared by the patient and ophthalmologist. Decisionmaking and caregiving should occur within the context of the bond of trust that develops between the patient and health professionals. Effective and sensitive communication concerning the impairment, treatment alternatives, benefits, and risks is essential. Continuity of professional care, including patient instruction, is another part of that bond of trust.

Diagnosis and Referral. The care of a patient with functional impairment due to cataract should begin when a disability is recognized. The diagnosis of cataract can be made by an ophthalmologist or by another health care provider (optometrist, internist, family physician, or registered nurse), who then refers the patient to an ophthalmologist. The decision to proceed with cataract surgery should be made only when the patient fully understands the potential benefits and possible risks.

Nonsurgical Options. Vision changes early in cataract development may be treated nonsurgically. The options include prescription changes, strong bifocals or magnifying lenses, appropriate lighting, and pupil dilation.

Cataract surgery should not be performed only because a cataract is present. It should not be performed when glasses or visual aids are satisfactory, when the patient's lifestyle does not require better vision, when the patient is medically unfit, or when the patient does not desire surgery.

Treatment Setting and Providers. The setting for cataract surgery should be convenient for the patient. If at all possible, the clinic or hospital outpatient setting should be close to home and the patient's social support system of family and friends. The ophthalmologist who performs the surgery is responsible for selecting the site and for providing follow up care. In meeting the patient's needs, the ophthalmologist may delegate care to other providers but should educate the patient concerning their roles in vision rehabilitation.

Preoperative Assessment. The purpose of cataract surgery is to eliminate or reduce functional impairment caused by a cataract. Only in unusual circumstances—when the lens is the source of other sight-threatening disease or when lens extraction is necessary for diagnosis of other eye conditions—is it performed for any other reason. The ultimate decision regarding whether cataract surgery should be performed and when it should be performed rests with the patient and the ophthalmologist who is to perform the surgery. The purpose of the ophthalmologist's preoperative evaluation is to confirm that vision has been reduced to the point of functional impairment and that cataract is the cause.

Cataract Surgery. The decision to perform surgery should be based on the patient's own assessment of functional impairment combined with the results of the eye examination and measurement of visual acuity using the Snellen test. When visual acuity is 20/40 or better, the potential for benefiting from the surgery decreases and the risk relative to potential benefit rises. In general the better the visual acuity is, the greater is the need for verification of functional disability before performing surgery.

In the past few years, the success of cataract surgery has increased dramatically because of advances in microsurgical techniques: the development of safe, effective intraocular lenses (IOLs); and the placement of the IOL behind the iris. The panel concluded that the two types of cataract surgery most often performed are equally effective in restoring vision. They are:

- Extracapsular surgery, in which the lens is removed and the back half of the capsule behind the lens (the posterior capsule) remains in the eye.

- Phacoemulsification, a type of extracapsular surgery in which the lens is softened with sound waves and removed through a needle. The posterior capsule remains.

- Intracapsular surgery is a third, rarely used, type of cataract surgery in which the surgeon removes the entire lens, including the capsule.

Cataract extraction is usually a nonemergency procedure. It can be performed under either local or general anesthesia.

Cataracts usually develop in both eyes, but surgery should not be done on both eyes at the same time. Surgery should not be performed on the second eye until the results of the first eye surgery are known, so that the benefits and risks can be weighed. The indications for cataract surgery in the second eye are the same as for the first eye.

Postoperative Care and Rehabilitation. The period of postoperative care extends from surgery until the goal of surgery is achieved and the patient has stable, improved vision. If complications arise—such as increased pressure, bleeding, or infection in the eye; damage or dislocation of the IOL; or swelling or clouding of the cornea—prompt care is crucial.

Optical correction (contact lenses or glasses) usually can be prescribed 6–17 weeks after surgery. The timing and frequency of refraction depend on patient needs, astigmatism, and consistency of measurement.

Overall planning for rehabilitation is the ophthalmologist's responsibility. A multidisciplinary team approach can be used, in which the ophthalmologist delegates certain aspects of postoperative care to older health professionals, such as optometrists, home health nurses, and social workers.

YAG Capsulotomy. Clouding of the capsule behind the lens is a natural consequence of modern cataract surgery (extracapsular surgery and phacoemulsification). If a patient begins to note decreased visual function or functional impairment, the ophthalmologist should confirm that the symptoms are caused by this posterior opacification. If so, outpatient laser surgery—called YAG (for yttrium aluminum garnet) capsulotomy—can restore visual function. YAG capsulotomy should never be performed as a preventive measure. As with cataract surgery, the patient should fully understand the benefits and risks involved.

For Further Information

Guideline information is available free of charge in several forms:

- *Clinical Practice Guideline: Cataract in the Adult: Management of Functional Impairment.* Prepared for the health practitioner, it includes discussion of the issue and the panel's findings and recommendations, plus fully referenced supporting evidence and an algorithm.

- *Quick Reference Guide for Clinicians: Management of Cataract in Adults.* This practitioner's companion to the *Clinical Practice Guideline* summarizes highlights of patient management.

- *A Patient's Guide: Cataract in Adults.* Published in English and Spanish, this brochure is a summary of information on cataract for consumers.

To order these publications, call toll free 800-358-9295, or write:

Agency for Health Care Policy and Research Publications Clearing-house
P.O. Box 8547
Silver Spring, MD 20907

Guideline Development

The Agency for Health Care Policy and Research convened a private-sector, interdisciplinary panel of health care professionals and a consumer active in the health care field. The panel members and selected expert consultants exhaustively reviewed the published literature on almost 8,000 basic science and clinical studies conducted since 1975. The panel then considered health policy issues, such as health care resources, patients' and practitioners' concerns, and ethical and legal questions. Through two public hearings, the panel received oral and written testimony from additional groups and individuals.

The results of both the literature review and the public hearings were incorporated in a draft guideline. A group of clinicians and other health professionals carefully chosen on behalf of the users who would benefit from the guideline evaluated the draft guideline for its validity, efficacy. and applicability in practice settings. The final recommendations combine the panel's guideline with the comments of reviewers representing professionals and patients around the country.

Key Points about Cataract

For the Practitioner

The goal of each stage of cataract treatment is to maintain or restore your patient's functional autonomy.

Cataract surgery is justified on the basis of both vision loss and your patient's perception of functional impairment due to cataract.

Successful rehabilitation depends on continuity of cares consultation and referral, and communication with your patient.

Find out more about cataract. Read the *Clinical Practice Guideline* and use the companion *Quick Reference Guide for Clinicians*. Give your patients *A Patient's Guide*.

For the Consumer

Cataracts occur as a normal part of aging. No medical treatment can prevent or slow their development.

Changes in vision due to cataract are important when they decrease your ability to lead a normal, independent life.

Whether to have cataract surgery is your decision. Talk with your eye doctor about the benefits and risks for you.

Read *Cataract in Adults: A Patient's Guide*. It gives the names of groups that can give you information on cataract. ANCPR also has a *Clinical Practice Guideline* and *Quick Reference Guide for Clinicians* for your doctor.

Chapter 45

Patient Guide to Cataracts in Adults

What Is a Cataract?

A cataract is a cloudy area in the lens of the eye.

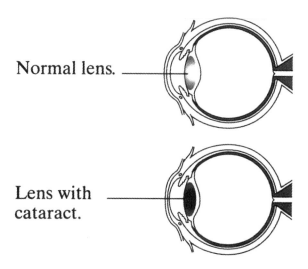

Normal lens.

Lens with cataract.

Figure 45.1. *Side view of the eye.*

AHCPR Pub. No. 93–0544.

A normal lens is clear. It lets light pass to the back of the eye. A cataract blocks some of the light. As a cataract develops, it becomes harder for a person to see.

Cataract is a normal part of aging. About half of Americans ages 65 to 74 have cataract. About 70 percent of those age 75 and over have this condition.

Most people with cataract have a cataract in both eyes. However, one eye may be worse than the other because each cataract develops at a different rate.

Some people with cataract don't even know it. Their cataract may be small, or the changes in their vision may not bother them very much. Other people who have cataract cannot see well enough to do the things they need or want to do.

This chapter can help you decide what to do if you have a cataract. Talk about it with your eye doctor so you can make the choices that are right for you.

What Are the Symptoms of Cataract?

Here are some signs of cataract:

- Cloudy, fuzzy, foggy, or filmy vision.
- Changes in the way you see colors.
- Problems driving at night because headlights seem too bright.
- Problems with glare from lamps or the sun.
- Frequent changes in your eyeglass prescription.
- Double vision.
- Better near vision for awhile only in farsighted people.

These symptoms also can be signs of other eye problems. See your eye doctor to find out what you have and how it can be treated.

How Is Cataract Diagnosed?

A regular eye exam is all that is needed to find a cataract. Your eye doctor will ask you to read a letter chart to see how sharp your sight is. You probably will get eye drops to enlarge your pupils (the round black centers of your eyes). This helps the doctor to see the inside of your eyes. The doctor will use a bright light to see whether your lenses are clear and to check for other problems in the back of your eyes.

Other eye tests may also be used occasionally to show how poorly you see with cataract or how well you might see after surgery:

- Glare test.
- Contrast sensitivity test.
- Potential vision test.
- Specular photographic microscopy.

Only a few people need these tests.

How Is Cataract Treated?

A change in your glasses, stronger bifocals, or the use of magnifying lenses may help improve your vision and be treatment enough. The way to surgically treat a cataract is to remove all or part of the lens and replace it with an artificial lens.

Just because you have a cataract does not mean it must be removed immediately. Cataract surgery can almost always be put off until you are unhappy with the way you see.

Your eye doctor will tell you whether you are one of a small number of people who must have surgery. For example, your doctor may need to see or treat an eye problem that is behind the cataract. Or surgery may be required because a cataract is so large that it could cause blindness.

How Do I Decide Whether to Have Surgery?

Most people have plenty of time to decide about cataract surgery. Your doctor cannot make your decision for you, but talking with your doctor can help you decide.

Tell your doctor how your cataract affects your vision and your life. Check (✓) the statements below that apply to you and share this list with your doctor:

❑ I need to drive, but there is too much glare from the sun or headlights.

❑ I do not see well enough to do my best at work.

❑ I do not see well enough to do the things I need to do at home.

381

❏ I do not see well enough to do things I like to do (for example, read, watch TV, sew, hike, play cards, go out with friends).

❏ I am afraid I will bump into something or fall.

❏ Because of my cataract, I am not as independent as I would like to be.

❏ My glasses do not help me see well enough.

❏ My eyesight bothers me a lot.

You may also have other specific problems that you want to discuss with your eye doctor.

What Should I Know about Surgery?

Your doctor will discuss the options with you before choosing the best kind of cataract removal and lens replacement for you. He or she will also explain how to prepare for surgery and how to take care of yourself after it is over.

Most people do not need to stay overnight in a hospital to have cataract surgery. You may go to an outpatient center or hospital, have your cataract removed, and leave when your doctor says you are fit to leave. However, you will need a friend or family member to take you home. You also will need someone to stay with you for at least a day to help you follow your doctor's instructions.

It takes a few months for an eye to heal after cataract surgery. Your eye doctor should check your progress and make sure you have the care you need until your eye recovers fully.

Removing the Lens

There are three types of surgery to remove lenses that have a cataract.

Extracapsular surgery. The eye surgeon removes the lens, leaving behind the back half of the capsule (the outer covering of the lens).

Phacoemulsification. In this type of extracapsular surgery, the surgeon softens the lens with sound waves and removes it through a needle. The back half of the lens capsule is left behind.

Intracapsular surgery. The surgeon removes the entire lens, including the capsule. This method is rarely used.

Replacing the Lens

A person who has cataract surgery usually gets an artificial lens at the same time. A plastic disc, called an intraocular lens, is placed in the lens capsule inside the eye. Other choices are contact lenses and cataract glasses. Your doctor will help you to decide which choice is best for you.

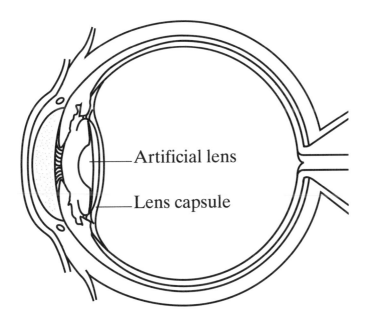

Artificial lens

Lens capsule

Figure 45.2. *Side view of eye with artificial lens.*

Can a Cataract Return?

A cataract cannot return because all or part of the lens has been removed. However, in about half of all people who have extracapsular surgery or phacoemulsification, the lens capsule becomes cloudy. This cloudiness of the lens capsule, if it occurs, usually develops a year or more after surgery. It causes the same vision problems as a cataract does.

The treatment for this condition is a procedure called YAG capsulotomy. The doctor uses a laser (light) beam to make a tiny hole in the capsule to let light pass. This surgery is painless and does not require a hospital stay.

Most people see better after YAG capsulotomy, but, as with cataract surgery, complications can occur. Your doctor will discuss the risks with you. *YAG capsulotomy should not be performed as a preventive measure.*

Is Cataract Surgery Right for Me?

Most people who have a cataract recover from surgery with no problems and improved vision. In fact, serious complications are not common with modern cataract surgery. This type of surgery has a success rate of 95 percent in patients with otherwise healthy eyes. But no surgery is risk free. Although serious complications are not common, when they occur they could result in loss of vision.

If you have a cataract in both eyes, experts say it is best to wait until your first eye heals before having surgery on the second eye. If the eye that has a cataract is your only working eye, you and your doctor should weigh very carefully the benefits and risks of cataract surgery.

You will be able to make the right decision for yourself if you know the facts. Ask your doctor to explain anything you do not understand. There is no such thing as a "dumb" question when it comes to your health.

Here are some questions you might ask:

- Do I need surgery right away?
- If not, how long can I wait?
- What are my personal risks?
- What benefits can I expect?
- If I choose surgery, which type is best for me?
- Which lens replacement is best for me?
- What are the chances of developing cloudiness in the lens capsule after cataract surgery?
- What are the benefits and risks of YAG capsulotomy?

You may wish to write down other questions to ask your doctor to help you make an informed decision about treatment.

Benefits and Risks of Cataract Surgery

Improvements in Activities

- Everyday activities
- Driving
- Reading
- Working
- Moving around
- Social activities
- Hobbies
- Safety
- Self-confidence
- Independence

Possible Complications

- High pressure in the eye
- Blood collection inside the eye
- Infection inside the eye
- Artificial lens damage or dislocation
- Drooping eyelid
- Retinal detachment
- Severe bleeding inside the eye
- Swelling or clouding of the cornea
- Blindness
- Loss of the eye

How Can I Learn More about Cataract?

Organizations that can provide additional information include:

American Academy of Ophthalmology
P.O. Box 7424
San Francisco, CA 94120-7424
Phone: (415) 561-8500

American Optometric Association
Communications Center
243 North Lindbergh Boulevard
St. Louis, MO 63141-7881
Phone: (314) 991-4100

National Eye Institute
National Institutes of Health
Bethesda, MD 20892
Phone: (301) 496-5248

National Society to Prevent Blindness
500 East Remington Road
Schaumburg, IL 60173
Phone: toll free 800-331-2020

For Further Information

This information was based on the *Clinical Practice Guideline on Cataract in Adults: Management of Functional Impairment*. The guideline was developed by an expert panel sponsored by the Agency for Health Care Policy and Research. Other guidelines on common health problems are available, and more are being developed.

For more information on guidelines or to receive more copies of this booklet, call toll free 800-358-9295 or write to:

Agency for Health Care Policy and Research
Publications Clearinghouse
P.O. Box 8547
Silver Spring, MD 20907

Chapter 46

Management of Cataracts in Adults

Abstract

Functional impairment due to cataract is prevalent in the adult population. Cataract extraction is the therapeutic surgical procedure performed most frequently on Americans age 65 and over. It is important to recognize the effect of cataract-related disability on a person's ability to function autonomously. The purpose of this guideline is to help ensure quality care for individual patients. This Quick Reference Guide for Clinicians deals with highlights of patient management, ranging from referral pathways and access to care through post-operative care, rehabilitation, and the possibility of posterior capsular opacification and YAG capsulotomy. This guideline is the work of the Cataract Management Guideline Panel, a multidisciplinary expert panel made up of ophthalmologists, nurses, optometrists, internists, a patient representative, and others. The panel, developed under the sponsorship of the Agency for Health Care Policy and Research, conducted an extensive literature review and employed science-based methodology and expert clinical judgment to develop specific statements on patient assessment and management of cataract.

Note: Clinicians should not rely on this Quick Reference Guide alone. Refer to the complete Clinical Practice Guideline for a more detailed analysis and discussion of the available research, critical evaluation of the assumptions and knowledge of the field, considerations for

AHCPR Pub. No. 93–0543. Feb. 1993.

387

patients with special needs, and references. The full Guideline Report
has a more complete discussion of relevant research.

Purpose and Scope

A cataract can cause a decrease in visual function, which in turn
can be classified as a visual disability. Thus, a cataract can be defined
in three ways. The first definition is an objective lens change. The
second is a lens opacity that is associated with a defined level of visual acuity loss. The third relates to the functional consequences of
lens opacification. This guideline focuses on the last definition. It deals
with care of the patient with functional impairment due to cataract
and improvement in function as a result of treatment for the condition.

The purpose of the guideline is to help ensure quality care for individual patients. Practitioners are encouraged to use the information provided here, but the recommendations may not be appropriate
for use in all circumstances. Decisions to adopt any particular recommendations must be made by the practitioner in light of available
resources and the circumstances presented by individual patients.

Functional impairment due to cataract refers to lost or diminished
ability to do any of the following:

- Perform everyday activities—Bathing, dressing, eating, using
  the toilet, walking, preparing meals, doing housework, doing
  laundry, shopping, taking medicine, getting around outside,
  driving or using other transportation, managing money, and using the telephone.
- Participate in hobbies or other leisure time activities—Reading,
  watching television, etc.
- Work in one's occupation.

It is important to recognize the impact of this disability on the
individual's ability to function autonomously. The goal of cataract
treatment is to maintain or restore autonomy through appropriate
treatment to remove the disability.

Functional impairment due to cataract in the adult is prevalent
in the U.S. population. Cataract extraction is the therapeutic surgical procedure performed most frequently on Americans age 65 and
over. About 1.35 million extractions are performed annually in the
United States.

Currently, there is no medical treatment to prevent the formation or progression of cataract in the otherwise healthy adult eye.

Multiple factors influence the risk of cataract: ultraviolet-B radiation, diabetes, drugs, smoking, diarrhea, alcohol, and low antioxidant vitamin status. Different risk factors are associated with different types of opacities. There are insufficient data to provide management guidelines on reducing the risk of cataract.

Highlights of Patient Management

Referral Pathways and Access to Care

The process of caring for a patient with functional impairment due to cataract should start when a disability is recognized. A diagnosis of cataract can be made by any of a number of health care providers, including ophthalmologists, optometrists, family physicians, and internists. However, in order to decide whether to have the cataract removed, a patient must understand the likely benefits and potential risks of undergoing cataract surgery. Such an understanding of the risks and benefits comes from a discussion with the ophthalmologist who might perform the surgery. The surgeon is responsible for ensuring that the patient understands the likely benefits and potential risks of cataract surgery in his or her case before making a decision about whether or not to proceed with surgery.

Setting and Providers of Care

Cataract surgery should be performed where the patient can receive quality care in a safe environment—close to home, if at all possible, or close to the best social support system of family and friends. Outpatient surgery can be performed in a hospital or an independent surgery center. The selection of the site is the responsibility of the ophthalmologist who performs the surgery. It is preferable that the perioperative care and surgery be performed in the same community.

The ophthalmologist who performs the surgery has the responsibility and ethical obligation to the patient for care during the postoperative period. The surgeon must examine the patient the day following surgery, initiate appropriate postoperative treatment, monitor the patient's recovery from the surgery, diagnose and treat postoperative complications (or refer the patient to an ophthalmologist better able to deal with those complications), and perform surgical revision when appropriate. In order to fulfill these responsibilities, the surgeon must examine the patient periodically until he or she is confident that the patient has fully recovered from surgery, a process that usually takes 6–12 weeks.

The surgeon cannot abrogate his or her responsibility for the patient's postoperative care. However, certain components of postoperative care can be delegated to one or more members of a team of appropriately trained professionals, including optometrists, community health nurses, social workers, and other health care professionals.

If anyone other than the operating ophthalmologist is to provide all or most of the postoperative care, then the operating ophthalmologist has an obligation to inform the patient prior to surgery of the arrangements and of the relative qualifications of the postoperative caregiver. If the patient with cataract is seeking surgery by an ophthalmologist located far from home, so that provision of postoperative care by that ophthalmologist is impractical, the surgeon should educate the patient about the importance of the continuum of the care process involved in cataract surgery. This includes the preoperative phase, the surgical procedure, and the period of postoperative care.

Diagnosis and Preoperative Ophthalmologic Testing

1. The decision to perform cataract surgery is generally made after judging the effect of the cataract on the patient's visual and overall function, after assessing the patient's visual needs, and after a thorough consideration of the potential risks associated with surgery.

2. Management decisions should be made primarily on the basis of a complete patient history and ocular examination.

3. Special preoperative tests are rarely of assistance in deciding whether to recommend cataract surgery.

Contrast sensitivity testing. At this time there is inadequate scientific evidence that contrast sensitivity testing provides information that is useful for determining whether a patient would benefit from cataract surgery beyond that obtained by history and ocular examination.

Glare testing. In general, there is inadequate evidence that glare testing provides useful information beyond that obtained by history and ocular examination. However, it may be useful for corroborating glare symptoms in a small percentage of cataract patients who complain of glare yet measure good Snellen acuity in office testing. Even in these patients, a positive glare test does not determine whether surgery should be recommended.

Potential vision testing. Adequate evidence is lacking to determine whether tests of potential vision assist the ophthalmologist in predicting the outcome of cataract surgery. Available data suggest that these tests may not be useful. There are no data to substantiate the value of potential vision testing in situations in which it is uncertain whether other diseases, particularly mild to moderate atrophic macular degeneration, might limit postoperative visual rehabilitation.

Specular photographic microscopy. There is currently no evidence or rationale to support routine use of specular microscopy in order to predict the response of the cornea to cataract surgery.

Treatment

Functional rehabilitation as a result of visual improvement is possible in the vast majority of patients and should be the goal at each stage of treatment.

Nonsurgical Management

1. Patients developing cataract should be educated and reassured about the cause of visual disability and the prognosis.

2. During early cataract development, visual impairment can often be reduced by nonsurgical means (changing the distance spectacle lens prescription; use of strong bifocals, magnification, or other visual aids; and appropriate illumination). Pupillary dilation may help patients with a posterior subcapsular cataract. However, the glare caused by such a cataract may be unacceptable, particularly when the intensity of ambient light is high or when facing high-intensity light, as in night driving.

Surgical Management

1. Cataract surgery is generally a nonemergency procedure.

2. Clinical judgment combined with Snellen acuity remains the best general guide to the appropriateness of surgery.

3. Individual functional and visual needs, environment, and risks may vary widely and must be taken into account. The likely degree of visual improvement and its impact on the quality of life must be weighed against the risk and cost of surgery.

Indications for Surgery

1. Cataract surgery is indicated when the cataract reduces visual function to a level that interferes with everyday activities of the patient.

2. Surgery is not necessary solely because the cataract is present.

3. The patient should make the decision to proceed with surgery after careful consideration of the ophthalmologist's recommendation and after considering subjective, objective, and educational criteria for various levels of visual impairment.

    *   *Visual disability with Snellen acuity of 20/50 or worse.*

        —*Subjective*: The ability to carry out needed or desired activities is impaired.
        —*Objective*: Ocular examination confirms that the best correctable visual acuity in the affected eye is 20/50 or worse and that the cataract is responsible for this.
        —*Educational*: After the ophthalmologist educates the patient about likely benefits and risks of surgery, including alternatives to surgery, the patient decides that expected improvement in function outweighs the potential risk, cost, and inconvenience of surgery.

- *Visual disability with Snellen acuity of 20/40 or better.* For patients with Snellen acuity of 20/40 or better, the indicators are the same as for patients with Snellen acuity of 20/50 or worse. However, it is especially important to document visual impairment for any of the following reasons:

    —Visual function fluctuates because of glare or dim illumination.
    —Patient complains of monocular diplopia or polyopia.
    —Visual disparity exists between the two eyes.
    —Patient needs but cannot obtain an unrestricted driving license.

- *Visual disability of the one-eyed patient.* A one-eyed patient with cataract is defined as a patient with a cataract in one eye and permanent legal blindness in the other eye. The indications for surgery for the one-eyed patient are the same as those for the two-eyed patient, except that the ophthalmologist should emphasize the risk of total blindness.

4. There are two other indications for cataract removal.

    - *Lens-induced disease*: Phacomorphic glaucoma, phacolytic glaucoma, and other lens-induced diseases may require cataract surgery, and the need for extraction may be urgent.

    - *Concomitant ocular disease that requires clear media*: Cataract extraction may be required to adequately diagnose or treat other ocular conditions, such as diabetic retinopathy.

Contraindications for Surgery

Surgery should not be performed solely to improve vision under the following circumstances:

- The patient does not desire surgery.

393

- Glasses or visual aids provide satisfactory functional vision.
- The patient's lifestyle is not compromised.
- The patient is medically unfit.

Preoperative Medical Evaluation

1. The primary purpose of the preoperative medical evaluation is to ensure a safe perioperative course for the patient. It also provides an opportunity to evaluate many patients who may not be receiving regular medical care.

2. The preoperative medical evaluation and appropriate testing should be done on all patients undergoing cataract surgery.

3. Preoperative medical management should be guided by consideration of the patient's age, the presence of concurrent medical illnesses, the patient's use of medicine, and the patient's proximity to the location where surgery is to be performed.

4. The preoperative medical evaluation should include screening for functional or emotional disability. Elderly patients should receive special screening of functional status, and particular attention should be given to the psychosocial and economic problems imposed by aging.

5. Prior to surgery, areas of special importance to the individual, such as cultural, ethical, and spiritual values, should be taken into consideration. The patient's own assessment of the quality of his or her life also should be considered to optimally prepare him or her for surgery and recovery.

Anesthesia

1. Anesthesia for cataract surgery can be either general or local.

2. General anesthesia is preferred in the following situations:

    - The patient has extreme anxiety that does not respond to counseling or sedation.

- The patient is unable to cooperate with the surgical team.
- Satisfactory local anesthesia cannot be provided.
- The patient has a known allergy to local anesthetic medications.
- Disorders are present that are best managed under general anesthesia (e.g., severe back pain or postural problems).

3. Monitored anesthesia care by an anesthesiologist or anesthetist is strongly preferred. Monitored anesthesia care includes physiologic monitoring with life-support systems available. It should include use of electrocardiogram, pulse oximetry, blood pressure, and respiration monitoring techniques.

4. Either peribulbar or retrobulbar injection is acceptable. The injection should be administered by an ophthalmologist or by an appropriately trained and qualified professional who has demonstrated competence in these techniques.

5. Peribulbar and retrobulbar anesthesia should be administered to properly monitored patients with intravenous access established. There should be access to oxygen with assisted respirations via mask ventilation apparatus.

Surgical Techniques and Complications

1. Phacoemulsification and extracapsular surgery appear to be equally effective in restoring vision. Inadequate data are available to determine if one technique is more effective than the other in reducing or eliminating functional impairment due to cataract.

2. It cannot be determined from existing data whether the smaller wound incision needed for phacoemulsification leads to more enhanced safety and more rapid postoperative rehabilitation than with extracapsular surgery.

3. Ophthalmologists should use their best judgment in selecting surgical techniques for individual patients after discussing the alternatives with the patient.

4. The ophthalmologist who is to perform the surgery is respon-
    sible for the following:

    •   Ensuring that the patient has had an appropriate general
        medical history and physical examination.

    •   If an intraocular lens is to be implanted, ensuring that
        the appropriate keratometry and A-scan measurements
        have been performed.

    •   If an intraocular lens is to be implanted, selecting the ap-
        propriate intraocular lens power after discussion with the
        patient.

    •   Reviewing the results of presurgical and diagnostic pa-
        tient evaluations and discussing the findings with the pa-
        tient or, in appropriate cases, with another responsible
        adult acting for the patient.

Second Eye Surgery

1. Indications for second eye surgery are the same as for first
    eye surgery.

2. In no case should surgery be done on both eyes at the same
    time. The time interval should be based on the following fac-
    tors:

    •   The patient is able to provide informed consent for sur-
        gery on the second eye after evaluating the visual results
        and postoperative course of surgery on the first eye.

    •   Adequate time has passed to detect and treat the most
        immediate vision-threatening complications of cataract
        surgery.

    •   Vision in the operated eye has recovered sufficiently that
        the patient is not at risk of injury due to functional im-
        pairment during second eye cataract surgery and the im-
        mediate postoperative period.

- In the event that vision has not recovered or is not recoverable, there is time to arrange for adequate assistance so that the patient is not at risk of injury due to functional impairment following second eye cataract surgery.

3. Surgery in the second eye is justified and appropriate when the subjective, objective, and educational criteria outlined under "Indications for Surgery" are met. An exception is the special case in which the opposite eye has no useful vision. In this case, the decision for surgery is determined by the degree of vision reduction at the time the patient enters into the evaluation process. In some cases, surgery may be delayed because of the greater potential for total blindness in the event of a serious complication of surgery. It is then the obligation of the ophthalmologist to inform and educate the patient about the potential risk of total blindness. Although the decreased visual acuity and level of disability may fall well within the guidelines for cataract surgery, the worse the vision is in the fellow eye, the greater the need is for caution in considering cataract surgery in a patient's only seeing eye.

Postoperative Care

Patient Education

The ophthalmologist who performs the surgery has an obligation to educate and instruct the patient about appropriate signs or symptoms of possible complications, as well as eye protection, level of activity permitted, medications, required visits, and details concerning access to emergency care. The patient likewise has an obligation during the postoperative phase to follow the advice and instructions of the surgeon and to notify the surgeon promptly if problems occur.

Patient's Condition at Discharge

Criteria for discharge after ambulatory surgery include:

- Stable vital signs.
- Return to preoperative mental state.
- Absence of nausea.

397

- Absence of significant pain.
- Availability of an escort.
- Review with the patient or escort of postsurgical care until the first postoperative visit on the day following surgery, including relief of pain, activity level permitted, and access to emergency care if needed.
- Prearranged followup appointment.
- Written postoperative instructions.
- Suitable home environment.
- Adequate home care support.

Unplanned Postoperative Hospitalization

1. Operative complications of an ocular or medical nature are possible indications for unplanned postoperative hospitalization.

2. Ocular complications can include hyphema, infection, wound dehiscence, endophthalmitis, uncontrolled elevated intraocular pressure, threatened or actual expulsive hemorrhage, retrobulbar hemorrhage, severe pain, or other ocular problems requiring acute management or careful observation.

3. Medical complications can include cardiac instability, respiratory instability, a cerebrovascular episode, diabetes mellitus requiring acute management, uncontrolled nausea or vomiting, acute urinary retention, acute psychiatric disorientation, or other medical conditions requiring acute management or careful monitoring.

Planned Postoperative Hospitalization

Indications for planned postoperative hospitalization are as follows:

- Medical conditions are present that require prolonged postoperative observation by a nurse or skilled personnel.
- Best correctable vision in the unoperated eye is 20/200 or worse.
- Patient is mentally debilitated, diagnosed as mentally ill, or functionally incapacitated so that a risk of injury exists in the immediate postoperative period.

- Physical disability prevents satisfactory immediate post-operative care.

Postoperative Visits

1. The frequency of examination during the postoperative period is based on the need to:

   - Diagnose and provide the most efficient treatment for complications when they arise.

   - Provide routine postoperative care as healing proceeds.

   - Educate and support the patient during the postoperative period.

2. The frequency of normal followup for a patient without signs or symptoms of possible complications is as follows:

   - The day following surgery.

   - Approximately 1 week, 3 weeks, and 6–8 weeks following surgery.

   - More frequently if unusual findings or complications occur.

Postoperative Examinations

1. The components of postoperative examinations include:

   - Visual acuity measurement each visit.
   - Intraocular pressure measurement each visit.
   - External examination each visit.
   - Slit lamp examination each visit.
   - Patient counseling and education each visit unless the patient's condition does not allow it. This should include medication instructions and information about progress toward healing, level of activity permitted, symptoms requiring emergency care, and access to emergency care.

399

- Ophthalmoscopy. A dilated fundus exam to include the peripheral retina should be done at least once during this postoperative period.

2. The timing and frequency of refraction will depend on patient needs, the amount of astigmatism, and the stability of the measurement. Sutures may be cut or removed by the ophthalmologist to reduce astigmatism. Usually, optical correction can be prescribed 6–12 weeks after surgery.

Long-Term Follow Up

Patients should be informed of the need for periodic eye examinations and of the possible need for YAG capsulotomy if a posterior capsular opacification develops.

Rehabilitation

1. Overall supervision of planning for postoperative rehabilitation is the responsibility of the surgeon. Appropriate planning for postoperative care and rehabilitation can be accomplished by office personnel interacting with the family and patient preoperatively and postoperatively or through a multidisciplinary approach utilizing optometrists, registered nurses, and/or social workers.

2. Successful rehabilitation involves numerous factors:

   - *Physician instructions*: The patient should understand and comply with physician instructions.

   - *Patient education*: Careful preoperative assessment of the abilities of the patient and family to understand and comply with instructions is critical to ensuring adequate postoperative care. Referral to a home health care agency can be appropriate for further education and to evaluate a patient's ability to follow discharge instructions.

   - *Timely management of postoperative complications*: Postoperative complications can occur unpredictably as a result of coexisting medical problems, physical limitations from a preexisting condition, difficulty in identifying labels on medications because of altered visual status, adverse systemic reactions from mixing medications by patients concurrently treated with other drug therapy, and premature discharge of a patient with delayed postanesthetic recovery or with unrecognized or delayed postanesthetic complications. Immediate intervention is necessary, particularly for the patient living alone.

- *Economic factors*: Attention should be given to the possible adverse economic impact of cataract on patients and their families.

- *Environmental factors*: The patient's home environment may pose safety risks that can profoundly influence rehabilitation.

- *Cultural and ethnic factors*: Recognizing the mores and belief systems of patients of diverse cultural and ethnic backgrounds aids in developing an appropriate plan for care. Non-English-speaking or deaf patients require the efforts of interpreters to ensure effective communication.

- *Psychosocial factors*: Learning how elderly people function in their daily lives is essential to understanding and caring for them. Referral for counseling should be made when indicated. When cataract patients who are considering surgery have the responsibility of being the primary caretaker for another individual, they should be referred to a home health care agency or family service agency for help in obtaining interim assistance in fulfilling those responsibilities.

Posterior Capsular Opacification and YAG Capsulotomy

1. Opacification of the posterior capsule is a consequence of modern cataract surgery. As the opacification increases, the patient begins to notice a decrease in visual function that can lead to functional impairment.

2.   The most commonly used technique for treating posterior capsular opacification is Nd:YAG capsulotomy, usually referred to as YAG or laser capsulotomy. YAG capsulotomy is performed as an outpatient procedure.

3.   The approach to the management of functional impairment due to posterior capsular opacification is similar to that for functional impairment due to cataract.

4.   The time of onset of capsular opacification following cataract surgery is variable, as is the frequency with which YAG capsulotomy is performed.

5.   Capsular opacification severe enough to require YAG capsulotomy should be a rare occurrence within 3 months of surgery and uncommon in the first 6 months. Data suggest that less than 25 percent of patients undergo YAG capsulotomy within 2 years following surgery. The optimum rate of YAG capsulotomy following cataract surgery is unknown.

Diagnosis

1.   The same general approach as outlined for cataract should be followed.

2.   Diagnosis of functional impairment due to capsular opacification is based on clinical judgment regarding the following:

- Visual loss and/or symptoms of glare.
- Symptoms of decreased contrast.
- The amount of posterior capsular opacification.
- Other possible causes of decreased vision following cataract surgery.
- The degree of functional impairment.

Indications for Surgery

1.   Laser capsulotomy is appropriate and justified when the following subjective, objective, and educational criteria are met.

- *Subjective*: The ability to carry out needed or desired activities is increasingly impaired.

- *Objective*: The eye examination confirms the diagnosis of posterior capsular opacification and excludes other ocular causes of functional impairment.

- *Educational*: The patient has been educated about the risks and benefits of surgery.

2. Occasionally, laser capsulotomy is indicated to diagnose and treat retinal detachment, macular disease, or diabetic retinopathy; to evaluate the optic nerve head; or to diagnose posterior pole tumors or other conditions requiring ophthalmological evaluation.

Contraindications for Surgery

1. Laser capsulotomy should never be scheduled at the time cataract surgery is scheduled or performed, and it should never be performed prophylactically because:

   - There is no predictable time at which laser surgery may be required,

   - Laser surgery is seldom indicated before 3 months following surgery,

   - Laser surgery carries its own risks.

2. Justification for performing the procedure should be well documented in the patient's record.

Preoperative Ophthalmic and Medical Evaluation

1. Fluorescein angiography and B-scan ultrasonography may be indicated in certain circumstances.

2. The preoperative ophthalmic evaluation should include a history and complete ocular examination.

3. The ophthalmologist who will perform the laser surgery is responsible for assessing the medical suitability of the patient for the procedure and the perioperative use of vasoactive drugs.

Complications

The major complications of YAG capsulotomy include:

- Elevated intraocular pressure.
- Retinal detachment.
- Cystoid macular edema.
- Damage to the intraocular lens.
- Hyphema.
- Dislocated intraocular lens.
- Corneal edema.

Postoperative Care

1. The ophthalmologist who performed the laser capsulotomy has an ethical and legal responsibility to provide postoperative care and to provide appropriate care if complications develop. Referral to another ophthalmologist should be made only with the patient's consent.

2. Following capsulotomy, patients must be observed for at least 1 hour for evidence of elevated intraocular pressure. If the pressure is elevated, appropriate treatment must be instituted and the patient followed until the problem is resolved.

3. Within 2 weeks of the procedure, the patient should be reexamined by the ophthalmologist who performed the surgery. The examination should include:

   - Measurement of intraocular pressure.

   - Slit lamp examination of the anterior segment to confirm the adequacy of the capsulotomy and stability of the intraocular lens.

- Indirect ophthalmoscopy for retinal tears or detachment.

- Refraction, if necessary.

- Instruction to patients about the risk and symptoms of retinal detachment, the slight risk of glaucoma and other long-term complications, and the need for periodic eye examinations.

Bibliography

American Academy of Ophthalmology. Policy statement on cataract surgery in the otherwise healthy adult second eye. San Francisco: American Academy of Ophthalmology; 1991.

American Academy of Ophthalmology, Quality of Care Committee, Anterior Segment Panel. Cataract in the otherwise healthy adult eye. San Francisco: American Academy of Ophthalmology; 1989. 12 p. A Preferred Practice Pattern approved by the Board of the Academy, September 16, 1989.

American College of Physicians, Clinical Efficacy Project. Clinical efficacy reports. Philadelphia: American College of Physicians;1987.

American College of Physicians, Medical Practice Committee. Periodic health examination: a guide for designing individualized preventive health care in the asymptomatic patient. Ann Intern Med 1981 Dec;95(6):729–32.

Canadian Task Force on the Periodic Health Examination. Periodic health examination, 1991 update: 1. Screening for cognitive impairment in the elderly. Can Med Assoc J 1991 Feb 15;144(4):425–31.

Cink DE, Sutphin JE. Quantification of the reduction of glare disability after standard extracapsular cataract surgery. J Cataract Refract Surg 1992 Jul;18:385–90.

Donnelly D. Instilling eyedrops: difficulties experienced by patients following cataract surgery. J Adv Nurs 1987 Mar;12(2):235–43.

Drummond MF. Measuring the quality of life of people with visual impairment. Proceedings of a workshop. Washington: National Institutes of Health;1990. NIH Pub. No. 90–3078.

Ederer F, Hiller R, Taylor HR. Senile lens change and diabetes in two population studies. Am J Ophthalmol 1981 Mar;91(3):381–95.

Holahan J, Berenson RA, Kachavos PG. Area variations in selected Medicare procedures. Health Aff (Millwood) 1990 Winter;9(4):166–75.

Javitt JC, Tielsch JM, Canner JK, Kolb MM, Sommer A, Steinberg EP National outcomes of cataract extraction: increased risk of retinal complications associated with Nd:YAG laser capsulotomy. Ophthalmology 1992 Oct;99(10):1487–98.

Klein BE, Klein R, Moss SE. Prevalence of cataract in a population based study of persons with diabetes mellitus. Ophthalmology 1985 Sep;92(9):1191–6.

Kupfer C. The conquest of cataract: a global challenge. Trans Ophthalmol Soc U K 1984;104(Pt 1):1–10. Leader S. (Public Policy Institute, Washington). The outpatient surgical experiences of aged Medicare enrollees. Washington: American Association of Retired Persons;1990 Aug.

Miller ST, Graney MJ, Elam JT, Applegate WB, Freeman JM. Predictions of outcomes from cataract surgery in elderly persons. Ophthalmology 1988 Aug;95(8):1125–9.

Pellegrino ED, Thomasma DC. For the patient's good. The restoration of beneficence in health care. New York: Oxford University Press;1988.

Slomovic AR, Parrish RK 2d. Acute elevations of intraocular pressure following Nd:YAG laser posterior capsulotomy. Ophthalmology 1985 Jul;92(7):973–6.

Sommer A, Tielsch JM, Katz J, Quigley H, Gottsch JD, Javitt JC, Martone JF, Royall RM, Whitt KA, Ezrine S. Racial differences in the cause-specific prevalence of blindness in East Baltimore. N Engl J Med 1991 Nov 14;325(20):1412–7.

Veatch RM. The foundations of justice: why the retarded and the rest of us have claims to equality. New York: Oxford University Press;1986.

Whitaker VB, Whitaker R. Cultural, ethnic, racial and religious factors: implications for ophthalmic nursing practice and research. Insight 1991 Jun;16(3):28–31.

Chapter 47

Cataracts in Children

What Is a Cataract?

A cataract is a clouding of the eye's normally clear lens. Located directly behind the iris, the lens focuses light on the retina, the light sensitive tissue at the back of the eye. A cloudy lens inhibits light rays from reaching the retina and results in hazy or blurred vision. The degree of visual impairment caused by a cataract varies and depends on how much of the lens is obstructed by the cataract.

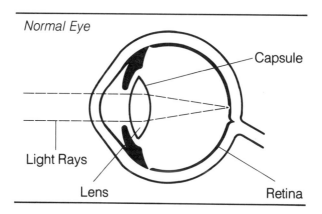

Figure 47.1. The lens focuses light on the retina.

American Academy of Ophthalmology, ©1988. Used by permission.

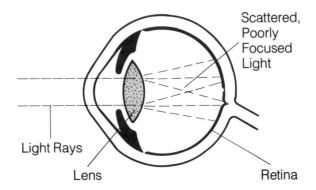

Figure 47.2. *As a cataract forms, the lens becomes opaque and light cannot easily be transmitted to the retina.*

What Causes Cataracts in Infants and Children?

Although most cataracts occur in older adults, infants and children can also be affected. Occasionally, an infant is born with a cataract. Although infant cataracts may be inherited or occur as a result of a viral infection such as German Measles contracted during pregnancy, it is usually impossible to determine the exact cause.

A cataract may develop during childhood, often as a result of an eye injury or a disease process involving other parts of the body. Other causes of childhood cataracts include abnormal lens growth or the late appearance of an inherited cataract.

How Are Cataracts Treated?

Some childhood cataracts may only partially cloud the lens and not interfere with vision. These small cataracts usually do not require treatment but should be observed periodically. Moderate size cataracts which do interfere with vision may require treatment with glasses or treatment for amblyopia ("lazy" eye). Larger cataracts which severely interfere with vision require immediate surgery.

Using microscopic surgical techniques, an ophthalmologist removes the entire lens or its cloudy contents. All cataract operations involve incisions into the eye and on children are usually performed under general anesthesia. Lasers cannot remove cataracts.

How Is Vision Corrected After Surgery?

Once the cloudy lens is removed, the child will need a substitute lens to focus images on the retina. There are four ways of restoring focusing power: eyeglasses, contact lenses, intraocular lenses, and corneal surgery (epikeratophakia). Regardless of which method of visual correction is used, the child will need bifocals to see near objects clearly.

Glasses

Glasses or contact lenses are the most commonly used means of correcting children's vision after cataract surgery. Glasses work well for children who have had cataracts removed from both eyes.

However a child with a cataract in only one eye presents a difficult problem. The lens necessary to correct vision in the operated eye magnifies the size of the image and creates a situation in which the child sees one magnified image and one normal sized image. The child's brain may correct this double image by suppressing (turning off) the image from the operated eye. This suppression results in an amblyopic or "lazy" eye. Children who have had cataract surgery in one eye only need a contact lens, an intraocular lens or epikeratophakia to restore binocular vision. Cataract glasses can be used to help maintain useful vision in the operated eye but they will not restore binocularity.

Contact Lenses

Several varieties of contact lenses are available: rigid, soft daily wear, and extended wear. The type of contact lens selected depends upon the shape of the eye, its ability to adapt to a contact, the power of the lens and the child's or parents' dexterity in handling the lenses. Several types of contact lenses may be tried before the proper one is selected. Since an infant's eye grows rapidly, frequent lens changes may be necessary.

Intraocular Lenses

Intraocular lenses are used to correct focus after cataract surgery in special cases. The plastic intraocular lens is placed inside the eye during the original cataract surgery or during a subsequent surgery.

The optical correction is constant, and the images seen by both eyes are of equal size.

Intraocular lenses are not usually inserted in young infants because the focusing power changes rapidly in the young eye and the power of the implanted lens does not. The long-term safety of intraocular implants in children has not been established.

Epikeratophakia

Focusing power can be corrected with an epikeratophakia corneal graft, a specially ground piece of cornea surgically stitched onto the surface of the eye. As with any surgical procedure, complications can occur.

Amblyopia: A Special Problem

Poor vision resulting from amblyopia ("lazy" eye) can be caused by an infant or childhood cataract. While the visual system is developing, the brain must receive clear images from both eyes. If this does not occur, the visual part of the brain for that eye will not develop properly.

For this reason, when a cataract develops in infancy or early childhood, surgery should be performed as soon as vision is threatened. When older children lose vision because of a cataract, they usually can be treated in the same way as adults because their visual development is complete.

When amblyopia is present, cataract removal is only the first step in treatment. Proper optical correction is necessary and the good eye must be patched until vision improves in the amblyopic eye. Patching the good eye forces use of the weaker eye. If patching is not done after cataract surgery, good vision usually fails to develop. Even after the weak eye has become stronger, patching may be continued on a part-time basis until the child is visually mature (about age 9).

Even with prompt therapy, some children develop only partial visual recovery due to the presence of other eye defects.

Strabismus

Children with cataracts often develop strabismus (misaligned eyes). This misalignment is usually treated with eye muscle surgery to straighten the eyes.

Chapter 48

National Eye Institute Report on Cataracts

To the researchers who are acquainted with this organ, the lens always has been a great source of excitement and interest. To the ophthalmologists and optometrists who are aware of the magnitude and ramifications of age-related cataract and presbyopia, the lens will continue to be a source of challenge and inspiration. However, it is important to realize that lens and cataract research encompasses a multitude of fields and disciplines.

According to some commonly held beliefs, the lens is "dead" tissue; but, on the contrary, it is one of the very few organs in the body that continues to grow throughout life. The lens always has been an excellent model system in the field of developmental biology. Where else can a researcher who is interested in aging find relatively large amounts of tissue as old (in the center of the lens) as the person or animal itself?

To the electrophysiologist and biophysicist, the lens architecture, with its elaborate membrane system and its highly specialized communication channels, offers an ideal system for studying various channel conductances as well as for studying active and passive transport systems. To the physicist and engineer trying to understand the basis of lens transparency or to design a better lens system, the living lens is without equal. Recent advances in molecular biologic techniques using transgenic animals and lens-specific promoters prove that the lens can be an ideal system for studying many biologic and

NIH Pub. No. 93–3186. Excerpt from *Vision Research: A National Plan*, pp. 155–159.

biomedical topics ranging from transparency to the complex processes of growth, development, and aging.

Program Description

Extent of the Problem

The eye lens is a complex, transparent, avascular organ whose function is to focus images on the retina. "Cataract" is generally defined as any opacity in the lens. It becomes clinically significant when visual acuity is affected. Although cataract generally appears in the elderly population, it can develop at any time in life and may be inherited or congenital in nature. It may develop or accelerate its progression as a consequence of metabolic diseases such as diabetes or develop in response to toxic and environmental agents such as various forms of electromagnetic radiation, drugs, or nutritional deficiencies. In general, cataract formation can result from multitudes of physical or chemical insults to the lens or from changes in lens metabolism associated with aging or the onset or progression of metabolic disorders. Cataract formation is generally accompanied by changes in various biochemical and biophysical parameters, including changes in ion and nutrient levels, redox potentials, and metabolic activity.

Age-related cataract, by far the most common type of cataract, is a major public health problem throughout the world. In developing countries where cataract surgery is often not widely available, cataract is the leading cause of blindness. In Western countries, an increasing demand for cataract surgery has placed a growing burden on medical resources. Cataract surgery is now the most frequently performed operation in the United States among persons over age 60.

Since 1987 more than 1 million cataract operations have been performed annually. Reimbursement for cataract surgery now accounts for 12 percent of the entire Medicare budget. The problem threatens to worsen in coming decades as the U.S. population ages and as technical advances extend the indications for cataract surgery. Population projections indicate that the number of persons older than age 55 will increase by 82 percent between 1980 and 2030. During this period the group of persons older than age 85 will increase by 150 percent. Population projections for less-developed regions in the world indicate that the number of persons older than age 55 in the year 2025 will exceed 1.1 billion.

Data on cataract blindness and cataract surgery provide incomplete information about the magnitude of the cataract problem. Large numbers of persons with visual impairment from cataract are not included in these data because their impairment is not sufficient to require surgical correction or to result in blindness. In the Framingham Eye Study cataract, defined as a lens change that cannot be ascribed to specific causes and is accompanied by a visual acuity of 6/9 or worse, was found in 5 percent of persons ages 52 to 64, 18 percent of persons ages 65 to 74, and 46 percent of persons ages 75 to 85. The 1971–72 National Health and Nutrition Examination Survey of the National Center for Health Statistics reported that 28.5 percent of persons ages 65 to 74 had lens opacities causing a decrease in visual acuity. Further evidence of the public health importance of cataract is provided by data from a national sample of office-based physicians—the National Ambulatory Medical Care Survey—that report an estimated 6.3 million physician visits because of cataract in 1985. In the National Health Interview Survey a continuing nationwide household interview of the civilian, noninstitutionalized population of the United States, 12 percent of persons between the ages of 65 and 74 and 25 percent of persons ages 75 and older report the presence of cataracts.

Cataract Treatment

Currently surgery to remove the opaque, nonfunctioning lens is the only effective treatment for cataract. The cataract may be removed by several methods, including intracapsular extraction (i.e., removal of the entire lens, including its surrounding capsule) with a cryoextractor that freezes the cataract to it, enabling the lens to be detached and extracted. This method is still widely used in many developing countries. A second approach for cataract removal is the extracapsular method (i.e., removal of the anterior capsule and lens substance while retaining the posterior capsule). Extracapsular cataract extraction coupled with posterior chamber intraocular lens implantation has been the method of choice in recent years. Techniques developed during the past three decades have made the process of cataract extraction and intraocular lens implantation one of the safest and most successful of all major operations.

Animal research and observational epidemiologic studies have provided preliminary data suggesting a protective role for antioxidant nutrients in the development of cataract. The hypothesis regarding the role of antioxidant nutrients in cataract development deserves further investigation. Recently in the United States various formulations of vitamins, antioxidants, and minerals have appeared on the market with claims of beneficial effects for various eye problems. To date, none of these drugs or vitamin formulations has been shown to be effective in preventing or slowing the formation of cataracts. Moreover, there is growing concern that excessive intake of vitamins and minerals can result in toxic reaction and interact adversely with other drugs and vitamins. As such, the development of well-designed studies of the safety and efficacy of any promising anticataract drugs including antioxidant nutrients is a goal of high priority in this program.

Highlights of Research Accomplishments

During the past 5 years the progress in all areas of cataract research has been remarkable. Techniques in molecular biology have revealed exciting new findings that profoundly affect our thinking on the structure and evolution of the genes encoding the crystallins, the major structural proteins of the lens. A striking finding is that certain lens crystallins are either identical or closely related to metabolic enzymes. For example γ-crystallin is enolase, ε-crystallin is lactate dehydrogenase, and δ-crystallin is argininosuccinate lyase. S-111 squid crystallin is related to glutathione S-transferase, and the list goes on. Not all of these crystallins have full enzymatic activity, but their structural similarities have important implications not only for evolutionary theory but also for our understanding of the stability and unique structural properties of these proteins in the lens. Utilizing one gene to express a functional enzyme in one instance and a structural protein in another certainly reduces the need for multiple genes. This gene-sharing hypothesis has opened a new area of research in which we now may look at the differential regulation of various lens genes.

Among other important recent contributions in the field of lens molecular biology is the finding that lens-specific crystallin promoters will target the synthesis of a nonlens-specific gene product to the lens. In addition, several groups have achieved the identification and characterization of various lens growth factors, the discovery that αB-crystallin is expressed in many nonlenticular tissues, the characterization and identification of lens cytoskeletal components, and the characterization of lens plasma membrane gap junctional and channel components.

Exciting progress is being made in studies of lens development and cataractogenesis using mouse models of human hereditary lens disorders. The mouse is ideally suited to this approach since its genome has been extensively mapped, and a comprehensive mouse-man homology map, which demonstrates remarkable congruence and conservation of sequence, is available. Screening studies of the large collection of existing mouse mutant strains at the Jackson Laboratory have identified and mapped seven different cataract markers. One particularly intriguing mutant, lop-10 (lens opacity), shows variable expressivity in the heterozygous lop-10 mouse. There appears to be a second site modifying gene which affects cataractogenesis, and the expression of cataract appears to require the loss of two separate functions. The identification and biochemical characterization of the modifying factor(s) is an obvious priority. Another set of lop markers defines a complex site on the small arm of the human-2/mouse-1 chromosome where several different loci affect the lens. Fine-structure analysis of this region is under way.

Another development in recent years is the successful culturing of human lens epithelial cells. Through improvements in tissue culture conditions, several groups of scientists are now able to grow human lens epithelial cells in culture. This opens the door for a variety of studies dealing with lens development, aging, and cataractogenesis.

Major emphasis has been placed in recent years on the growing attractiveness of the oxidative stress model to explain maturity-onset cataract. Many studies are focusing on characterizing various oxidative insults to the lens and on rationales to prevent oxidative stress. It is now commonly believed that oxidative insults are among the prime causes of lens cataractogenesis.

Significant advances have been made in our understanding of the structure and expression of aldose reductase (AR), an important enzyme that may be involved in many diabetic complications, including cataract. AR now has been cloned from various tissues and species, and the information obtained is indispensable for the future design of highly effective AR inhibitors—a high-priority goal for many investigators who are studying the various diseases caused by diabetic complications.

With recent advances in cataract surgery, it is very difficult at present to obtain whole, intact human lenses. Progress in sample retrieval and application of various microbiochemical techniques have shown that even small amounts of lens fragments obtained during cataract surgery are very useful. Thus, pieces of lens capsular epithelium obtained during routine cataract surgery have been used to study various enzymes in the epithelium. Similarly, capsular epithelium fragments have been successfully used for tissue culture studies.

Significant advances have been made in the areas of cataract classification and epidemiology. The Lens Opacities Classification System II (LOCS II) has proven to be a useful system that now opens the door for reliable epidemiologic studies.

Recommended Program Structure

The 1994–98 recommended program structure essentially encompasses most of the aims and goals of the current program structure. The format of the new program was changed to better reflect the recent advances in the molecular and developmental biology of the lens as well as our present understanding of the etiology of cataract. Whereas in the 1983–87 program, diabetic cataract, senile cataract, and cataract induced by environmental and toxic effects were each dealt with separately, our present understanding of the etiology of cataract points to common pathogenic mechanisms for all the different insults that may cause cataract. This knowledge has led to the formulation of a new program structure with the following six closely interrelated subprograms:

- Lens Development and Aging
- Cell Biology of the Lens
- Molecular Genetics
- Lens Biochemistry and Biophysics
- Pathogenesis of Cataract
- Epidemiology of Cataract.

Program Goals

The overall goal is to find the means of preventing or slowing cataract development. To achieve this, it is important to increasingly focus on studies of the human lens and meet the following supplemental goals:

- To understand, on the cellular and molecular level, the development, biochemistry, and biophysics of the normal and the cataractous lenses.

418

- To determine the causes and mechanisms of cataract formation.

- To evaluate the safety and efficacy of anticataractous drugs and methods of clinical management of cataract.

Chapter 49

National Eye Institute Report on Lens Development and Aging

Introduction

The lens is an excellent model for aging, as it is formed early in embryonic development and grows throughout life. Consequently, "lens development" is a lifelong process, not something that is over before birth. Cataract marks a transition between this normal developmental program and the expression of pathology. This means that abnormalities in developmental processes may be important contributors to age-related cataract.

Disturbances of early lens development lead to congenital cataracts. The accurate formation and function of the entire visual system require proper light transmission to the retina in the first few years of life. Consequently, congenital cataract can have effects that are not cured simply by removal of the defective lens. A thorough understanding of lens formation in the embryo and its growth and function before birth is needed to reduce the incidence and consequences of congenital cataract. Important progress has been made in understanding the events of early lens development. Advances in cell and molecular biology are expected to add to these gains.

Subprogram Objectives

- To understand the events of normal lens development and aging in order to identify the defects or pathologic interactions that

NIH Pub. No. 93–3196. Excerpt from *Vision Research: A National Plan*, pp. 159–63.

lead to congenital, early-onset, and age-related cataracts in humans.

- To identify interventions that can prevent or delay the developmental changes that lead to cataract formation.

Current Level of National Eye Institute Support

In Fiscal Year (FY) 1992 the National Eye Institute (NEI) supported nine grants for a total of $1,366,656 for research on lens development and aging.

Recent Accomplishments

The embryonic tissue interactions that lead to the formation of the lens have been an area of longstanding interest to developmental biologists. Recently the role of embryonic tissues involved in lens formation has been reexamined. Studies show that the optic vesicle plays a much less important role in lens induction than was formerly believed. Tissue interactions that occur long before the presumptive lens ectoderm contacts the optic vesicle are essential for generating a lens-forming bias in the head ectoderm. These advances provide the foundation upon which studies of the molecules involved in cell-cell signaling during lens formation can proceed. Such studies will be important not only because a better understanding of lens development is needed but also because defects in lens formation are associated with severe disruptions in the development of the entire anterior segment of the eye.

Another important aspect of lens development is an understanding of how the expression of certain genes is selectively targeted to the lens. Most research in this area has dealt with the lens-specific expression of the crystallin genes. DNA sequences located near or within the crystallin genes have been shown to be necessary for the efficient expression of these genes in lens cells. Current experiments are extending these observations and identifying proteins that bind to these sequences.

Although the gene products responsible for lens development are currently unknown, a powerful approach for their identification is through correlation of chromosomal aberrations with disease. The first indication of a human lens chromosomal map assignment came from the study of patients with aniridia, a developmental failure in the formation of the iris associated with cataract and dislocated lens. A subset of children with aniridia were observed to suffer a variety of embryonic defects, including Wilms' nephroblastoma, genitourinary tract defects, and mental retardation (WAGR syndrome). Children with WAGR have a large interstitial deletion on the short arm of chromosome 11, and this locus has been intensively studied by cytogeneticists and oncologists interested in the molecular details of tumorigenesis. The WAGR locus is large and phenotypically complex, but localization of the aniridia locus has been greatly aided by the recent discovery of three key patients with aniridia isolated from other WAGR symptoms. Somatic cell mapping of these loci will permit identification of the aniridia gene(s) and give important insights into early ocular development.

Study of the factors that control the growth of cultured cells has led to the purification, sequencing, and cloning of the genes for a number of growth factors. It is now evident that at least three of these play important roles in lens development and growth. Early work demonstrated the presence of an eye-derived growth factor in the retina. This activity was later shown to be due largely to the presence of basic and acidic fibroblast growth factor (FGF). Recently it has been shown that in addition to causing cell division, this family of growth factors can stimulate lens epithelial cells to differentiate into lens fibers. Thus, FGFs may play important roles in both lens growth and differentiation.

Another family of growth factors, the insulin-like growth factors (IGFs), have also been shown to stimulate lens growth and differentiation. IGF-1 could fully restore lens growth in animals in which the growth of the lens had been halted by removal of the pituitary gland. Later studies showed that IGF-like substances in the vitreous humor could stimulate embryonic lens epithelial cells to differentiate into lens fibers. Study of the role of FGFs and IGFs in lens fiber formation continues and is likely to provide important information on the control of lens growth and differentiation in the future.

One additional growth factor appears to play a role in lens growth. Platelet-derived growth factor could stimulate the growth of lenses from newborn rats. Interestingly, pulsatile release of this growth factor helps maintain the transparency of the lens in culture, whereas lenses grown without the factor or in its continued presence become cloudy and do not grow.

Recent information suggests that growth in lens thickness and curvature over many years of life may contribute to presbyopia in older individuals. Studies on the structure of the lens sutures in aging humans have raised the possibility that the pattern in which the new lens fibers are laid down is frequently altered in older lenses. These changes may be related to an increased risk for cataract formation. Thus, it is possible that the continuing growth of the lens is responsible for some of the deleterious changes that occur in older persons.

Another change in the function of the human lens that occurs with increasing age is a gradual decrease in its transmembrane potential. It has been suggested that this is due to an increase in the permeability of the lens to $Na+$ ions. Whether this change in ion permeability increases the risk of cataract formation is not known. However, the function and regulation of lens ion channels are under active investigation, and the relevance of this observation to lens function appears accessible to future study.

Important Research Questions to Be Addressed

Questions to be addressed include the following:

How do cells acquire the competence for lens formation?

The tissue interactions that result in lens formation have been redefined recently. Lens "induction" is clearly not a single event, and it appears that the distribution of cells that are competent to form a lens is more restricted than was previously believed. This new view could lead to the identification of the signals that establish lens competence.

What factors direct lens formation in the early embryo?

Purified growth factors and molecular probes for the messenger RNAs that encode them are now widely available. This may provide new information on the stimulation of lens formation from competent ectoderm. Culture systems are needed to permit the study of lens induction in a reliable manner and to allow intervention by the investigator. Such systems would permit important advances in this central problem in lens development.

Significant progress has been achieved in identifying at least two families of growth factors that are able to stimulate lens fiber differentiation from cultured lens epithelial cells. Although there may be

424

additional factors yet to be discovered, additional information about the distribution of the FGFs and IGFs in the eye and their relative role in lens development and disease is needed. Obtaining this information may be aided by accurately describing the distribution of FGFs and IGFs in the normal eye and by studying their interaction in vitro. The study of changes that occur in the levels of these agents with development and aging is an important area for future research. It will be particularly interesting to determine whether their concentration or distribution in the ocular media differs in cataract patients or those at risk for cataract formation. Both the FGFs and IGFs bind to extracellular matrix molecules or extracellular carrier proteins. The role of these binding activities in regulating the distribution or activity of the growth factors is also likely to be important. There is relatively little information on intracellular signaling pathways for either class of molecule. Cultured lens cells may provide an important model for studying "second messengers" generated by these factors. The pathways by which lens-fiber differentiation is controlled and lens-fiber-specific genes are activated would then be available for direct investigation.

What are the unique aspects of aging in the lens?

The study of aging in human lenses presents several difficulties. Few experimental approaches are possible on ethical grounds, and although epidemiologic studies can provide important information about the risk factors associated with cataract, these studies are expensive and have limitations on the kinds of questions that can be addressed. Post mortem human lens material is a valuable asset. However, satisfactory material for experimental studies is not always available, and lenses often must be used immediately upon receipt, preventing many kinds of experimental studies.

Animal models like the Emory mouse, which develops cataracts at later stages of life, have provided important insights into the early events in cataract formation. However, neither the Emory mouse nor other animal models of age-related cataract develop cortical cataracts in their early stages, as is most frequently seen in age-related cataract in humans. This observation suggests that established models of cortical cataract, such as radiation- or steroid-induced cataract, could be used to better understand human cortical cataract and that new models of age-related cataract should be sought.

Few attempts have been made to relate the changes seen during age-related cataract formation with other aspects of aging in the rest of the body. One exception to this is the recent work showing that restricting caloric intake can slow or prevent the formation of cataracts in the Emory mouse strain, just as caloric restriction slows other aspects of the aging process in experimental animals. Investigators should be encouraged to apply promising ideas generated by research on the aging of other organ systems or cell types to studies of cataract etiology and progression.

Chapter 50

National Eye Institute Report on the Pathogenesis of Cataract

Introduction

Cataracts have traditionally been described and categorized in a variety of ways on the basis of the location of the opacity in the lens (nuclear, cortical, or subcapsular) or of the agent or condition thought to be responsible for initiation of the cataract (e.g., radiation, diabetes, and steroids). This approach gives the impression that each such category represents a unique pathogenic mechanism and that each should be studied as a distinct entity. In fact, present evidence suggests that while cataractogenesis may be potentiated by a great variety of environmental, physiologic, or genetic factors, the cascade of events that follows that initiating insult and culminates in opacification of the lens is probably similar in most cataracts. Additionally, the initiating insult can be identified for only a minority of cataracts—for instance, those opacities associated with specific metabolic abnormalities or exposure to particular drugs or environmental agents. The vast majority of cataracts are of the age-related type for which no such initiating factor can be identified. Such cataracts undoubtedly can be potentiated by a number of different factors interacting additively or synergistically. Some of the factors are the result of normal aging processes, whereas others derive from individual differences in metabolism, genetic background, and environmental exposure.

NIH Pub. No. 93–3186. Excerpt from *Vision Research: A National Plan*, pp. 184–91.

In view of these considerations, cataract will be treated here as a single disease entity rather than subdivided into etiologic types, as has typically been done in the past. Although in a small percentage of cases the disease can be prevented or potentially prevented by the elimination of a specific initiating factor, in general, the most efficacious means of preventing or retarding the development of cataracts will come through the development of therapeutic agents that act on the pathologic processes that follow the initiating events. In general, these processes appear to follow a limited number of common pathways in which oxidative reactions are very important. The role of oxidation is not surprising, since in any tissue undergoing cellular disruption, oxidative damage will occur because of the loss of the normal compartmentalization of reactive species. An extensive body of evidence supports the concept that, with respect to human age-related cataract, there are, in fact, two major forms of the disease with different biochemical characteristics.

Consequently, separate consideration of these two types—namely cortical and nuclear—seems warranted. The cortical type is characterized by changes in the content of electrolytes, leading to osmotic swelling of the cells in the outer portions of the lens. Such swelling damages membranes, changing their permeability characteristics and ultimately producing liquefaction of the lens cortex. In nuclear cataracts the proteins in the central region of the lens undergo extensive modification. These proteins are the oldest in the lens and also turn over very slowly, allowing accumulation of a variety of structural modifications, including oxidation of amino acid side chains, glycation, racemization, deamidation, and limited proteolysis. Ultimately, the proteins undergo an aggregation process to form species of very high molecular weight. In both nuclear and cortical cataracts, the normal refractive index gradient through the lens is disrupted, producing light scattering and thus cataract. During the past several years, a number of investigations have produced results that have significantly increased understanding of the mechanisms involved in lens opacification. At the same time, many questions remain to be clarified. In addition, it cannot be overemphasized that, for understanding cataractogenesis, a better understanding of the biology of the normal lens, particularly with respect to its development, growth, aging, and metabolism, is a primary need.

Subprogram Objectives

- To determine the initiating factors for age-related cataract and the pathogenic mechanisms responsible for the subsequent development of such cataract.

- To determine the events in the process of development of age-related cataract that are amenable to therapeutic intervention and develop appropriate agents for such intervention.

- To elucidate the genetic contribution to the pathogenesis of both age-related cataract and congenital cataract.

- To establish better model systems for studying the pathogenesis of cataract.

Current Level of National Eye Institute Support

In FY 1992 the NEI supported 21 grants, for a total cost of $3,491,672, in the areas of the natural history, initiation, and treatment of lens opacities.

Recent Accomplishments

One of the research areas of greatest activity has been the elucidation of the role of oxidative stress in the pathogenesis of cataract. Although it is widely believed that oxidation plays a major role in the development of cataract, there has been little agreement on the mechanisms responsible. Recently evidence from both experimental and epidemiologic studies have added to our knowledge in this area. Numerous investigators have used a variety of model systems to study the effects of activated species of oxygen on the lens or its constituents. Using intact lenses in organ culture, lens cell cultures, or lens protein solutions, the effects of singlet oxygen ($^{1}O_{2}$), hydroxyl radicals, and other oxidants should be determined. Oxidative modifications to lens crystallins, enzymes, and membranes that are similar to those found in the aging and cataractous human lens have been detected. Light-mediated processes, both direct and photosensitized, have been implicated as probable contributors to the oxidation occurring *in vivo*.

429

Additionally, the probable importance of metal-catalyzed oxidation reactions involving the high levels of H_2O_2 in the eye has been demonstrated. A model system of particular interest is hyperbaric oxygen, which is the first such system in which the primary damage is found in the lens nucleus. Analysis of the protein-thiol mixed disulfides in human cataracts and in lenses exposed to various oxidative stresses *in vitro* suggests that these may be important intermediates in the oxidative effects on proteins. Recent studies have also demonstrated that quite low levels of H_2O_2 can induce significant DNA damage in cultured lens epithelial cells. Single strand breaks and other types of damage have been quantified, and rates of repair have been studied.

From both the studies on DNA damage and those on metal-catalyzed oxidative effects on proteins, it is dear that activated species of oxygen derived from the H_2O_2, rather than H_2O_2 itself, actually produce the oxidative damage. Those studying oxidation as a cause of cataract have a major need for sensitive new assays for quantitation of oxygen radicals in the lens.

An epidemiologic study of Chesapeake Bay watermen has reported an association between cortical cataract and exposure to UV radiation, specifically UV-B radiation. Although it is unclear whether the findings of this study would apply to individuals with more normal exposure to UV-B radiation, the data do give some support to several earlier studies that reported a higher incidence of cataract in individuals living in areas of high levels of ambient UV radiation. A number of animal studies also have demonstrated cataract development induced by elevated exposure to UV radiation.

The importance of the various antioxidant systems in the lens also has been investigated. Although the lens contains several enzyme systems that may be involved in protection of the tissue from oxidation, it has been clearly established that the glutathione redox system is of primary importance in this regard.

Inhibition of this system has been shown to potentiate cataract formation in some experimental models. Further evidence that antioxidant status may be an important determinant of age-related cataract comes from epidemiologic studies, suggesting that plasma levels of the antioxidant nutrients vitamin E, ß-carotene, and vitamin C affect the susceptibility to cataract development. Additionally, there are reports that certain experimental cataracts can be prevented, or their development slowed, by administration of antioxidants such as ascorbic acid, butylated hydroxytoluene, or the monoethylester of glutathione.

There have been two advances that facilitate study of human lens epithelial cell function. First, methods to extend the growth of primary cell cultures of human lens epithelial cells have been improved. The growth potential is still quite limited in comparison with the success in growing lens cells from some other species, but it has been demonstrated that the cells can be made to undergo differentiation to form lenslike structures and that expression of crystallins and the lens-specific intrinsic membrane protein does occur. The use of epithelial cells from very young, normal lenses is most desirable for such culture. However, limited success with epithelial cells from clinically extracted cataracts also has been achieved. With respect to utilization of clinical samples, progress has been made in the development of methods for the microanalysis of enzyme activities and protein composition from the anterior capsule epithelium samples recovered from the operating room. Analysis of several enzymes can now be done on a single epithelial sample. Specifically, the activity of glutathione reductase was found to be significantly reduced in some cataract samples, and in a portion of these, addition of the obligate cofactor flavin adenine dinucleotide restored normal activity. Improvements in the techniques for fixation of the lens and for its analysis by light and electron microscopy make it possible now to study and compare the structure of all the cells throughout the entire lens. This has greatly facilitated the study of the plasma membrane and its interaction with the various cytoskeletal elements found in the lens. Cell fusion has been demonstrated to occur between lens fibers, and very recent studies of the architecture of the lens sutures have demonstrated that the normal symmetrical suture structure is altered in cortical cataracts. These alterations are evident in tissue laid down long before the cataract formed. In contrast, pure nuclear cataracts have the symmetrical suture structure characteristic of normal lenses.

With respect to hereditary cataracts, a large family with "Coppock-like" cataract has been shown to have a mutation closely linked to the γ-crystallin genes. Very recent data indicate that the mutation is in the promoter region of γE, a truncated pseudogene, and appears to result in markedly increased expression of this polypeptide. How the mutation causes the cataract is unclear, but this is the first human cataract family shown to have a mutation involving a lens crystallin. Previous linkage studies by several groups have consistently failed to find linkage with known crystallin genes. These studies indicate considerable heterogeneity in the loci responsible for human hereditary cataracts. Recent advances also have been made

431

in the study of animal models of hereditary congenital cataracts in which mutations have been demonstrated in the genes of major crystalins. In the Philly mouse, an internal deletion of four residues is present in the major ß-crystallin polypeptide ßB2. Although it remains to be determined how this change causes cataract, it has been demonstrated that the mutant protein has lost the unique heat stability characteristic of normal ßB2. In the congenital nuclear cataract present in the strain 13/N guinea pig, a mutation has occurred in the gene for the taxon-specific protein ζ-crystallin. Deletion at a splice site causes the loss of a complete exon from the transcript and produces a protein with an internal deletion of 34 residues. ζ-crystallin has been shown to be an NADPH-dependent oxidoreductase, and the mutant has lost the ability to bind NADPH. These systems represent opportunities for investigating the effects of specific structural modifications on the critical protein-protein interactions in the lens.

While the "function" of the lens crystallins remains largely speculative at present, it is thought that they play a pivotal role in the formation of at least some types of cataract. The past few years have seen a rapid increase in knowledge on the evolutionary origins of crystallins. As an outgrowth of the increasing emphasis on the molecular biology of the crystallin genes, it is now known that the major vertebrate crystallins are related to protein families that in other systems function as "stress" proteins.

The α-crystallins recently have been reported to possess molecular chaparonin activity *in vitro*. They inhibit the aggregation of other crystallins and thus may play an *in vivo* role in maintaining functional interactions between lens proteins. The class of "taxon-specific" crystallins has been greatly expanded and shown to represent metabolic enzymes recruited by the lens to function as structural proteins. The concept of "gene sharing" in which a single protein may have completely different functions in different tissues has been proposed to account for the enzyme crystallins. These major changes in our conception of the crystallins should move us closer to elucidation of their true function and the structural basis underlying that function.

In addition to the anticataract effects that have been reported in certain model systems for various antioxidants and the prevention of sugar cataracts in animals by AR inhibitors, there recently have been several other reports of prevention of cataracts by drugs. Both x-ray-induced cataract in rabbits and the selenite cataract in rats have been reduced in severity by administration of an agent that lowers the phase-transition temperature (Tc) in the lens. Although it remains to be definitely proven that the lowering of Tc is responsible for this effect, the results may represent an important advance in the area of cataract prevention. The fact that a single agent has an inhibitory effect on two cataracts that have very different morphological and biochemical characteristics and are initiated by completely different factors supports the hypothesis that inhibition of the cataractogenic process subsequent to its initiation is a viable approach to cataract prevention.

An additional instance of prevention of an experimentally induced cataract is the action of the AR inhibitor AL-1576 on the naphthalene-induced cataract in rats. This effect has been shown not to result from inhibition of AR. Rather, the agent may inhibit another oxidoreductase that is involved in the metabolic conversion of naphthalene to the compound responsible for toxic effects in the lens.

Important Research Questions to Be Addressed

Although the past several years have clearly seen considerable progress toward our understanding of many aspects of the biology of the normal lens and the mechanisms involved in the pathogenesis of cataract, we still have a long way to go before the problem of cataract is solved. Additional research is needed in virtually all areas. The following questions need to be addressed in future research efforts:

Is oxidative insult important in cataractogenesis?

Further studies of the impact of oxidation on the lens and its contribution to the pathogenesis of cataract are needed. The relationship between the generation of active species of oxygen in the lens and loss of transparency needs to be clarified. Which activated species are present and how are they formed? What are the specific target molecules for the free radicals or other oxidants? Which oxidative modifications are truly relevant to the formation of cataract? How do the various antioxidants in the lens and in the surrounding fluids interact to defend the lens against the chronic oxidative stress to which it is exposed? How can these defenses be augmented therapeutically? How important are transition metal ions in the lens as contributors to the formation of oxidants via mixed function oxidation systems? What is the true level of H_2O_2 in the aqueous humor, and does it play a major role in the causation of cataract?

These questions apply to oxidative damage to all the constituents of the lens, including the structural proteins, enzymes, membranes, and nucleic acids. The specific sites of damage need to be determined for each class of macromolecule. Also, the capacity of the lens to repair or replace such oxidized molecules needs to be established. To prove the hypothesis that oxidation causes cataract, appropriate model systems need to be developed in which antioxidants can be tested. Only by demonstrating the efficacy of such agents in preventing oxidation and cataract can the hypothesis be proven. Desirable systems would include animal models; improved lens organ culture systems providing long-term maintenance, growth, and differentiation; and human lens epithelial cell cultures with improved growth and better retention of lens characteristics.

What are the mechanisms and factors that control transparency in the lens?

Since the transparency of the lens is thought to depend upon precise protein-protein interactions within the highly concentrated and highly ordered protein matrix, there is a great need to elucidate the nature of these interactions and determine the effects of protein modifications on these interactions and on transparency. The forces that stabilize the protein matrix in the normal lens need to be understood, as do the forces involved in the protein aggregation phenomena that produce high molecular weight species. Both disulfide and nondisulfide cross-links are known to be involved in this aggregation process, as well as noncovalent interactions such as hydrophobic attractions. The relative importance of such processes needs to be carefully examined. Determination of the nature of the nondisulfide covalent cross-links should be a high priority because it would give direct evidence concerning the mechanism responsible. Several cross-linking mechanisms have been proposed and are known to occur in model systems. These include oxidation of amino acid side chains (probably histidine) by activated species of oxygen, with subsequent reaction of the modified side chain with another amino acid residue; cross-linking as a consequence of glycation; or cross-linking by malondialdehyde or other bifunctional aldehyde products produced by lipid peroxidation. The same processes also are known to produce pigmented and fluorescent material similar to that present in aging and accelerated mouse, may yield valuable insight cataractous human lenses.

The question of the role of glycation should be reexamined in light of recent data on glycation by ascorbate and the discovery of fructose-3 phosphate and sorbitol-3-phosphate in the lens. The contribution of glycation and other post translational modifications, such as carbamylation, racemization, and deamidation, should be investigated in cataracts of various types.

What is the role and significance of phase transitions in the lens?

The significance of the phase transition phenomenon as a general factor in lens opacification needs to be determined. An increase in phase-separation temperature seems to be a consistent feature in cataracts, and an agent believed to act by lowering the phase-separation temperature can prevent certain experimental cataracts. Is this physical principle strictly applicable to a complex interactive biologic system? What lens constituents are important in the phase-transition phenomenon, and how do the phase-transition inhibitors interact with these constituents?

What is the role of genetics in the development of cataracts?

Determination of genetic factors influencing congenital and age-related cataracts deserves higher priority and increased support. With respect to age-related cataracts, there is strong evidence that genetic differences can represent important risk factors. Individuals heterozygous for enzymes, such as those that metabolize galactose, are statistically more likely to develop age-related cataracts. There are also families that are predisposed to develop such cataracts at an earlier age than is usually expected (presenile cataracts). Linkage studies of such families might well reveal candidate genes responsible for this condition. Additionally, further analysis of the process of cataractogenesis in animal models, such as the Emory mouse, the inherited cataract rat, or the senescence into the factors involved in formation of age-related cataract.

With respect to genetic congenital cataract, linkage studies should still be rigorously pursued in families with appropriate pedigrees. Although success thus far has been very limited, both the technology used in such investigations and the base of knowledge on the human genome will rapidly expand in the next few years. Good animal models of congenital cataracts with defined mutations are now being described. These systems should be actively investigated to determine the precise mechanisms responsible for producing opacification. Not only the initiating mutation but also the entire sequence of molecular events that culminates in opacification needs to be elucidated.

Finally, the role of genetics should be investigated through the use of transgenic animals. Cataracts already have been produced in a number of transgenic mice. Lens-specific promoters are available to drive expression of transgenes; therefore, studies of the introduction of altered genes can be performed. In the case of congenital cataract animal models, gene replacement therapy using these techniques can be explored.

How can we improve our studies of human normal and cataractous tissues?

There is a need for new techniques and increased emphasis on studies of human lens tissue—both normal eye bank material and surgical specimens. Such studies are complicated by limitations on material due to the extracapsular cataract extraction techniques that are now employed and, except in the case of some congenital cataract samples, the degree of post-translational modification and heterogeneity present. These factors make determination of correlations between biochemical abnormalities and specific cataract types difficult. Improved means of analyzing lens protein composition need to be developed.

Since the lens epithelium undoubtedly plays a primary role in maintenance of homeostasis throughout the lens, studies of its metabolic and physiologic status in both normal lenses and cataracts need to be undertaken or extended. Additionally, human lens epithelial cell culture should be utilized to investigate processes such as oxidative effects on DNA and other cellular constituents as well as to expand studies on differentiation and regulation of crystallin expression.

What is the role of AR in human cataractogenesis?

Although the primary role of AR in the initiation of sugar cataract formation in various animal models is established, it is unclear whether it is important in the causation of cataract in human diabetics. It would be important to know whether the lower amount of AR present in the human lens represents a significant factor in the generation of such cataracts. A clinical trial may be necessary to resolve this question.

436

Chapter 51

National Eye Institute Report on Epidemiology of Cataract

Introduction

A growing awareness of the magnitude of the cataract problem throughout the world has stimulated interest in epidemiologic studies of cataract. Descriptive epidemiologic studies can provide data on the number and characteristics of persons affected by cataract, particularly in relation to person, time, and place. Analytic epidemiologic studies test hypotheses, often generated by descriptive studies or laboratory studies, about particular factors that may influence the risk of developing cataract. One of the most powerful analytic tools—clinical trials—can be used to evaluate preventive, diagnostic, and therapeutic techniques.

Subprogram Objectives

- To develop and evaluate cataract measurement techniques and classification systems.
- To determine the clinical course and prognosis of specific types of age-related lens opacities.
- To assess the incidence and prevalence of cataract.
- To identify factors that influence the risk of developing cataract.

NIH Pub. No. 93–3186. Excerpt from *Vision Research: A National Plan*, pp. 191–197.

- To evaluate diagnostic and therapeutic techniques in cataract management.

Current Level of National Eye Institute Support

In FY 1992 the NEI provided support for four epidemiologic studies of cataract at a total cost of $1,127,088. The various studies provided data on the incidence and prevalence of cataract, traced the natural history of specific types of lens opacities, identified factors that influence the risk of developing cataract, and developed and evaluated the reproducibility of cataract classification systems. Also, the NEI partially funded a clinical trial which had a secondary objective of determining whether aspirin use affected the risk of cataract development. In FY 1990 the NEI started a large, multiyear, multicenter study that will trace the clinical course and prognosis of age-related cataract.

Recent Accomplishments

Until recently a major obstacle to clinical studies of cataract had been the lack of adequate measurement and classification schemes for lens opacities. Differences in methods of examination and diagnostic criteria have made it difficult to know whether reported differences between studies are real. In recent years systems that reliably grade cataracts in vivo have been developed. One system, LOCS II, uses a series of photographic standards (four nuclear cataract standards for grading nuclear opalescence and color, six cortical cataract standards, and four posterior subcapsular cataract standards) to diagnose the presence and severity of the three major types of cataract. The standard photographs can be used to grade cataracts at the slit lamp or to grade slit lamp and retroillumination photographs. LOCS II and similar grading systems have been used successfully in cross-sectional studies and are now being evaluated in longitudinal studies of cataract.

Techniques with potential for grading smaller amounts of cataractous change than can be detected with LOCS II have been developed and are being evaluated. These techniques involve the analysis of images produced by the Topcon SL-45 slit camera, the Zeiss Video Image Analysis System, the Neitz CTR retroillumination camera, Sasaki's combination retroillumination/Scheimpflug system, and conventional photoslit and retroillumination photography as well as measurement of quasielastic light scattering in the lens.

Little is known about the incidence of age-related cataract in the population and the natural history of lens opacities. Attempts have been made to calculate incidence rates based on age-specific prevalence data. On the basis of Framingham Eye Study data, the 5-year incidence estimates for the development of lens changes for ages 55, 60, 65, 70, and 75 are 10, 16, 23, 31, and 37 percent, respectively. The 5-year incidence of age-related cataract (i.e., visual acuity of 6/9 or worse and lens opacities that entirely account for the vision loss) ranged from 1 to 15 percent for these same age groups. These rates may be underestimates if, as suggested by some, there is a differential mortality for persons with and without cataracts.

Studies that will provide additional data on the frequency and natural history of age-related cataract are under way. These studies are useful for measuring the magnitude of cataract as a cause of morbidity, describing the distribution of cataracts in the population according to demographic and other characteristics, monitoring trends in occurrence, and providing leads on etiologic factors. Surviving members of the Framingham Eye Study cohort, who were originally examined in 1973 to 1975, were reexamined in 1986 to 1989. Data from the two Framingham Eye Studies are being used to estimate incidence rates for lens opacities. Additional data on cataract prevalence will be derived from a population-based study currently being conducted in Beaver Dam, Wisconsin. Other studies funded by the NEI that will evaluate the rates of progression of lens opacities and the risk factors associated with progression are under way. It now seems likely that age-related cataract does not have a single etiology but can result from a variety of insults to the lens. A large number of possible risk factors for cataract have been suggested, but the strength of the epidemiologic evidence in support of the reported associations varies. There is a well-established relationship between increasing age and risk of cataract. While visually significant cataracts are rare before the fifth decade, one-half of the population has visually significant lens opacities by the eighth decade. There also is a small but consistently reported excess risk of cataract for women. The longstanding clinical impression that cataracts are more common among diabetics has been substantiated by epidemiologic studies. Diabetics under age 70 have an excess prevalence of age-related cataract; among those over age 70, the excess risk appears to be less. Less clearly established is the relationship between age-related cataract and a number of other possible risk factors that have been the subject of recent studies.

Animal studies have shown that a variety of nutritional deficiencies can lead to cataract formation. However, the importance of nutrient status in human cataractogenesis remains unclear. Two of three large, case-control studies that used food frequency interviews to estimate dietary intake of selected nutrients reported a decreased risk of cataract in persons with a higher intake of a number of micronutrients. One of the studies also reported a decreased risk of cataracts among persons who used multiple vitamin supplements regularly. A smaller case-control study found fewer cataracts in persons taking supplementary vitamin C or supplementary vitamin E. One additional observational study reported that persons with "high" plasma levels of at least two of three vitamins with antioxidant characteristics (vitamin E, vitamin C, or carotenoids) were at reduced risk of cataract compared with persons with "low" levels of these vitamins. No association was found between the risk of cataract and erythrocyte levels of superoxide dismutase and glutathione peroxidase, enzymes important in antioxidant systems of red blood cells as well as the lens. Potential problems caused by unadjusted confounding, bias, and lack of information about the relationship between nutrient levels in the blood and in the lens make it difficult to evaluate the results of these observational studies. Studies currently under way in the United States and Italy are attempting to examine further the relationship between nutritional factors and specific types of cataract.

Radiation from almost all regions of the electromagnetic spectrum is capable of damaging the lens. In recent years attention has been directed toward investigating whether exposure to ultraviolet light, in particular UV-B radiation, is an important factor in cataract development. Several correlational studies have suggested a higher prevalence of cataract in areas with greater UV exposure. Results from case-control studies also suggest that increased sunlight exposure may increase the risk of cataract. A study that attempted to quantify individual, lifetime UV-B exposure reported that fishermen with the highest amount of exposure were at increased risk of cortical and posterior subcapsular cataracts. Better evidence is needed to establish an association between cataract and exposure to ultraviolet light magnitude of any increased risk in the general population. The importance of UV exposure relative to other risk factors remains unclear.

An increased risk of cataract has been reported for nonwhites and persons with myopic refractive errors, episodes of severe diarrhea,

440

higher levels of systolic blood pressure, and various blood biochemistry markers. An association between nuclear lens opacities and smoking has been reported. Observational studies also have suggested a protective effect of aspirin and "aspirin-like analgesics" on cataract development. Other observational studies and two clinical trials seem to have excluded any large protective effect on cataract development from low aspirin dosage.

The NEI recently initiated the Age-Related Eye Disease Study (AREDS). AREDS is a 10-year, multicenter cohort study designed to assess the clinical cause, prognosis, and risk factors of age-related macular degeneration and of cataract. Various risk factors, such as medication use, medical conditions, demographic factors, and nutritional factors, will be evaluated. In addition, the effects of high-dose antioxidants (vitamin C and E and ß-carotene) on the development and progression of lens opacities will be assessed in randomized clinical trials.

Important Research Questions to Be Addressed

Important questions to be addressed include the following:

Are current grading systems suitable for follow-up studies of cataract?

A major research priority is to determine whether currently available systems for grading the type and severity of lens opacities in vivo will be suitable for cataract follow-up studies. The LOCS II and similar grading systems require an examiner to grade opacities subjectively at the slit lamp or on photographs using standardized techniques. These grading systems have been shown to be highly reproducible in cross-sectional studies. However, since the rate of change of lens opacities is not known, testing is needed to determine whether the grading systems are sufficiently sensitive to detect changes in lens status in relatively short time periods—a requirement for use in follow-up studies.

Under investigation are other techniques that have the potential for grading smaller amounts of cataractous change than can be detected with LOCS II and related systems. These techniques involve the analysis of images produced by the Topcon SL-45 slit camera, the Zeiss Video Image Analysis System, the Neitz CTR retroillumination camera, Sasaki's combination retroillumination/Scheimpflug system, and conventional photoslit and retroillumination photography as well as measurement of quasi-elastic light scattering in the lens. The ability to reliably detect small amounts of change could increase the efficiency of longitudinal studies of cataract should current systems prove to be unable to detect changes in lens status in relatively short time periods. Follow-up studies also could benefit from techniques for reliably identifying lens characteristics that predict the development of opacities before opacities become manifest.

What is the clinical course and prognosis of specific types of lens opacities?

Incidence and prevalence data would permit investigators to predict more accurately sample size requirements and the likely durations of follow-up studies of cataract. Limited data are available on the incidence and prevalence of the different types of cataract in the general population, characteristics of persons affected, extent of their visual impairment, existence of possible geographic differences, and time trends. Such data are important for public health planning. Information on the distribution of cataracts in the population may generate hypotheses about cataract etiology.

What risk factors are important in cataract etiology?

A major need is the identification of risk factors for age-related cataract. Analytic studies are needed to evaluate further the relationship between age-related cataract and possible risk factors such as nutritional status, exposure to UV and microwave radiation, family history of cataract, smoking, exposure to drugs with cataractogenic potential, metabolic factors, and a variety of other factors suggested by the literature. The identification of risk factors can lead to understanding etiology—a major goal of the Lens and Cataract Program.

What is the value of new diagnostic and therapeutic techniques in cataract management?

Epidemiologic input will be needed to evaluate proposed forms of cataract prevention and medical treatment as they become available. Well-designed clinical trials will be needed to assess the efficacy and long-term advantages of proposed preventive and therapeutic modalities.

Appropriate evaluation of the new devices and procedures used in the preoperative, operative, and postsurgical periods is required. Studies of the comparative value of the various options available for managing patients with cataract are needed to allow clinicians to make informed decisions about optimum patient management. Such studies could also provide information on cost-effectiveness. Because of the magnitude of the cataract problem, even small savings could have large overall effects.

Part Seven

Macular Disorders

Chapter 52

Macular Pucker

What is the macula?

The macula is the special area at the center of the retina which is responsible for clear, detailed vision. The retina is the light sensing layer of tissue that lines the back of the eye. If your macula is damaged, your sight will be blurred.

What is macular pucker?

The macula normally lies flat against the back of the eye, like film lining the back of a camera. If macular pucker is present, the macula becomes wrinkled.

This condition is also known as cellophane maculopathy, or premacular fibrosis.

What are the symptoms of macular pucker?

Vision becomes blurred and distorted, just as one would expect a picture to appear from a camera with wrinkled film. Straight lines, like doorways or telephone poles, often appear wavy.

Vision loss can vary from barely noticeable to severe. One or both eyes may be involved. For most people, vision remains stable and does not get progressively worse.

American Academy of Ophthalmology, ©1994. Used by permission.

What causes macular pucker?

A thin, transparent membrane grows over the macula. When the membrane stops growing, it contracts and shrinks, wrinkling the macula. Eye conditions that may be associated with macular pucker include:

- vitreous detachment (aging of gel inside eye);
- torn or detached retina;
- inflammation inside eye;
- severe injury to eye;
- retinal blood vessel disorders.

Macular pucker is not usually related to any medical problem outside the eye.

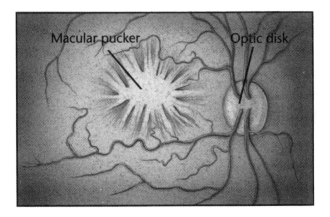

Figure 52.1. *Macular Pucker*

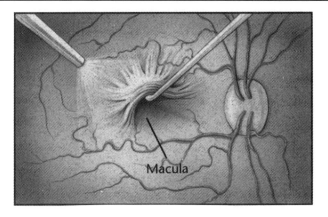

Figure 52.2. Surgical instruments removing membrane

How is it detected?

Your ophthalmologist can detect macular pucker by examining your retina. A photographic test called a fluorescein angiogram may be done in order to tell the extent of damage to the macula.

Does macular pucker need to be treated?

Treatment is not necessary if your symptoms are mild. Eyedrops, medicines, or laser surgery do not improve vision. Strengthening your bifocals or using a magnifier may improve near vision if both eyes are involved.

Vitrectomy surgery is the only treatment that can remove macular pucker. During this outpatient procedure, your ophthalmologist uses tiny instruments to remove the membrane which is wrinkling the macula.

Usually, the macula flattens out and the symptoms slowly improve. Vision does not usually return all the way to normal. Cataracts (clouding of the eye's lens) may develop sooner.

Complications are uncommon, but may include:

- infection;
- bleeding;
- retinal detachment;
- re-occurrence of macular pucker.

Surgery is not necessary for everyone who has macular pucker. Many people who have mildly blurred vision are not bothered enough to need surgery. You should consider surgery if your blurred vision is interfering with your daily activities.

Why are regular medical eye examinations important for everyone?

Eye disease can strike at any age. Many eye diseases do not cause symptoms until the disease has done damage. Since most blindness is preventable if diagnosed and treated early, regular medical examinations by an ophthalmologist are very important.

Chapter 53

Macular Degeneration

What is macular degeneration?
What causes it?
What can be done?
Will I go blind?

If you or a family member have been diagnosed with macular degeneration, you may be asking some of these questions. Although there is no "cure" for this condition, there is much that can be done. This brochure provides a basic explanation of the disease and answers some of your questions.

Understanding Macular Degeneration

Macular degeneration affects the macula, the central part of the retina. The macula is responsible for central vision and the ability to see detail.

When the macula is damaged, the eye loses its ability to see detail, such as small print, facial features, or small objects. The damaged parts of the macula often cause scotomas, or localized areas of vision loss. When you look at things with the damaged area, objects or parts of objects may seem to fade or disappear. Straight lines or edges may appear wavy.

The Lighthouse ©1995. Pub. No. P680. Used by permission.

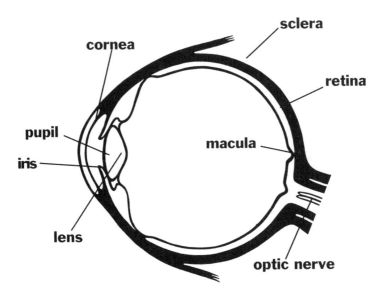

Figure 53.1. Cross section of the eye, visible structures.

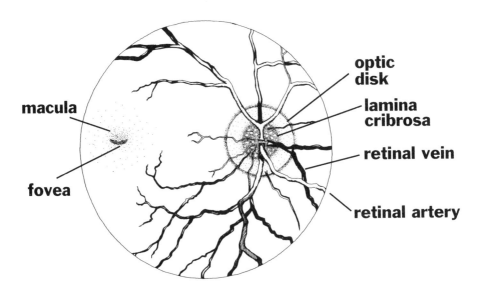

Figure 53.2. Internal structures of the eye.

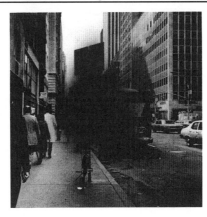

Figure 53.3. *Central vision is decreased because of a scotoma. Peripheral (side) vision is unaffected.*

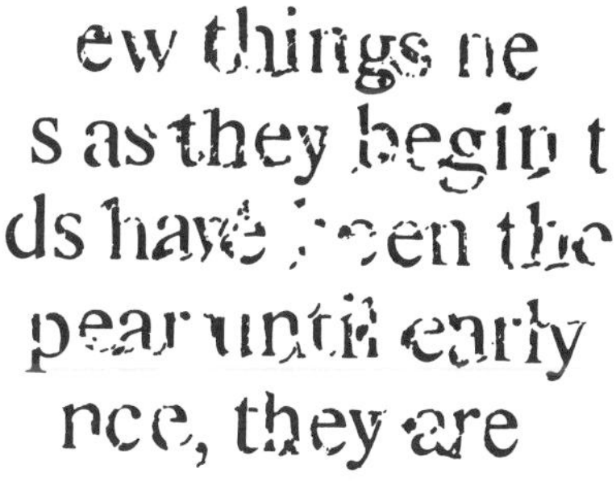

ew things ne
s as they begin t
ds have een the
pear until early
nce, they are

Figure 53.4. *Print appears distorted and parts of words may be missing.*

What Causes Macular Degeneration?

Age-related macular degeneration usually occurs in people over 60, and is found in two forms, atrophic, or "dry" macular degeneration, and exudative, or "wet" macular degeneration.

As people age, certain layers of the retina may deteriorate. Nowadays, because people live longer, more people are diagnosed with macular degeneration. What is not clear is why this happens as people age. Possible causes include:

- a lack of certain vitamins and minerals needed by the retina
- breakdown in the circulation to the retina

- excessive levels of cholesterol or sugar in our diets that, over time, may contribute to the degenerative process
- untreated general health problems such as hypertension
- excessive exposure to ultraviolet light, the harmful radiation from the sun
- heredity may also be a factor

"Dry" vs "Wet" Macular Degeneration: What's the Difference?

Dry

Origin: Degeneration and atrophy of one of the retinal layers
Progress: No leakage or bleeding unless disease progresses into the wet form.
Symptoms: Loss of detail vision
Identified by: Ophthalmoscopy, a simple procedure that allows the doctor to view the back of the eye.
Further Diagnosis by: Fluorescein angiogram test. Dye injected into a vein in the arm travels to the eye, where it highlights the damaged areas. This test indicates what type of macular degeneration is present.
Treatment: Laser treatment is not appropriate; however, in recent years there have been a number of promising research developments in medical and surgical treatment.
Outcome: Vision loss varies depending on location and extent of damage to the macula. Since peripheral (side) vision is not affected, some useable vision remains.

Wet

Origin: Fluid leaks into the space under the retina
Progress: New blood vessels may grow in or under the retina, and may leak or bleed. This is sometimes called hemorrhagic macular degeneration.
Symptoms: Diminished central vision
Identified by: Ophthalmoscopy, a simple procedure that allows the doctor to view the back of the eye.
Further Diagnosis by: Fluorescein angiogram test. Dye injected into a vein in the arm travels to the eye, where it highlights the areas

where there is leakage. This test indicates what type of macular degeneration is present.

Treatment: Laser treatment can seal off leaking areas, but it does not repair existing damage. A number of promising alternatives to laser treatment are under study.

Outcome: Vision loss varies depending on location and extent of the damage to the macula. Wet macular degeneration often leads to more extensive vision loss than dry macular degeneration. Since peripheral (side) vision is not affected, some useable vision remains.

What Can Be Done?

Although no surgical or medical treatment for macular degeneration has been found to be widely effective, there is still much that can be done. Vision rehabilitation agencies like The Lighthouse Inc. offer a variety of services that help people with macular degeneration.

Doctors specializing in low vision care perform a comprehensive evaluation of your vision and then prescribe optical devices to help you use your remaining vision more effectively. These may include high-powered spectacles, magnifiers, or telescopes. A Closed-Circuit Television (CCTV), which displays text on a screen in a magnified form, can help with reading. Training is necessary to help you use these devices.

You can learn new ways to perform daily activities such as cooking, managing finances, and grooming. Vision Rehabilitation Teachers can suggest ways to mark clothes, groceries, and medications so they are recognizable and easily found; to modify the home for safety and comfort; and to improve lighting and reduce glare.

Training is also available to help you get around in your home or outdoors; Orientation and Mobility Instructors can teach you to travel safely and confidently.

There are many devices and products that can make it possible to do things for yourself. Clocks and telephones with large numbers, bold-lined paper, signature guides, and black felt-tipped pens are simple and inexpensive products that make daily tasks easier. Talking or large-print books are also an important resource. These are called adaptive devices. These products and other useful items are available from The Lighthouse Consumer Products Catalog.

General Eye Care and Health

It is important to continue regular eye examinations to monitor the macular degeneration and to check for other conditions such as glaucoma and cataracts. If you experience any sudden vision changes, you should contact your doctor immediately. In addition, take good care of your general health including diet, control of cholesterol, high blood pressure, diabetes, or any other medical condition that could affect your vision.

Further Information and Resources

Contact The Lighthouse Information and Resource Service at (800) 334-5497 to:

- Find low vision centers, vision rehabilitation agencies, or support groups in your locale
- Learn more about adaptive devices and products
- Request a Consumer Products Catalog.

> —*By Eleanor E. Faye, MD, FACS,*
> *Michael Fischer, OD, FAAO*
> *and Martha Schulman, MAT.*

Chapter 54

Don't Lose Sight of Age-Related Macular Degeneration

What is age-related macular degeneration (AMD)?

AMD is a common eye disease associated with aging that gradually destroys sharp, central vision. Central vision is needed for seeing objects clearly and for common daily tasks such as reading and driving. In some people, AMD advances so slowly that it will have little effect on their vision as they age. But in others, the disease progresses faster and may lead to a loss of vision in one or both eyes.

How does AMD damage vision?

The retina is a paper-thin tissue that lines the back of the eye and sends visual signals to the brain. In the middle of the retina is a tiny area called the macula. The macula is made up of millions of light-sensing cells that help to produce central vision.

AMD occurs in two forms:

Dry AMD. Ninety percent of all people with AMD have this type. Scientists are still not sure what causes dry AMD. Studies suggest that an area of the retina becomes diseased, leading to the slow breakdown of the light-sensing cells in the macula and a gradual loss of central vision.

Wet AMD. Although only 10 percent of all people with AMD have this type, it accounts for 90 percent of all blindness from the disease.

NIH Pub. No. 93-3462.

As dry AMD worsens, new blood vessels may begin to grow and cause "wet" AMD. Because these new blood vessels tend to be very fragile, they will often leak blood and fluid under the macula. This causes rapid damage to the macula that can lead to the loss of central vision in a short period of time.

Who is most likely to get AMD?

The greatest risk factor is age. Although AMD may occur during middle age, studies show that people over age 60 are clearly at greater risk than other age groups. For instance, a large study found that people in middle-age have about a 2 percent risk of getting AMD, but this risk increased to nearly 30 percent in those over age 75.

Other AMD risk factors include:

- Gender: Women tend to be at greater risk than men.
- Race: Whites are much more likely to lose vision from AMD than Blacks.
- Smoking: Smoking may increase the risk of AMD.
- Family History: Those with immediate family members who have AMD are at higher risk of developing the disease.

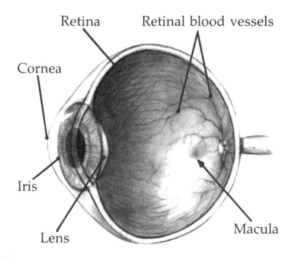

Figure 54.1.

What are the symptoms?

Both dry and wet AMD cause no pain. The most common early sign of dry AMD is blurred vision. As fewer cells in the macula are able to function, people will see details less clearly in front of them, such as faces or words in a book. Often this blurred vision will go away in brighter light. If the loss of these light-sensing cells becomes great, people may see a small—but growing—blind spot in the middle of their field of vision.

The classic early symptom of wet AMD is that straight lines appear crooked. This results when fluid from the leaking blood vessels gathers and lifts the macula, distorting vision. A small blind spot may also appear in wet AMD, resulting in loss of one's central vision.

How is it detected?

Your eye care professional may suspect AMD if you are over age 60 and have had recent changes in your central vision. To look for signs of the disease, he or she will use eye drops to dilate, or enlarge, your pupils. Dilating the pupils allows your eye care professional to view the back of the eye better.

You may also be asked to view an Amsler grid, a pattern that looks like a checkerboard. Early changes in your central vision will cause the grid to appear distorted, a sign of AMD.

How can it be treated?

No treatment now exists for dry AMD. It has been suggested that taking certain extra vitamins and minerals may slow the progress of the disease. But this treatment needs much more research before scientists can know for sure if it's helpful.

Eye care professionals can treat some cases of wet AMD with laser surgery. This treatment involves aiming a strong light beam onto the new blood vessels to destroy them. Laser surgery is done in a doctor's office or in an eye clinic and lasts a short period of time. Although a person may go home the same day, he or she will need to return for follow-up exams.

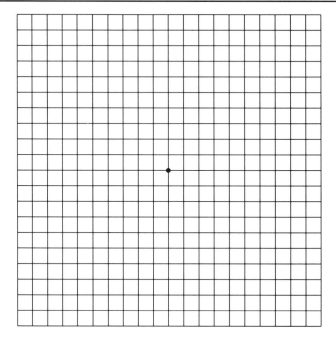

Figure 54.2. *While covering one eye, look at dot in center of grid. If lines around the dot are wavy or distorted, you should see your eye care professional.*

What research is being done?

The National Eye Institute is funding a number of research studies to learn what causes AMD and how it can be better treated. For instance, in the Age-Related Eye Diseases Study (AREDS), researchers are assessing the aging process in the eyes of thousands of older people to discover the earliest signs of AMD. The same study is also evaluating the effects of certain vitamins and minerals in preventing or slowing the progress of AMD.

At the same time, other scientists are trying to learn more about how the cells in the retina work. This knowledge will allow them some day to pinpoint the cause of the disease and design methods to prevent it.

What can you do to protect your vision?

Although there is no effective treatment for dry AMD at this time, it is crucial that those who progress to wet AMD and need laser surgery have it before the disease destroys central vision. For this reason, if you have dry AMD or are age 60 or older, you should have your eyes examined through dilated pupils at least once a year. You may also want to get an Amsler grid from your eye care professional to check your vision at home.

Chapter 55

Macular Degeneration and Nutrition

Do vitamins or zinc supplements help macular degeneration?

Good Nutrition

Good nutrition requires a diet with a healthy mixture of proteins, carbohydrates, fats, vitamins and minerals. Probably no part of our diet has been as misused or misunderstood as our requirement for vitamins and minerals.

Protein is needed for the building blocks and chemical machinery of our bodies; carbohydrates are needed for immediate fuel and energy; fats are needed for long term storage of fuel and energy. Vitamins are organic compounds that our bodies cannot manufacture and are essential for maintaining good health. Minerals, in small amounts, are required for the body's enzyme system (enzymes assist chemical reactions such as the breakdown of food into energy).

What do vitamins and minerals (particularly zinc) have to do with macular degeneration?

There are different kinds of macular problems, but the most common is age-related macular degeneration. Exactly why it develops is not known, and no treatment has been uniformly effective.

American Academy of Ophthalmology, ©1991. Used by permission.

Macular degeneration is the leading cause of severe visual loss in people over 65.

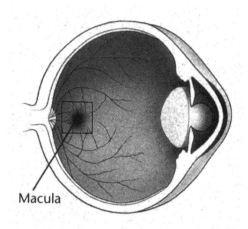

Macula

Figure 55.1. *Cross section of eye*

Zinc

Zinc, one of the most common trace minerals in our body, is highly concentrated in the eye, particularly in the retina and tissues surrounding the macula. Zinc is necessary for the action of over 100 enzymes, including chemical reactions in the retina.

Studies have shown that some older people have low levels of zinc in their blood, either because of poor diet or poor absorption of zinc from food. Because zinc is important for the health of the macula, some doctors think that supplements of zinc in the diet may slow down the process of macular degeneration. But the scientific studies are not complete and there is no agreement among doctors concerning the value of zinc supplements. It is possible that too much zinc may interfere with other trace minerals such as copper.

Vitamins

Normal chemical reactions from light in the eye activate oxygen which may cause macular damage. Some vitamins function as antioxidants, chemicals which work against this activated oxygen, and perhaps protect the macula from damage. It is claimed that antioxidant vitamins (vitamin A, C and E) can help slow down macular degeneration and other aging factors. As in the controversy over zinc, there is no agreement that these antioxidants actually help macular degeneration.

Should I take antioxidant vitamins or zinc for macular degeneration?

The first step to overall good health is a balanced diet. Vitamins and minerals are commonly given as supplements to the diet in amounts determined by recommended daily allowances. These supplementary dosages cause no apparent harm and are commonly available. But large doses of vitamins, called therapeutic doses, in amounts many times the daily recommended allowances, may not be completely safe.

Research is still in progress about nutrition and macular degeneration. It is best to consult with your ophthalmologist to decide whether it is advisable for you to begin such treatment.

Why are regular medical eye examinations important for everyone?

Eye disease can occur at any age. Many eye diseases do not cause symptoms until the disease has done damage. Since most blindness is preventable if diagnosed and treated early, regular medical examinations by an ophthalmologist are very important.

Chapter 56

National Eye Institute Report on Macular Degeneration

Introduction

Light passing into the eye is focused on a patch of central retina called the macula. Within the macula, a central avascular specialization, the fovea, contains only cone photoreceptors, which provide the high resolution and color vision to which we are accustomed. Unfortunately, in some disorders, the macula becomes diseased, and vision is dramatically impaired. Degenerative changes to the macula (maculopathy) can occur at any time after maturity, but they are by far most prevalent with advancing age. Ophthalmic signs of AMD include the appearance of opaque yellow spots (drusen) located between Bruch's membrane and the RPE; reduced pigmentation of the RPE and imputed changes in RPE physiology and biochemistry; changes in choroidal capillary permeability, and degeneration of photoreceptors, with corresponding loss of the central visual field. Factors that cause maculopathy are thought to arise from either the abnormal trafficking of material through Bruch's membrane or a disruption in cell-cell interactions that support the structure and function of the macula. Within the macula, cone photoreceptors reciprocally communicate via ions and macromolecules with retinal glial cells and the RPE. Moreover, the RPE, which screens the photoreceptors from body fluids, also must interact with the vascular capillaries that

NIH Pub. No. 93–3186. Excerpt from *Vision Research: A National Plan*, pp. 55–65.

feed the macula. These morphological relationships are discussed in more detail in the Photoreceptors and Pigment Epithelium section.

What is special about the macula that renders it susceptible to degeneration? Are these changes due to genetic, immunologic, systemic, or environmental factors? Uncertainties about the etiology of MD reflect the sparsity of information about factors that cause maculopathy, the absence of animal models for studying macular disease, and the limited amount of information about cell-cell communication within the retina/RPE/choroid complex.

Of the estimated 33.9 million people in the United States who will be ages 65 or older in 1995, approximately 1.7 million will have some visual impairment as a result of AMD, with approximately 100,000 experiencing a devastating, rapid loss of vision due to subretinal neovascularization (SRNV). The remaining 1.6 million will inevitably become affected with slow, progressive retinal atrophy and with severe visual handicaps; most may have difficulty performing routine visual tasks such as driving, reading printed material, or recognizing the faces of friends.

As the U.S. population ages, more elderly persons will become blind from AMD than from glaucoma and diabetic retinopathy combined. In AMD with SRNV, blindness almost always results from scarring in the macular region, with scars resulting from the ingrowth of blood vessels from the choriocapillaris through breaks in Bruch's membrane. Clinical research shows that laser treatment can reduce the risk of extensive scarring in selected "classic" cases. The treatment effect lasts, however, for only 1 or 2 years in at least 50 percent of the treated cases because of the development of recurrent choroidal neovascularization on the foveal edge of the laser scar, which can be accompanied by subsequent scarring of the foveal center and severe visual loss. Furthermore, laser treatment does not apply to more than 75 percent of patients at risk of going blind from macular disease with SRNV. Many of the latter patients are at risk of developing scarring from "occult" or "poorly defined" choroidal neovascularization, which often progresses to severe visual loss.

Because the number of individuals with the SRNV form of AMD is large, effective treatment of even 25 percent of all cases can lead to significant savings to society and decreases in the number of Social Security and other disability payments, with savings far out weighing the costs of clinical management and treatment.

MD is associated with a group of disorders, some of which include the following:

- AMD, a major cause of blindness in the United States and the leading cause of new cases of blindness in people ages 65 and older. In 85 to 90 percent of cases, discrete drusen accumulate and vision is impaired slowly; in other cases, however, drusen become confluent, and new blood vessels from the choroid penetrate the RPE to proliferate or bleed beneath the fovea, resulting in rapid loss of sight.

- Central serous choroidopathy, a disorder in which fluid accumulates beneath the neurosensory retina, producing retinal detachment in the macula. Predominantly afflicting individuals ages 20 to 40, this disorder results in distorted vision and, with repeated episodes, severe loss of vision.

- Hereditary (juvenile) MD, a group of genetically transmitted degenerations of the macula affecting the young. These include vitelliform MD and fundus flavimaculatus.

MD also can be associated with other ocular or systemic conditions and with cytotoxic drugs. This category includes macular edema, which may occur following cataract surgery, retinal detachment surgery, as well as vascular or inflammatory disorders. MD also occurs in ocular histoplasmosis syndrome, measles maculopathy, autoimmune maculopathy, and ischemic maculopathy. Moreover, the macula is susceptible to damage by radiant energy (e.g., visible, ultraviolet, or x-ray) or by mechanical impact. In addition, the macula has a speciasusceptibility to the toxic effects of several types of drugs and chemicals.

Subprogram Objectives

- To develop a universally accepted classification of MD based on clinically and histopathologically relevant features of MD.

- To support epidemiologic studies characterizing the influence of genetics, nutrition, and systemic disease on MD.

- To establish a registry for patients with clinically documented MD and to collect blood and solid tissue samples from patients and donors for future biochemical and genetic investigations.

- To discover noninvasive techniques for the early diagnosis of MD and devise prevention and treatment paradigms for MD.

- To ascertain whether the RPE and/or the choroid overlying the macula are different from the RPE/choroid of the peripheral retina in paracrine, metabolic, or functional capabilities.

- To characterize further the physiology of cone photoreceptors and define their interrelationship with the RPE/choriocapillaris complex.

- To prepare cDNA/genomic libraries and molecular probes for a systematic analysis of the inherited forms of MD.

- To determine the normal course of aging in the retina/RPE/choroid complex and identify the causative factors for SRNV and for slow, progressive macular atrophy.

Current Level of National Eye Institute Support

During FY 1992 the NEI funded 37 research projects related to macular disease at a total cost of $5,503,403. Funds were allocated to investigator-initiated grants and the MPS.

Investigator-initiated research grants included investigations of the aging retina, cone photopigments, and the effect of light or chemical factors on the integrity of the photoreceptor/RPE complex. The MPS evaluates the usefulness of laser photocoagulation in the treatment of AMD and the presumed ocular histoplasmosis syndrome and documents the natural history of both diseases. The study has demonstrated a beneficial effect of confluent laser treatment for well-defined, classic choroidal neovascularization in which the posterior edge of the neovascularization was at least 1mm from the foveal center.

Recent Accomplishments

The MPS and its natural history followup have contributed to our understanding of how the fundus of the eye changes with advancing age, and it is exploring whether laser treatment can be beneficial for the many cases of vascularization occurring within the fovea. From the laboratory has come a steady stream of discoveries that document how cone photoreceptors respond to light, how the RPE nurtures the photoreceptors and phagocytizes their daily sheddings, and how proteins and lipids accumulate in Bruch's membrane with age.

Cone photoreceptor cells respond to light by initiating a neuronal message that is transmitted to the brain for processing. Three cone types respond to red, green, and blue light, respectively. Each cone type has a different, but molecularly related, photosensitive protein that is coded by its respective gene. Genes for the red and green photosensitive proteins are located on the X-chromosome, and those for blue cones are on chromosome 7. Blue cone monochromasy is a rare, X-linked disorder of color vision characterized by red-green color blindness. Analysis of the respective genes for color sensitivity has shown that red-green color blindness results from either point mutations/deletion or rearrangement of X-chromosome genomic DNA, without alteration to the gene encoding the blue photosensitive protein.

The visual process of cones utilizes many unique proteins. Light absorbed by a photosensitive protein triggers the isomerization of 11-*cis* retinal, and protein-structure adjustments activate a cascade of reactions that culminate in the closure of ion channels at the surface of the cell. Molecular analysis reveals that the phototransduction cascade of cones is similar to that of rod photoreceptors and also to the transduction cascade of many hormonesensitive cells. Cones contain cell-specific proteins, and normally these proteins are isolated from the immune system; however, with disease and perhaps aging, antigens escape to the blood. Immunologically competent cells have been identified in SRNV lesions, and immunoreactive antibodies to retinal proteins have been identified in the serum of patients with AMD. The antibodies recognize a protein doublet of 58 to 62 kd that has been localized by immunocytochemistry to photoreceptor outer segments.

Only the 11-*cis* retinaldehyde form of vitamin A is useful for human vision. Specific binding proteins have been identified in photoreceptors, Muller cells, the RPE, and the interphotoreceptor matrix that aid in the metabolism, stabilization, and translocation of this retinoid. All-*trans* retinal is released from opsin during light exposure, and it is converted to the 11-*cis* isomer for the regeneration of visual pigments by a novel mechanism in the RPE. Dietary pigments (i.e., zeaxanthin and lutein) that are antioxidants and blue light absorbers also accumulate in the macula; they are believed to increase visual acuity and protect against photodamage.

Cone and rod photoreceptor outer segments protrude into the subretinal space and shed their tips daily. The shed outer segment fragments are phagocytized by the RPE. The shedding/phago-cytosis process may be driven by an internal clock that also regulates the synthesis of melatonin. Molecular analysis suggests that protein synthesis and the assembly of new outer segment membranes are linked to the daily rhythm. The outer segments are surrounded by a sheath of extra-cellular material that differs in composition from that of rod photoreceptors. Cone matrix sheaths are interdigitated with the apical processes of RPE cells and may contribute to the adhesion of the macula and RPE.

RPE acts as a selective, polarized complex that mediates the transport of fluids, ions, macromolecules, and metabolites between the choroid and the retina. RPE pumps and cell-cell junctions are essential for maintaining the protected environment of photoreceptors. Bruch's membrane, which separates the RPE from the choriocapillaris, is a five-layered structure composed of matrix material, glycoproteins, glycosaminoglycans, collagen, and elastin. Drusen accumulate within Bruch's membrane during aging, possibly as a byproduct of phagocytosis in the RPE. Retrospective studies suggest that large or confluent drusen are an important risk factor for vision loss in AMD. Cytochemical studies show that lipids accumulate with age in Bruch's membrane, disrupting its structure and altering its permeability to fluid. Recent advances in photocoagulation suggest that mild laser burns stimulate the removal, possibly by choroidal pericytes, of drusen from monkey eyes and that comparable treatment also might be beneficial for human drusen.

Photoreceptor outer segment renewal is tied to RPE cell phagocytosis of shed photoreceptor discs. The RPE cell's phagocytosis system involves cell surface recognition, internalization, lysosomal enzymic digestion, and accumulation of residual material or export of residual material from the cell. In the RCS rat, failure of phagocytosis leads to photoreceptor degeneration; transplantation of RPE from normal eyes rescues the photoreceptors. Over time the aging human RPE accumulates residual bodies (i.e., undigested substances), also known as lipofuscin (i.e., aging pigment), and some of this material is removed apparently via a mechanism of exocytosis (i.e., apoptosis) of debris onto Bruch's membrane.

The effects of the phagocytic load and internal accumulation of undigested material on the function of the aging RPE need investigation, for there is compelling evidence that lipofuscin-laden RPE cells are unhealthy. Moreover, highly significant correlations have been found between the amount of debris in Bruch's membrane and the amount of lipofuscin in the overlying RPE; still, any relationship between lipofuscin and drusen remains elusive. The dynamics of Bruch's membrane and the chemical composition of drusen require further study, including the effect by vitamin E and other antioxidants on the phagocytic process. Punctate "hard" drusen seem to cause micro-detachments of the RPE from Bruch's membrane, whereas the diffuse "soft" drusen appear to overlay accumulations of fluid, possibly resulting from active pumping of ions and fluid from the retina by the RPE.

The RPE does not normally proliferate, but it can be activated by injury (i.e., photocoagulation) or after isolation in culture. In culture RPE of the macula differs from that of the peripheral retina, and aging reduces the RPE potential for cell division. It is suggested that the RPE produces factors that influence the development and maintenance of photoreceptors and other factors that prevent the growth of capillaries into Bruch's membrane and the RPE. These and other RPE-specific proteins are now being sought in complementary DNA libraries because they may be a component of the MD sequela.

Capillaries of the choroid normally are denied access to the subretinal space and the neural retina, possibly by antiangiogenic factors from the photoreceptors and/or RPE. These factors are now being assessed in co-cultures of RPE and choroidal endothelium. The process by which the barrier to capillary ingrowth is maintained or broken by physical/enzymatic means probably depends upon a balance of signals directing cellular movement and vascularization. A sign of communication between the RPE and choroid is the presence of fenestrae (windows) on the RPE side of the choriocapillaris. Fenestrae appear as the choriocapillaris matures, and they are lost in some disorders that affect the RPE/choroid complex.

The clinical pathology of MD is poorly understood. Perhaps AMD and normal aging are only points on a continuum in the natural history of the macula. Pathologic changes, including development of soft, confluent drusen, choroidal neovascular membranes, choroidal atrophy, and depigmentation of the RPE, either continue the aging process or are superimposed on it. Study of diseases that are clearly inherited and affect young or mature individuals may help differentiate the disease process from aging. Reasonable candidates are Sorsby's pseudoinflammatory macular dystrophy, which is accompanied by neovascularization and has an autosomal dominant mode of inheritance; Stargardt's disease, a recessive macular dystrophy of juvenile onset; and dominant MD of early onset, in which the accumulation of drusen is lacking.

Whereas no completely effective treatment is available now for MD, randomized clinical trials have established that argon or krypton laser photocoagulation of carefully defined eyes with neovascular membranes can be beneficial. The high rate of recurrent choroidal neovascularization in AMD diminishes the treatment effect in many eyes 1 to 2 years after laser treatment. Hypertension is an overlying variable with adverse impact on treatment of choroidal neovascularization in AMD. Nevertheless, the treatment effect is significant even after 5 years, and the cumulative savings to society are immense when it is realized that in the next decade at least 150,000 elderly citizens will be enabled through treatment to continue independent and productive lives.

Epidemiologic factors affecting the macula encompass a range of potential hazards. Speculation about causes of MD has focused on hereditary and environmental factors such as light exposure, diet, and drugs. Eyes with only a few small drusen are almost ubiquitous and do not appear to be age related. On the other hand, the presence of large, soft, confluent drusen as well as atrophy of the RPE do appear to be age related. Exposure to ultraviolet light has not been shown to be associated with any stage of AMD in patients with lenses, although blue light may be a risk factor. The human diet and its mineral content also may influence the probability of development of MD; it is unknown whether the macular accumulation of lutein and zeaxanthin are impaired in MD. Reanalysis of the 1971 to 1972 data from the first national health and nutritional survey of 10,000 subjects noted that the frequent consumption of fruits and vegetables rich in carotene and vitamin A is negatively associated with prevalence of AMD, even after adjustment for demographic and medical factors. Finally, inherited factors cannot be excluded because African-Americans and Asians appear to have a low incidence of AMD with SRNV. Very few African-Americans are in any of the MPS trials; their absence in this trial and inclusion in many diabetic retinopathy trials imply that SRNV is less common in African-Americans. Moreover, some types of MD are clearly inherited, and characterization of the early-onset heritable forms may provide some insight into the diseases that present later in life.

Important Research Questions to Be Addressed

Advances in medical science are escalating, with new concepts emerging from genetics and cell/molecular biology and novel methodology incorporating state-of-the-art technology. Still, an understanding of MD awaits an imaginative leap in concept that will unify the diverse pieces of pathologic and clinical evidence. As a focus for the current plan, the following set of representative questions may stimulate new investigations and facilitate the formulation of concepts that explain the etiology of any of the types of MD:

Is it possible to develop a uniform classification of MD that will facilitate the identification of eyes that are candidates for AMD with SRNV?

Funduscopic, angiographic, and pathologic studies should address why laser treatment of choroidal neovascularization is less effective in patients with hypertension; why some neovascular lesions are prone to reoccur; and why significant disciform scarring occurs only in some patients. The analysis of fundus photography needs rapid processing of information and computer automation, with software utilized to reduce interobserver variation. Is cone function an informative tool for diagnosis; can the development of SRNV be predicted on the basis of diminished foveal sensitivity to light? Whether light or dark eye color enhances risk for MD should be resolved. These observations may provide information useful in both future treatment procedures and cell biology studies of macular disease. New laser technology may be developed for the treatment of now unsuitable candidates, and the cytopathology may give clues to the mechanisms of disease. Is there an enhanced role in the future for the scanning laser ophthalmoscope? It is imperative that efforts be made to pass beyond phenomenology to address directly the cause of AMD with SRNV.

Are the genetic defect(s) of juvenile MD expressed in the RPE?

Families can be identified, and the genetic and clinical manifestations of the disease can be characterized. RPE cells from the macula and periphery can be isolated from normal and affected donor eyes and analyzed directly or cultured for *in vitro* analysis of protein and lipid metabolism. mRNA can be prepared and analyzed directly or used to prepare cDNA libraries. Genes corresponding to proteins, expressed, repressed, or altered only in affected RPE can be identified in the cDNA library. Characterization of the cell biology of these proteins can provide a clue to both the normal function of the RPE and a defect in affected RPE. Corresponding DNA probes can be developed for mapping the chromosomal location of genes that encode specific RPE proteins and, if the aberrant gene is identified, for diagnosing affected individuals before the development of macular pathology. Resolution of the cause of juvenile MD would provide a prototype for investigating AMD.

Is the accumulation of drusen related to the accumulation of lipofuscin in RPE cells?

What factors lead to the accumulation of lipofuscin, and is the level of accumulated lipofuscin related to the phagocytic load, to the composition of material that is phagocytized, or to the inability of RPE cells to jettison unphagocytized material? Are capillary pericytes involved in the removal of jettisoned material? There is a need for an animal model in which lipofuscin and drusen develop so that the pathway for processing photoreceptor outer segment material can be traced and in which the turnover rate of phagocytized material can be determined as a function of age, diet, and environmental factors. Whereas the formation of rodent drusen may differ from that of humans, the intravitreal injection of aminoglycoside antibiotics in rabbits induces RPE/choroid changes that resemble drusen. Imaging microscopy of cultured RPE might be useful in mapping in real time the phagocytic process and the suspected apoptosis of residual bodies. In culture, the effect of ions (e.g., zinc and copper) and antioxidants (e.g., glutathione and vitamins E and C) could be evaluated with RPE from different regions of the retina and from animals of different ages. If hard drusen are transformed to soft drusen, which in turn favor neovascularization, it is imperative that the mechanisms that produce both hard and soft drusen be identified.

What activities of cone photoreceptors are driven by an intrinsic oscillator, and are they modulated by diet, light, or age?

A diurnal shedding event may synchronize the RPE to photoreceptor activities. A diurnal clock may become defective with age or be modulated by dietary or environmental factors. A role for melatonin in photoreceptor activities needs clarification. A barrier to the direct assessment of cone activities exists because conditions have not been established for the maintenance of cultured photoreceptors in the differentiated state. There is also the possibility that MD arises from cone dysfunction and that the macular RPE cells display functional abnormalities as a secondary response to cone pathology.

What genetic or cell-cell interactions induce and maintain the structure of foveal cones?

The fovea of humans and primates is a specialized structure that contains cones with long, thin outer segments but no neurons of the inner retina or retinal blood vessels. Forces controlling the postnatal development of the fovea are unknown; supplemental knowledge about regionalization might be derived from the analysis of cone-rich retinal regions in birds, reptiles, and some fishes. Gene expression may be essential for the induction of a fovea, and these gene products can be identified. Antineovascular factors or surface-receptor-mediated responses from photoreceptors may discourage the ingrowth of blood vessels. If photoreceptors release antineovascular factors, are they different from those proposed for the RPE to retard neovascularization from the choroid?

Do cones produce their extra cellular matrix sheaths, and does the sheath function in retinal adhesiveness or outer segment shedding/phagocytosis?

Cones may secrete proteoglycans and other constituents of the interphotoreceptor matrix, and these compounds may be both self-protective for cones and informative to the RPE. The cone sheath is an outward expression of cone specialization; it should be determined whether the sheath is lost with age or disease, whether drugs or diet alter its composition and function, and whether cones survive in its absence. Sheaths are associated with all mammalian cones. Genetic disorders affecting proteoglycan metabolism in animals should be identified, and macula function and structure examined. A complementary DNA library for cones can be prepared, and unique proteins of the sheath can be identified and utilized as probes for the study of MD.

How do genetic, biochemical, metabolic, and immunologic factors vary in different forms of MD?

Longitudinal studies of normal subjects and those with MD should include a parallel analysis of nutrition, genetics, and immunologic factors. Attention should be given to vitamins and trace minerals, since some human and several animal studies indicate that a benefit can be derived from dietary intake of these substances. The drusen content and foveal sensitivity to light should be scored, and the effect of photocoagulation on neovascularization documented. Subjects with different genetic or acquired forms of MD may respond differently to photocoagulation, and this may be informative. The appearance of and/or morphologcal changes in drusen may be related to an autoimmune response. Both the retina and the RPS: must be considered likely sources of autoantigens, and the blood of normal and affected subjects should be screened against proteins from these tissues. Immunosuppressive drugs may be useful in treating at least some forms of MD.

What are the factors that control proliferation of vessels from the choroid into the retina?

The growth of choroidal capillaries into the space between the RPE and the retina occurs frequently in AMD. Animal models of neovascularization are now in place and should be exploited. The RPE has been shown to produce growth-regulating factors, but their role in neovascularization is unclear. Moreover, the environmental, hormonal, or cell-cell interactions that control the production and release of such factors are unresolved. From understanding of neovascularization comes the possibility of countering capillary growth with drugs, hormones, or dietary factors. This one accomplishment would preserve the vision of countless individuals.

What are the mechanisms that cause fluid to accumulate in the subretinal space?

Much is known about the kind and location of electrolyte pumps within the polarized RPE, but not as much is known about their regulation. A compositional abnormality in Bruch's membrane cannot be excluded in some disorders, particularly those in which the RPE appears to produce the fluid for its own detachment. The phenomenology suggests that the entire retina/RPE/choroid complex may be involved and that an appropriate animal model that mirrors the pathology of human disease is needed.

In summary, the preceding questions are mere examples of the abundance of opportunities for investigations into the factors that may contribute to MD. They stress the importance of both clinicopathologic studies and cellular/molecular biologic investigations of MD. The questions are predicated on the belief that investigations of the multiple forms of MD must progress beyond phenomenology to address the underlying mechanisms of disease.

Chapter 57

Age-Related
Eye Disease Study

Purpose

- To assess the clinical course, prognosis, and risk factors of age-related macular degeneration (AMD) and cataract.

- To evaluate, in randomized clinical trials, the effects of pharmacologic doses of (1) antioxidants and zinc on the progression of AMD and (2) antioxidants on the development and progression of lens opacities.

Background

AMD and cataract are the leading causes of visual impairment and blindness in the United States. The prevalence of both diseases increases dramatically after age 60. The Framingham Eye Study conducted from 1973 to 1975 found the overall prevalence of AMD to be 11.6 percent (8.1 percent for men and 15.1 percent for women). Framingham Eye Study data also documented that the prevalence of lens changes accompanied by visual acuity limitation increased from 4.5 percent for ages 52–64 to 45.9 percent for ages 75–85. The number of AMD cases in the aging U.S. population is expected to increase from 2.4 million in 1970 to 6.3 million in 2030.

Excerpt from NIH Pub. No. 93-3960. *Clinical Trails Supported by the National Eye Institute*, pp. 7–11.

Neither the etiology nor the natural history of AMD and cataract is known. Epidemiologic studies suggest that a number of risk factors may be associated with AMD and cataract, but the strength of the evidence in support of these hypotheses varies. Possibly associated with AMD are personal characteristics such as age, race, height, family history, and strength of hand grip; ocular characteristics such as hyperopia and color of iris; and cardiovascular diseases, smoking, lung infections, and chemical exposures. Clinical and laboratory studies suggest the following factors may be associated with progression of AMD: drusen type, choroidal vascular diseases, and photic injury.

Epidemiologic studies of cataract suggest that associated risk factors may include personal characteristics such as age, sex, race, occupation, and educational status; ocular characteristics such as iris color; diabetes mellitus, hypertension, drug exposure, smoking, and sunlight exposure. Animal studies and observational epidemiologic studies suggest that deficiencies in vitamins C and E, carotenoids, and the trace elements zinc and selenium also may be associated with the development of the two diseases, especially cataract. Although surgical treatment to remove cataract is very effective, cataract surgery carries risks as does any other surgery. Therefore, many research efforts focus on prevention or slowing cataract development as well as on determining the causes of cataract formation.

Description

The Age-Related Eye Disease Study (AREDS) is a major research program to improve our understanding of the predisposing factors, clinical course, and prognostic factors of AMD and cataract.

Participant Eligibility

Men and women between the ages of 55 and 78 years whose macular status ranges from no evidence of AMD in either eye to relatively severe disease with vision loss in one eye but good vision in the fellow eye, are eligible for the study, provided that their ocular media are clear enough to allow good fundus photography.

Participant Recruitment Status

Ongoing. Identification of potentially eligible study participants began on September 1, 1990. Randomization of the 4,600 study participants has begun and will continue into 1994. Seven years of participant followup is projected.

Current Status of Study

Ongoing.

Results

None.

Publications

None.

Clinical Centers

Georgia

Antonio Capone, Jr., M.D.
Department of Ophthalmology
Emory Eye Center
Emory University
1327 Clifton Road, N.E., Room 4901
Atlanta, Georgia 30322
Telephone: (404) 248-5224
Fax: (404) 248-5128

Illinois

David H. Orth, M.D.
Irwin Retina Center
Ingalls Memorial Hospital
One Ingalls Drive
Harvey, Illinois 60426
Telephone: (708) 333-2300, ext. 6814
Fax: (708) 596-9820

Maryland

Susan B. Bressler, M.D.
Wilmer Ophthalmological Institute
The Johns Hopkins Medical Institutions
Wilmer Building, Room 205
600 North Wolfe Street
Baltimore, Maryland 21287-9022
Telephone: (410) 955-3648
Fax: (410) 955-0869 (call before sending)

Michael J. Elman, M.D.
Elman Retina Group
University of Maryland
9101 Franklin Square Drive, Suite 108
Baltimore, Maryland 21237
Telephone: (410) 686-3000
Fax: (410) 686-3690

Emily Y. Chew, M.D.
Frederick L. Ferris III, M.D.
National Eye Institute
Building 10, Room 10C420
Bethesda, Maryland 20892
Telephone: (301) 496-6583
Fax: (301) 496-2297

Massachusetts

Johanna M. Seddon, M.D.
Massachusetts Eye and Ear Infirmary
Epidemiology Unit, First Floor
243 Charles Street
Boston, Massachusetts 02114
Telephone: (617) 573-3285
Fax: (617) 573-3570

Michigan

Raymond R. Margherio, M.D.
Associated Retinal Consultants, P.C.
3535 West Thirteen Mile Road, Suite 636
Royal Oak, Michigan 48073
Telephone: (810) 288-2280
Fax: (810) 288-5644

New York

Aaron Kassoff, M.D.
Albany Eye Associates
The Eye Center at Memorial
63 Shaker Road
Albany, New York 12204
Telephone: (518) 434-1042
Fax: (518) 434-4327

Oregon

Richard F. Dreyer, M.D.
Devers Eye Institute
1040 N.W. 22nd Avenue, N-200
Portland, Oregon 97210-3065
Telephone: (503) 229-7746
Fax: (503) 725-1734

Pennsylvania

Thomas R. Friberg, M.D.
The Eye and Ear Institute of Pittsburgh
203 Lothrop Street
Pittsburgh, Pennsylvania 15213
Telephone: (412) 647-2214
Fax: (412) 647-5880

Wisconsin

Suresh R. Chandra, M.D.
Department of Ophthalmology
University Station Clinics
University of Wisconsin
2880 University Avenue, Room 224
Madison, Wisconsin 53705
Telephone: (608) 263-9338
Fax: (608) 263-1466

Frank L. Myers, M.D.
Department of Ophthalmology
University Station Clinics
University of Wisconsin
2880 University Avenue, Room 224
Madison, Wisconsin 53705
Telephone: (608) 263-1468 or 263-1480
Fax: (608) 263-7694

Resource Centers

Chairman's Office

Frederick L. Ferris III, M.D.
Robert Sperduto, M.D.
Emily Y. Chew, M.D.
National Eye Institute
Building 31, Room 6A24
Bethesda, Maryland 20892
Telephone: (301) 496-6583

Coordinating Center

Fred Ederer, M.A., F.A.C.E.
Anne S. Lindblad, Ph.D.
The EMMES Corporation
11325 Seven Locks Road, Suite 214
Potomac, Maryland 20854
Telephone: (301) 299-8655

Central Laboratory

Eric Sampson, Ph.D.
Dayton Miller, Ph.D.
Centers for Disease Control
NHANES Laboratory
Building 17, Room 2814, MS F18
4770 Buford Highway, N.E.
Atlanta, Georgia 30341-3724
Telephone: (404) 488-4026

Drug Distribution Center

Tom Shaffer
U.S. Public Health Service
Perry Point, Maryland 21902
Telephone: (410) 642-2244

NIH Contract Office

Mollie Shea
National Institutes of Health
Division of Contracts Administration
Building 31, Room 1B44
Bethesda, Maryland 20892
Telephone: (301) 496-4487

Ophthalmic Photograph Reading Center

Matthew D. Davis, M.D.
Barbara Klein, M.D.
Ronald Klein, M.D.
Department of Ophthalmology
University of Wisconsin - Madison
WARF Building, Room 417
610 North Walnut Street
P.O. Box 5240
Madison, Wisconsin 53705
Telephone: (608) 263-6071

Storz Ophthalmic Pharmaceuticals

Lorraine J. Brancato, M.D.
American Cyanamid Company
Middleton Road
Building 190, Room 112C
Pearl River, New York 10965
Telephone: (914) 732-5000

NEI Representative

Natalie Kurinij, Ph.D.
National Eye Institute
Executive Plaza South, Suite 350
6120 Executive Boulevard
Rockville, Maryland 20892
Telephone: (301) 496-5983

Data and Safety Monitoring Committee

Janet Wittes, Ph.D., Chair
Washington, DC

Gladys Block, Ph.D.
University of California
Berkeley, CA

Stuart L. Fine, M.D.
Scheie Eye Institute
Philadelphia, PA

Curt D. Furberg, M.D.
Bowman Gray School of Medicine
Winston-Salem, NC

M. Cristina Leske, M.D., M.P.H.
SUNY - Stony Brook
Stony Brook, NY

Giovanni Maraini, M.D.
University of Parma
Parma, Italy

Donald Patrick, Ph.D., M.S.P.H.
University of Washington
Seattle, WA

Robert Veatch, Ph.D.
Georgetown University
Washington, DC

Ex Officio Members

Barbara Bowman, Ph.D.
Centers for Disease Control
Atlanta, GA

Lorraine J. Brancato, M.D.
American Cyanamid Company
Pearl River, NY

Wiley Chambers, M.D.
Food and Drug Administration
Rockville, MD

Emily Y. Chew
M.D. National Eye Institute
Bethesda, MD

Matthew D. Davis
M.D. University of Wisconsin
Madison, WI

Fred Ederer, M.A., F.A.C.E.
The EMMES Corporation
Potomac, MD

Frederick L. Ferris III, M.D.
National Eye Institute
Bethesda, MD

487

Natalie Kurinij, Ph.D.
National Eye Institute
Bethesda, MD

Anne S. Lindblad, Ph.D.
The EMMES Corporation
Potomac, MD

Mollie Shea
National Institutes of Health
Bethesda, MD

Robert Sperduto, M.D.
National Eye Institute
Bethesda, MD

Chapter 58

Endophthalmitis Vitrectomy Study

Purpose

- To determine the role of initial pars plana vitrectomy in the management of postoperative bacterial endophthalmitis.

- To determine the role of intravenous antibiotics in the management of bacterial endophthalmitis.

- To determine which factors, other than treatment, are predictors of outcome in postoperative bacterial endophthalmitis.

Background

Endophthalmitis is a serious ocular infection that can result in blindness. Approximately 70 percent of cases occur as a direct complication of intraocular surgery. Current management requires culture of intraocular contents and intravitreal antibiotic administration. Vitrectomy surgery may be beneficial in the management of endophthalmitis by removing infecting organisms and their toxins and has been shown to be of value in various animal models of endopthalmitis. However, human studies have not shown an advantage to vitrectomy with intraocular antibiotics compared to intraocular antibiotics alone.

Excerpt from NIH Pub. No. 93–3960. *Clinical Trials Supported by the National Eye Institute*, pp. 29–32.

In all large comparison studies to date, eyes with the worst initial presentations were those selected for vitrectomy. Because of the selection bias involved in determining which cases received vitrectomy, existing clinical information on the efficacy of the procedure for treating endophthalmitis is inconclusive. Determining the role of initial vitrectomy and whether certain subgroups of patients may benefit, will help the clinician in the management of endophthalmitis.

In addition, although systemic antibiotics historically have been used in the management of endophthalmitis, there has been little evidence to support their efficacy, but many reports of toxic systemic effects. In view of this, the role of systemic antibiotics will be assessed in the management of endophthalmitis.

Description

Endophthalmitis Vitrectomy Study (EVS) patients are randomized to one of two standard treatment strategies for the management of bacterial endophthalmitis. Eyes receive either (1) initial pars plana vitrectomy with intravitreal antibiotics, followed by retap and reinjection at 36–60 hours for eyes doing poorly as defined in the study, or (2) initial anterior chamber and vitreous tap/biopsy with injection of intravitreal antibiotics, followed by vitrectomy and reinjection at 36–60 hours in eyes doing poorly. In addition, all eyes are randomized to either treatment or no treatment with intravenous antibiotics.

Study endpoints are visual acuity and clarity of ocular media, the latter assessed both clinically and photographically. Each patient's initial endpoint assessment occurs at 3 months, after which procedures to improve vision, such as late vitrectomy for nonclearing ocular media, may be performed. The final outcome assessment occurs at 9 months. Multiple centers are cooperating by enrolling 420 eyes during a proposed 42-month recruitment period.

Patient Eligibility

Men and women are eligible for entry into the EVS if they have clinical signs and symptoms of bacterial endophthalmitis in an eye that has had cataract surgery or lens implantation within 6 weeks of onset of infection. The involved eye must have either hypopyon or enough clouding of anterior chamber or vitreous media to obscure clear visualization of second-order arterioles, a cornea and anterior chamber in the involved eye clear enough to visualize some part of the iris, and a cornea clear enough to allow the possibility of pars plana vitrectomy. The eyes should also have a visual acuity of 20/50 or worse and light perception or better.

Patients are ineligible when the involved eye is known at the time of study entry to have had any preexisting eye disease that limited best-corrected visual acuity to 20/100 or worse prior to development of cataract, any intraocular surgery prior to presentation (except for cataract extraction or lens implantation), treatment for endophthalmitis prior to presenting at the study center, or any ocular or systemic condition preventing randomization to any of the study groups.

Patient Recruitment Status

Recruitment began in February 1990.

Current Status of Study

Ongoing.

Results

None.

Publications

None.

Clinical Centers

California

Richard R. Ober, M.D.
Department of Ophthalmology
University of Southern California
450 San Pablo Street, DOH 4703
Los Angeles, California 90033
Telephone: (213) 342-6450

Lon S. Poliner, M.D.
4150 Regents Park Row, Suite 200
La Jolla, California 92037
Telephone: (619) 558-9666

District of Columbia

Howard P. Cupples, M.D.
Department of Ophthalmology, PHC7
Georgetown University Medical Center
3800 Reservoir Road, N.W.
Washington, D.C. 20007
Telephone: (202) 687-4755

Florida

Mark E. Hammer, M.D.
617 Lakeview Road, Suite B
Clearwater, Florida 34616
Telephone: (813) 875-6373

Robert Mames, M.D.
Hillis Miller Medical Center
Box J-284
Department of Ophthalmology
University of Florida College of Medicine
Gainesville, Florida 32610-0284
Telephone: (904) 392-3451

Scott E. Pautler, M.D.
Tampa Bay Vitreo-Retinal Associates
4600 North Habana Avenue, Suite 3
Tampa, Florida 33614
Telephone: (813) 879-5795

Peter Reed Pavan, M.D.
Eye Institute
University of South Florida
12901 B. B. Downs Boulevard
Tampa, Florida 33612-9400
Telephone: (813) 974-3820

Georgia

Antonio Capone, Jr., M.D.
Emory Eye Center, 5th Floor
Emory University
1327 Clifton Road, N.E.
Atlanta, Georgia 30322
Telephone: (404) 248-3956

Illinois

Kirk H. Packo, M.D.
Illinois Retina Associates, S.C.
71 West 156th Street, Suite 400
Harvey, Illinois 60426
Telephone: (708) 596-8710

Kentucky

Charles C. Barr, M.D.
Department of Ophthalmology
Kentucky Lions Eye Research Institute
University of Louisville
301 East Muhammad Ali Boulevard
Louisville, Kentucky 40202
Telephone: (502) 588-5466

Maryland

Peter Campochiaro, M.D.
Wilmer Eye Institute
Maumenee 719
The Johns Hopkins Medical Institutions
600 North Wolfe Street
Baltimore, Maryland 21218-9277
Telephone: (410) 955-5106

Richard A. Garfinkel, M.D.
Retina Group of Washington
5454 Wisconsin Avenue, Suite 1540
Chevy Chase, Maryland 20815
Telephone: (301) 656-8100

Vinod Lakhanpal, M.D.
Eye Associates
University of Maryland
419 West Redwood Street
Baltimore, Maryland 21201
Telephone: (410) 328-5906

Massachusetts

Donald D'Amico, M.D.
Massachusetts Eye and Ear Infirmary
243 Charles Street
Boston, Massachusetts 02114
Telephone: (617) 573-3291

Michigan

Raymond R. Margherio, M.D.
Associated Retinal Consultants, P.C.
Royal Oak Center
3535 West Thirteen Mile Road, Suite 636
Royal Oak, Michigan 48073
Telephone: (810) 288-2280

Andrew K. Vine, M.D.
Kellogg Eye Center
University of Michigan
1000 Wall Street
Ann Arbor, Michigan 48105
Telephone: (313) 763-0482

Minnesota

Herbert L. Cantrill, M.D.
6363 France Avenue South, Suite 570
Edina, Minnesota 55435
Telephone: (612) 929-1131

Mark W. Balles, M.D.
Department of Ophthalmology
University of Minnesota
Box 493 UMHC, Room 9-240 PWB
516 Delaware Street, S.E.
Minneapolis, Minnesota 55455
Telephone: (612) 625-4400

New Jersey

David L. Yarian, M.D.
Retina-Vitreous Center, P.A.
Medi-Plex Suite 310
98 James Street
Edison, New Jersey 08820
Telephone: (908) 906-1887

Ohio

Robert B. Chambers, D.O.
Ohio State University
456 West 10th Avenue
Columbus, Ohio 43210
Telephone: (614) 293-8041

Phillip T. Nelsen, M.D.
Retina Consultants of NW Ohio
JOBST Tower, Suite E
2109 Hughes Drive
Toledo, Ohio 43606
Telephone: (419) 479-6180

Thomas A. Rice, M.D.
Retina Associates of Cleveland
26900 Cedar Road, Suite 303
Beachwood, Ohio 44122
Telephone: (216) 831-5700

Oklahoma

Reagan H. Bradford, Jr., M.D.
Dean A. McGee Eye Institute
University of Oklahoma
608 Stanton L. Young Boulevard
Oklahoma City, Oklahoma 73104
Telephone: (405) 271-7232

Pennsylvania

Bernard H. Doft, M.D.
Retina-Vitreous Consultants
3501 Forbes Avenue, Suite 500
Pittsburgh, Pennsylvania 15213
Telephone: (412) 683-5300

Thomas Gardner, M.D.
Department of Ophthalmology
College of Medicine
The Pennsylvania State University
Hershey, Pennsylvania 17033
Telephone: (717) 531-8783

Gary C. Brown, M.D.
Retinovitreous Associates
910 East Willow Grove
Philadelphia, Pennsylvania 19118
Telephone: (215) 233-4300

Texas

H. Michael Lambert, M.D.
Alkek Eye Center
Smith Tower, Suite 1501
6550 Fannin Boulevard
Houston, Texas 77030
Telephone: (713) 798-6100

Wisconsin

Dennis P. Han, M.D.
Eye Institute
Milwaukee County Medical Complex
Medical College of Wisconsin
8700 West Wisconsin Avenue
Milwaukee, Wisconsin 53226
Telephone: (414) 257-5341

Resource Centers

Chairman's Office

Bernard H. Doft, M.D.
Retina-Vitreous Consultants
3501 Forbes Avenue, Suite 500
Pittsburgh, Pennsylvania 15213
Telephone: (412) 683-5300
Fax: (412) 621-4833

Coordinating Center

Sheryl F. Kelsey, Ph.D.
Department of Epidemiology
The University of Pittsburgh
127 Parran Hall
130 DeSoto Street
Pittsburgh, Pennsylvania 15261
Telephone: (412) 624-1607

Fundus Photograph Reading Center

Matthew D. Davis, M.D.
Department of Ophthalmology
University of Wisconsin
WARF Building, Room 417
610 North Walnut
Madison, Wisconsin 53705
Telephone: (608) 263-4538
Fax: (608) 263-0525

NEI Representative

Donald F. Everett, M.A.
National Eye Institute
Executive Plaza South, Suite 350
6120 Executive Boulevard
Rockville, Maryland 20892
Telephone: (301) 496-5983
Fax: (301) 402-0528

Data and Safety Monitoring Committee

Kathryn Davis, Ph.D., Chair
University of Washington
Seattle, WA

Stanley P. Azen, Ph.D.
University of Southern California
Los Angeles, CA

Preston Covey, Ph.D.
Carnegie Mellon University
Pittsburgh, PA

Brooks W. McCuen, M.D.
Duke University
Durham, NC 27710

Andrew Packer, M.D.
Consulting Ophthalmology, P.C.
Hartford, CT

Ex Officio Members

Matthew D. Davis, M.D.
University of Wisconsin
Madison, WI

Bernard H. Doft, M.D.
Retina-Vitreous Consultants
Pittsburgh, PA

Donald F. Everett, M.A.
National Eye Institute
Bethesda, MD

Sheryl F. Kelsey, Ph.D.
University of Pittsburgh
Pittsburgh, PA

Chapter 59

Vitrectomy Surgery

What is a vitrectomy?

Vitrectomy is a type of eye surgery that treats disorders of the retina and vitreous.

The retina is the light-sensing tissue at the back of the eye. The vitreous is the clear, jelly-like substance that fills the middle of the eye.

The vitreous is removed during vitrectomy surgery and usually replaced by a saltwater solution.

Why do you need a vitrectomy?

Your ophthalmologist (medical eye doctor) may recommend vitrectomy surgery to treat the following eye problems:

- Diabetic retinopathy, where there is bleeding and scar tissue;
- Some retinal detachment;
- Infection inside the eye;
- Severe eye injury;
- Wrinkling of the retina (macular pucker);
- Macular hole (partial loss of vision for fine details);
- Certain problems after cataract surgery.

American Academy of Ophthalmology, ©1993. Used by permission.

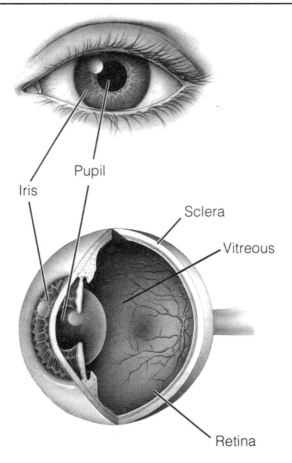

Iris

Pupil

Sclera

Vitreous

Retina

Figure 59.1. *Anatomy of the eye*

How can a vitrectomy improve your vision?

Vitrectomy surgery often improves or stabilizes your vision. The operation removes any blood or debris (from infection or inflammation) that may be blocking or blurring light as it focuses on the retina.

Vitrectomy surgery removes scar tissue that can displace, wrinkle or tear the retina. Vision is poor if the retina is not in its normal position. A foreign object may be stuck inside the eye as the result of an injury. Most foreign objects will damage vision if they are not removed.

What happens if you decide to have vitrectomy surgery?

Before surgery

Your ophthalmologist will decide whether local or general anesthesia is best for you. You may have to stay overnight in the hospital. Before surgery you will need to have a physical examination to alert your ophthalmologist to any special medical risks.

A painless ultrasound test may be performed before the surgery to view the inside of the eye.

Vitrectomy surgery

The length of the operation varies from one to several hours, depending on your condition. In certain situations, your ophthalmologist may do another surgical procedure at the same time, such as repairing a detached retina or removing a cataract.

Your ophthalmologist does the operation while looking into your eye with a microscope. Various miniature instruments are placed into the eye through tiny incisions in the sclera (white part of the eye).

In order to get the best possible vision for you, your ophthalmologist will do one or more of the following:

- Remove all cloudy vitreous;
- Remove any scar tissue present, attempting to return the retina to its normal position;
- Remove any foreign object that might be in the eye;
- Treat the eye with laser to reduce future bleeding, or to fix a tear in the retina;
- Place an air or gas bubble in the eye to help the retina remain in its proper position. The bubble will slowly disappear on its own.
- Inject a special fluid that is later removed from the eye.

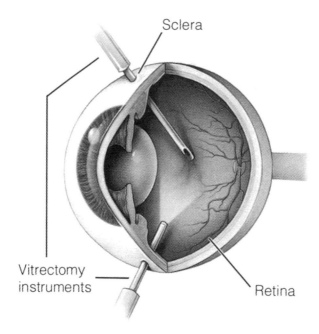

Figure 59.2. Vitrectomy surgery removes vitreous clouded with blood that might be causing blurry vision.

After surgery

You can expect some discomfort after surgery. You will need to wear an eye patch for a short time. Your ophthalmologist will prescribe eye drops for you and advise you when to resume normal activity.

If a gas bubble was placed in your eye, your ophthalmologist may recommend that you keep your head in special positions until the gas bubble is gone. Do not fly in an airplane or travel up to high altitudes until the gas bubble is gone! A rapid increase in altitude can cause a dangerous rise in eye pressure.

What are the risks of your vitrectomy surgery?

All types of surgery have certain risks, but the risks are less than the expected benefits to your vision.

Some of the risks of vitrectomy include:

- Infection;
- Bleeding;
- Retinal detachment;
- Poor vision;
- High pressure in the eye;
- Cataract is uncommon right after surgery—elderly patients often develop cataract over many months.

How much will your vision improve?

Your vision after surgery will depend on many variables, especially if your eye disease caused permanent damage to your retina before the vitrectomy. Your ophthalmologist will discuss your situation with you and how much improvement in your eyesight is possible.

Part Eight

Other Ophthalmic Problems

Chapter 60

Answers to Your Questions about Color Deficiency

What is color deficiency?

Color deficiency occurs when your ability to distinguish colors and shades is less than normal. The term "color blind" is often used, but usually incorrectly. Only a very small number of people are completely unable to identify any colors.

What causes color deficiency?

Color deficiency is usually inherited, but can also result from certain diseases, trauma or as a side effect of certain medications. It happens when the color-sensitive cone cells in the retina of your eye do not properly pick up or send to the brain correct color signals.

What types of color deficiency exist?

There are several. Red-green deficiency is by far the most common and results in the inability to distinguish between certain shades of red and green. In very rare cases, color deficiency exists to an extent that no colors can be detected. This person sees all things in shades of black, white and grey.

American Optometric Association Q15/990. Used by permission.

How is color deficiency detected?

People who are color deficient are generally unaware of their condition. They assume that everyone sees things the way they do. As a result, a complete optometric examination, including a test for color vision, is recommended. The test for color deficiency is a relatively simple one typically involving the viewing of a series of colored designs. The designs have been created in such a way that a person with normal color vision can see certain figures in the designs. A color deficient person will not be able to distinguish the figures.

When should a person be tested for color deficiency?

Every child should be checked for color deficiency by at least age five. It is important to detect color deficiency early because color coded learning materials are used extensively in the primary grades. In addition, color deficiency may affect the career path of an individual, since the ability to distinguish colors is an important aspect of some jobs, such as pilots, electricians, some military personnel, police officers and others.

Can color deficiency be cured?

Unfortunately a cure for color deficiency has not yet been discovered. A person with color deficiency can, however, be taught to adapt to the inability to distinguish colors. For example, you can be taught to recognize the brightness and location of a traffic light rather than the color itself. It is also possible to increase the ability to distinguish colors with the use of special filters. A special red tinted contact lens, used in one eye, and other devices are used, in some cases, to aid persons with certain color deficiencies.

Chapter 61

Aging and Your Eyes

Poor eyesight is not inevitable with age. Some physical changes occur during the normal aging process that can cause a gradual decline in vision, but most older people retain good eyesight into their 80's and beyond.

Older people generally need brighter light for such tasks as reading, cooking, or driving a car. In addition, regular household light bulbs (incandescent bulbs) are better for older eyes than tubular overhead (or fluorescent) lights.

Certain eye disorders and diseases occur more frequently in old age, but a great deal can be done to prevent or correct these conditions. Here are some suggestions for protecting your eyes:

- Have regular health checkups to detect such treatable diseases as high blood pressure and diabetes, both of which may cause eye problems.

- Have a complete eye exam every 2 or 3 years since many eye diseases have no early noticeable symptoms. The exam should include a vision (and glasses) evaluation, eye muscle check, check for glaucoma, and an exam looking at the retina through dilated pupils.

National Institute on Aging, Age Page, 1991.

- Seek eye health care more often if you have diabetes or a family history of eye disease. Make plans for care at once if you have signs such as loss or dimness of vision, eye pain, discharged fluids from the eye, double vision, or redness or swelling of the eye or eyelid.

Common Eye Complaints

Presbyopia—a gradual decline in the ability to focus on close objects or to see small print—is common after the age of 40. People with this condition often hold reading materials at arm's length, and some may have headaches or "tired eyes" while reading or doing other close work. There is no known prevention for presbyopia, but the focusing problem can be relieved with glasses.

Floaters are tiny spots or specks that float across the field of vision. Most people notice them in well-lighted rooms or outdoors on a bright day. Although floaters are normal and usually harmless, they may be a warning of certain eye problems, especially when occurring with light flashes. If you notice a sudden change in the type or number of spots or flashes, call your doctor.

Dry eyes occur when the tear glands produce too few tears. The result is itching, burning, or even reduced vision. An eye specialist can prescribe special eyedrop solutions ("artificial tears") to correct the problem.

Excessive tears may be a sign of increased sensitivity to light, wind, or temperature changes. In these cases, protective measures (such as sunglasses) may solve the problem. Tearing may also reflect more serious problems such as an eye infection or a blocked tear duct—both of which can be treated and corrected.

Eye Diseases Common in Older People

Cataracts are cloudy or opaque areas in part or all of the transparent lens located inside the eye. The lens is normally clear and allows light to pass through. So when a cataract forms, light cannot easily pass through the lens and this affects vision. Cataracts usually develop gradually and without pain, redness, or tearing in the eye. Some remain small and do not seriously affect vision. However, if a cataract becomes larger or denser, it can be surgically removed. Cataract surgery (in which the clouded lens is removed) is a safe procedure that is almost always successful. Cataract patients should discuss the risks and benefits of this optional procedure with their doctor. After surgery, vision is restored by using special eyeglasses or contact lenses or by having an intraocular lens implant (a plastic lens that is implanted in the eye during surgery).

Glaucoma occurs when there is too much fluid pressure in the eye, causing internal eye damage and gradually destroying vision. The basic cause of glaucoma is not known but, with early diagnosis and treatment, it can usually be controlled and blindness prevented. Treatment consists of prescription eyedrops, oral medications, laser treatments, or in some cases surgery. Glaucoma seldom produces early symptoms; and usually there is no pain from increased pressure. For these reasons, it is important for eye specialists to test for the disease during routine eye examinations in those over 35.

Retinal disorders are a leading cause of blindness in the United States. The retina is a thin lining on the back of the eye made up of nerves that receive visual images and pass them on to the brain. Retinal disorders include macular degeneration, diabetic retinopathy, and retinal detachment.

- Age-related **macular degeneration** is a condition in which the macula (a part of the retina responsible for sharp central and reading vision) stops functioning efficiently. The first signs may include blurring of reading vision, distortion or loss of central vision (for example, a dark spot in the center of the field of vision), and distortion in vertical lines. Early detection of macular degeneration is important since some cases may be handled well with laser treatments.

- **Diabetic retinopathy**, one of the possible problems of diabetes, occurs when the small blood vessels that feed the retina fail to do so properly. In the early stages of the condition, the blood vessels may leak fluid, which distorts vision. In the later stages, new vessels may grow and release blood in the center of the eye, resulting in serious loss of vision.

- **Retinal detachment** is a separation between the inner and outer layers of the retina. Detached retinas can usually be surgically reattached with good or partial renewal of vision. New surgical and laser treatments are being used today with increasing success.

Low-Vision Aids

Many people with visual impairments can be helped by using low-vision aids. These are special devices that provide more power than regular eyeglasses. Low-vision aids include telescopic glasses, light-filtering lenses, and magnifying glasses, along with a variety of electronic devices. (Some are designed to be hand-held; others rest directly on reading material.) Partially sighted individuals often notice surprising improvements with the use of these aids.

Resources

Your area agency on aging can refer you to organizations providing services for people with visual impairments. Most libraries have books with large print. In many areas, libraries for those with special needs are equipped with magnifying lamps, machines which enlarge the print of books, and "talking" books on cassettes, records, and computer disks.

A number of organizations can send you more information. The National Eye Institute, part of the National Institutes of Health, supports research on eye disease and the visual system. They can send you free brochures on eye disorders. Write to the NEI, Building 31, Room 6A32, Bethesda, MD 20892.

The National Society to Prevent Blindness has several free pamphlets on specific diseases affecting the eyes. They also have Home Eye Test for Adults, which is available for $1.25 (to cover the cost of postage and handling). Contact the Society at 500 East Remington Road, Schaumburg, IL 60173; or call (800) 221-3004.

The American Foundation for the Blind can send a list of their free publications on vision. Contact the Foundation at 15 West 16th Street, New York, NY 10011; or call (800) 232-5463.

The National Association for the Visually Handicapped is a voluntary health agency that works with people who can partially see. Their address is 22 West 21st Street, New York, NY 10011.

The Vision Foundation publishes the Vision Resource List, which includes information on special products and services for visually impaired people. There is no charge for the List. Write to the Foundation at 818 Mt. Auburn Street, Watertown, MA 02172.

The National Eye Care Project of the American Academy of Ophthalmology has a helpline number to refer callers to a local eye doctor or surgeon (ophthalmologist) who has volunteered to provide needed medical care. This public service program brings medical eye care and information to disadvantaged older people. Write to the AAO at P.O. Box 6988, San Francisco, CA 94120-6988; or call (800) 222-EYES.

Chapter 62

Pstosis in
Children and Adults

What Is Ptosis?

Ptosis is a Greek word meaning downward displacement. In Ophthalmology, it refers to a drooping upper eyelid. The lid may droop only slightly or it may droop enough to partially or completely cover the pupil, restricting or obscuring vision.

Ptosis may be inherited. It can affect one or both eyelids, be present at birth, or occur later in life. Ptosis which is present at birth is called congenital ptosis.

When an infant is born with moderate to severe ptosis, treatment is necessary to allow normal visual development. If the ptosis is not corrected, a condition called amblyopia ("lazy eye") may develop. If untreated, amblyopia can lead to permanent suppression of sight in one eye.

When ptosis is mild, treatment may be desired for cosmetic reasons but is not medically necessary. When ptosis is severe enough to obstruct vision, treatment is usually beneficial.

Congenital Ptosis

What Causes Congenital Ptosis?

Ptosis which is present at birth is often caused by poor development of the eyelid-lifting muscle, called the levator. Although usually

American Academy of Ophthalmology, ©1988. Used by permission.

517

occurring as an isolated problem, children born with ptosis may also have eye movement abnormalities, muscular diseases, lid tumors or neurological disorders. Congenital ptosis usually does not improve with time.

What Are The Signs And Symptoms Of Congenital Ptosis?

A drooping upper eyelid is the primary sign of ptosis. Children with ptosis will often tip their heads back into a chin-up posture to see underneath their eyelids, or raise their eyebrows in an effort to raise their lids.

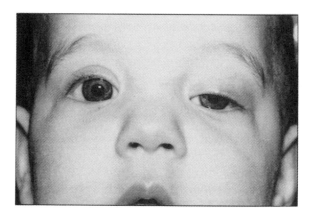

Figure 62.1. A young child with ptosis of the left eyelid.

What Problems Can Occur As A Result Of Childhood Ptosis?

The most serious problem associated with childhood ptosis is amblyopia. Amblyopia is poor vision in an eye that failed to develop normal sight in the early years of life. This may occur in a child with ptosis if the lid is drooping severely enough to block vision or cause astigmatism. Ptosis can also hide a misalignment or crossing of the eyes which can itself cause amblyopia. If not treated early in childhood, amblyopia persists throughout life. Other problems which can occur as a consequence of uncorrected childhood ptosis include astigmatism and blurred vision. Finally ptosis may negatively affect a child's appearance.

How Is Congenital Ptosis Treated?

The treatment for ptosis is surgery, although there are a few rare disorders that may be treated non-surgically with medications. In determining whether surgery is advisable, an ophthalmologist considers the individual's age, the severity of the ptosis, and whether one or both eyelids are involved. Measurement of the eyelid height, evaluation of the eyelid's lifting and closing muscle strength, and observation of the eyes' movements aid your ophthalmologist in determining what surgical procedure is most appropriate.

During surgery the levators, the eyelid lifting muscles, are tightened. In severe ptosis, when the levator muscle is extremely weak, the lid can be attached or suspended from the brow so that the forehead muscles do the lifting.

Severe congenital ptosis may require prompt surgery to avoid amblyopia and to allow proper visual development. Mild or moderate ptosis in children usually does not require surgery early in life, but does require periodic eye exams to monitor visual development and check for refractive errors which may need correcting with glasses. Surgery can be performed at any age for cosmetic reasons.

Any child with ptosis, whether they have had surgery or not, should be examined annually by an ophthalmologist for amblyopia, refractive errors and other associated conditions. Even after surgery, focusing problems may develop as the eyes grow and change shape.

Adult Ptosis

What Causes Adult Ptosis?

The most common type of adult ptosis is caused by the separation of the levator muscle tendon from the lid. This can occur as a result of aging, after cataract or other eye surgery, or from an injury. Adult ptosis may also occur as a complication of other diseases involving the levator muscle or its nerve supply, such as diabetes. Or, it may occur when movement of the levator muscle is restricted as may happen in the case of an eyelid tumor. Finally, an adult with untreated childhood ptosis will still have the condition as an adult.

What Are The Signs And Symptoms Of Adult Ptosis?

The most obvious sign is a drooping upper eyelid. There may be some vision loss in the upper field of vision or fatigue from attempting to elevate the drooping lid. Adults with ptosis will often tip their heads back to see past their eyelids, or raise their eyebrows in an effort to raise their lids An adult with severe ptosis. The pupil in the right eye is completely covered by the drooping lid and nearly so in the left.

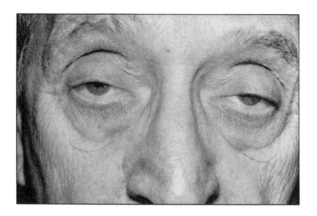

Figure 62.2. *An adult with severe ptosis. The pupil in the right eye is completely covered by the drooping lid and nearly so in the left.*

How Is Adult Ptosis Treated?

Your ophthalmologist may use blood tests, X-rays or other tests to determine the cause of the ptosis and plan the best treatment. Treatment, when necessary, is usually surgical. When the levator tendon has separated from the lid, reattachment of the muscle can correct the ptosis. Sometimes a small tuck in the lifting muscle and eyelid can lift the lid sufficiently. More severe Ptosis requires greater tightening of the levator muscle.

An ophthalmic consultation can provide a comprehensive assessment of your ptosis, a discussion of the available treatment methods, and information about possible risks and complications.

What Are The Risks Of Ptosis Surgery?

The risks of ptosis surgery include infection, bleeding and reduced vision but these complications occur very infrequently. A temporary inability to fully close the eye after ptosis surgery is not uncommon. Lubricant drops and ointments are frequently useful in this situation. It is also important to know that although improvement of the lid height is usually achieved, perfect symmetry in the height of the two eyelids and full eyelid movement is sometimes not achieved.

Summary

Ptosis in both children and adults can be successfully treated with surgery to improve visual function as well as cosmetic appearance. Children with ptosis should have ophthalmic examinations early in life to protect them from the serious consequences of untreated amblyopia.

Chapter 63

Blepharitis

What is blepharitis?

Blepharitis is a common and persistent inflammation of the eyelids. Symptoms include irritation, itching, and occasionally, a red eye.

This condition frequently occurs in people who have oily skin, dandruff, or dry eyes. Blepharitis can begin in early childhood, producing "granulated eyelids," and continue throughout life as a chronic condition, or develop later in life.

Bacteria reside on the surface of everyone's skin, but in certain individuals they thrive in the skin at the base of the eyelashes. The resulting irritation, sometimes associated with overactivity of the nearby oil glands, causes dandruff-like scales and particles to form along the lashes and eyelid margins.

For some people the scales or bacteria associated with blepharitis produce only minor irritation and itching, but in others they may cause redness, stinging or burning. Some people may develop an allergy to the scales or to the bacteria which surround them. This can lead to a more serious complication, inflammation of the eye tissues, particularly the cornea (the clear "front window" of the eye).

How is blepharitis treated?

Blepharitis can be a stubborn problem. Although there is no specific cure, it can be controlled through a careful, regular program of hygiene. First, you should obtain the necessary equipment:

American Academy of Ophthalmology, ©1994. Used by permission.

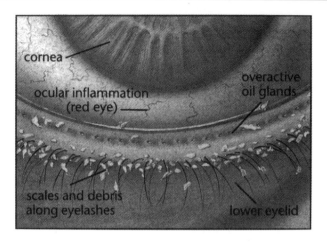

Figure 63.1. *In blepharitis, both upper and lower eyelids become coated with oily debris and bacteria near the base of the eyelashes. The eye feels irritated and may become inflamed. Regular, thorough cleansing of the lid margin helps control blepharitis.*

- A concave or "cosmetic" mirror (available in most drug stores);
- Cotton balls, a clean washcloth or commercial lint-free pads;
- Cotton-tipped applicators ("Q-tips");
- A mild baby shampoo, soap which doesn't sting the eyes, or a commercial eyelid cleansing solution;
- A small, clean glass or jar.

The cleansing routine below should be followed at least twice a day at first; perhaps less often as the condition improves.

1. Take a clean washcloth, wet it with warm water, wring it out and place it over your closed eyelids for five minutes. This will help to soften the crusts and loosen the oily debris. Rewet as necessary to maintain the desired temperature.

2. If you are not using one of the ready-made eyelid cleansing solutions, prepare your own by filling the small glass or jar with 2–3 ounces of warm water and adding three drops of baby shampoo.

3. Moisten a cotton ball, clean cloth or lint-free pad in the solution and then gently scrub the eyelids for about two minutes.

Your eyes should not be squeezed tightly shut, but closed softly as if you were sleeping.

4. Looking into the magnifying mirror, gently use a Q-tip moistened in the cleansing solution to brush the scales away from the eyelids. You can brush either in a horizontal or vertical direction, as long as the granular debris trapped in the eyelashes is effectively loosened and removed. This procedure should take approximately half a minute for each eyelid.

5. Thoroughly rinse your eyes with cool tap water and dry gently with a clean towel.

6. Discard any cleansing solution left in the small glass and rinse it clean.

7. If medication has been prescribed it should be applied to the eyes and/or eyelids along the lashes, following your ophthalmologist's instructions.

Will medication help?

Many medications are available for the treatment of blepharitis, including antibiotics and steroid (cortisone) preparations in drop or ointment form. While cortisone medications often hasten relief of symptoms, long-term use can cause some harmful side effects.

Once the acute phase of the condition is overcome—a process which may take several weeks—milder medications, if any, may be helpful to control your blepharitis. However, medications alone are not sufficient; the daily cleansing routine described above is essential.

Why are regular medical eye examinations important for everyone?

Eye disease can occur at any age. Many eye diseases do not cause symptoms until damage has occurred. Since most blindness is preventable if diagnosed and treated early, regular medical examinations by an ophthalmologist are very important.

Chapter 64

Dry Eyes

An estimated 12 million Americans have dry eyes. This condition is the inability to produce enough tears to keep the surface of the eyes lubricated and comfortable.

Tears are made by tissue in the lacrimal glands. The major lacrimal glands lie under the skin and extend into the eye socket. Tears reach the surface of the eye via small openings from the gland. Tears drain from the eye's surface by flowing into other tiny openings (lacrimal puncta), then into canals in the eyelids (lacrimal ducts), into a small pouch (lacrimal sac) and finally into the nose.

Normally, blinking helps the eyelids spread a tear film over the eye. If blinking is prevented, dry spots develop on the surface of the eye and vision decreases.

The continuous production and drainage of tears is very important. Tears keep the eyes moist, help ocular wounds heal and protect against eye infections. Persons with dry eyes are at greater risk of developing eye infections.

What Causes Dry Eyes?

Dry eyes occur:

- With age. Dry eyes are more common in women, especially after menopause.

From *Eye Facts*, Sept./Oct. 1991. ©1991 Board of Trustees of the University of Illinois, Chicago, Illinois. Used by permission.

- With the use of some drugs, including antihistamines, nasal decongestants and sedatives.
- Sometimes after eye surgery.
- In some persons with malpositioned lower eyelids.
- Infrequently after irradiation to the eye.
- In climates with dry air.
- Sometimes with vitamin A deficiency or after a chemical burn to the eye.
- In dry eye syndromes, called keratoconjunctivitis sicca. These syndromes usually affect both eyes, causing dryness, redness, swelling, itching and burning of the eyes and often reduced vision.
- In autoimmune diseases such as Sjögren's syndrome.
- In connective tissue diseases such as rheumatoid arthritis.

What Are the Symptoms of Dry Eyes?

The main symptom of dry eyes is usually a scratchy or sandy feeling that something is in the eyes. Other symptoms may include:

- Stinging, burning and itching of the eyes.
- Episodes of excess tearing that follow periods of very dry sensations.
- A stringy discharge from the eyes.
- Heaviness of the eyelids.
- Pain and redness of the eyes.
- Blurred, changing or decreased vision. Loss of vision usually is not severe.

How Are Dry Eyes Diagnosed?

The patient's historical information often gives the most reliable clues to the diagnosis of dry eyes. A careful examination of all the eye tissues usually provides more documentation for making a diagnosis. Also, a number of tests may help confirm the diagnosis.

The main test for dry eyes is the Schirmer test. This test involves placing a strip of filter paper over part of the eye (conjunctival sac) for up to five minutes. Less than the normal amount of wetting, on repeated examinations, indicates decreased tear production. Unfortunately, this test misses detecting many patients with dry eyes. Other tests should also be done before ruling out a diagnosis of dry eyes.

528

Other diagnostic tests include applying a drop of special dye (rose bengal stain) onto the eye. If there is a tear deficiency, the dye forms a characteristic pattern on the surface of the eye.

What Treatments Help Dry Eyes?

The main goal in the treatment of dry eyes is relief of symptoms. Usually this is achieved with artificial tears. These tear substitutes lubricate and wet the eyes. They are available over-the-counter as eye drops. Since artificial tears have short-lasting effects, they need to be applied often.

There are many brands of artificial tears on the market, and you may need to try several brands to find the one that works best for you. Sometimes combinations of different artificial tears are most helpful. Some types have preservatives, which may trigger allergic reactions with long-term use.

Sterile ointments containing petrolatum are sometimes used at night to help lubricate and prevent the eye from drying. In some people, however, they may irritate their eyes. These ointments usually do not require a prescription.

Other approaches to increasing moisture for the surface of the eve are available. There are different types of "inserts" that slowly dissolve in the eye and release artificial tears. These inserts are not suitable for everyone and usually require a prescription.

Preventing tears from evaporating also may help dry eyes. Using a humidifier in winter to add moisture to the air may be helpful. Also, moisture chamber glasses are available, which have a tight-fitting plastic shield on the sides to keep moisture inside.

In severe cases of dry eyes, if artificial tears do not control the symptoms, other treatments may be needed. One method is closing the opening to the lacrimal ducts to prevent drainage of tears from the eyes. This involves cauterizing the tissue (using heat or electric current), laser treatment or surgery. A possible complication of closing the tear ducts is an overflow of tears. Thus, some eye surgeons first close or plug the tear ducts temporarily to test how effective this procedure would be.

When a malposition of the lower eyelids causes dry eyes, eyelid surgery may help the dryness.

For drug-induced dry eyes, stopping the medication sometimes relieves the symptoms.

There is no cure for dry eye syndromes, so treatment with artificial tears is long term. The severity of the condition, however, often fluctuates and may improve. A major part of treatment also involves preventing the complications of eye infections.

Research at the UIC Eye Center is trying to find the best treatments of dry eyes. Investigators are testing different types of artificial tears as well as chemicals that may stimulate tear secretion. They are also testing immunologic-mediating drugs that may decrease the dry eye complications in some diseases. Additionally, our researchers are studying what causes dry eye conditions and are developing new medical and surgical treatments.

—by John W. Chandler, M.D.

Part Nine

Ophthalmic Disorders Related to Other Diseases

Chapter 65

National Eye Institute Report on Diabetic Retinopathy, Sickle Cell Retinopathy and Other Vascular Abnormalities

Introduction

The retina is supplied by two major systems of blood vessels. Its inner layers of nerve and supporting (glial) cells are supplied by the retinal circulation, which in humans consists of branches of one main feeder trunk called the central retinal artery and one main collecting trunk called the central retinal vein. Branches of these major vessels are arterioles; venules; and capillaries, the smallest blood vessels of all, which have a caliber only wide enough to allow passage of blood cells in single file. The capillary wall is composed of basement membrane and two types of cells. The endothelial cells which line the lumen and the pericytes which are embedded in the basement membrane are thought to perhaps play a role in regulating blood flow.

The outer layer of cells of the neural retina (the rods and cones) and the RPE are nourished by the choroidal circulation. This system consists of three layers of vessels. The innermost vascular layer, the choroidal capillaries (or choriocapillaris), is adjacent to the pigment epithelium. These capillaries are wider and much more closely packed than the capillaries of the retina, and their volume flow of blood is much greater than that in the retinal circulation. Moreover, it can be shown by electron microscopy that their lining cells (endothelial cells) have multiple holes (fenestrae) to allow ready passage of even rather large molecules. By contrast, the retinal capillaries, like those of the

NIH Pub. No. 93–3186. Excerpt from *Vision Research: A National Plan*, pp. 16–27.

brain, have a tight endothelial lining that normally serves as a barrier to large molecules. External to the choriocapillaris are two additional layers of choroidal vessels consisting of arteries and veins.

Normally a tight barrier prevents the free exchange of blood components between the circulatory system and other retinal tissues. This blood-retinal barrier, which appears to be essential for normal retinal function, is formed by the endothelial cells lining the retinal blood vessels, by the cells of the RPE, and by their associated basement membranes.

Three major pathologic processes characterize retinal vascular disorders: (1) excessive permeability, (2) vascular closure, and (3) the proliferation of newly formed blood vessels. Excessive permeability of retinal capillaries can lead to edema of the retina, resulting in blurring of vision if the center of the macula is involved. Diseases causing excessive permeability include diabetic retinopathy, retinal venous occlusions, and other less common vascular and inflammatory disorders. Microaneurysms, saccular dilatations of the retinal capillaries, are typical of diabetic retinopathy and certain other retinal vascular disorders. These microaneurysms provide one important site of excessive permeability, and diffusely leaking capillaries provide another.

Closure of the central retinal artery usually leads to complete or nearly complete loss of vision in the affected eye from ischemic infarction of the inner layers of the retina. Occlusion of the central retinal vein or of one of its branches also may cause rapid diminution of vision from macular edema or retinal hemorrhage. Later sequelae of retinal venous occlusion may include retinal neovascularization, vitreous hemorrhage, and neovascularization of the anterior segment of the eye. This latter condition can block aqueous humor drainage and cause intractable glaucoma.

Closure of retinal capillaries does not produce such dramatic symptoms, but the long-term effects may be equally harmful to vision. Because the retina has the highest oxygen requirement of any tissue in the body as well as high requirements for glucose and other metabolites, loss of blood supply to even a small region of the retina may have serious consequences. One important, current hypothesis (amplified below) is that extensive areas of retinal capillary nonperfusion in some way may stimulate the growth of abnormal new blood vessels. Capillary nonperfusion may be demonstrated in diabetic retinopathy, sickle cell retinopathy, retinal vein occlusions, retinopathy of prematurity, and other diseases.

Newly formed blood vessels arising in the retina or on the optic disc, presumably in response to retinal ischemia, have a tendency to break through the inner limiting membrane of the retina and grow along its inner surface. Then hemorrhage may occur from the new vessels into the vitreous, and/or traction retinal detachment may result from contraction of fibrous or glial tissue accompanying the vessels.

Subprogram Objectives

- To develop greater understanding of the pathogenesis of diabetic retinopathy and other vascular diseases of the retina and choroid.

- To develop better methods of preventing, diagnosing, and treating these disorders.

- To understand the anatomy, biochemistry, and physiology of the retinal and choroidal vasculature in normal and diseased states.

- To understand how blood flow is regulated in the retina.

Recent Accomplishments

Clinical Research

Diabetic retinopathy. Diabetic retinopathy is one of the most important causes of visual loss and accounts for approximately 12 percent of new cases of blindness each year in the United States. Diabetes increases the risk of blindness 25-fold over that of the general population, and it is estimated that 8,000 Americans become blind each year as a result of diabetic eye disease.

The scientific basis for the management of diabetic retinopathy was provided during the 1970s by the NEI's first large-scale, randomized clinical trial entitled the Diabetic Retinopathy Study (DRS). The DRS has been expanded during the 1980s by additional NEI-sponsored multicenter trials. The Diabetic Retinopathy Vitrectomy Study demonstrated that the prognosis for maintenance or recovery of good vision could be improved in eyes with very severe proliferative diabetic retinopathy by prompt vitrectomy rather than vitrectomy deferred until traction retinal detachment involving the center of the macula developed or until severe vitreous hemorrhage failed to clear after a waiting period of 6 to 12 months. The ETDRS found that, for eyes with nonproliferative or early proliferative retinopathy careful follow up and deferral of laser photocoagulation surgery until retinopathy progressed to the high-risk stage (defined in the DRS) were highly effective in preventing severe visual loss and were almost as effective as early treatment (5-year rates of 4 percent and 2.5 percent, respectively). They also were attended by lower rates of complications. The ETDRS also provided the following strong evidence for the efficacy of focal photocoagulation for diabetic macular edema: reduction of the 3-year rate of moderate visual loss (in eyes with the center of the macula involved) from 33 percent for untreated eyes to 13 percent for treated eyes. The ETDRS found no evidence that aspirin (650 mg/day) influenced the course of retinopathy. Data from this study have demonstrated that currently recommended treatments are 90 percent effective in preventing blindness in patients with proliferative retinopathy.

Population-based epidemiologic studies have provided a wealth of new information on the prevalence and incidence of diabetic retinopathy and risk factors for the severity and progression of retinopathy. Additional evidence for the possible importance of blood sugar levels in the genesis of diabetic retinopathy was provided by one such study. This study found a strong dose-response relationship between the 4-year risk of retinopathy progression and the baseline level of glycosylated hemoglobin, a relationship that held across broad ranges of baseline nonproliferative retinopathy severity and diabetes duration. A definitive assessment of the importance of blood glucose control in slowing the development of retinopathy and other complications is being addressed by the Diabetes Control and Complications Trial. This study, sponsored by the National Institute of Diabetes and Digestive and Kidney Diseases, is a long-term comparison of standard treatment versus intensive insulin treatment.

Another promising medical approach to preventing or slowing the progression of diabetic retinopathy is the inhibition of aldose reductase (AR), a principal enzyme of the polyol pathway by which hexoses such as glucose and galactose are converted to sugar alcohols (sorbitol and galactitol, respectively) with damaging metabolic consequences to the cells involved. In a randomized clinical trial in insulin-dependent diabetic patients, one such inhibitor, sorbinil, was found not to have a clinically important effect on retinopathy progression over a 3-year period. This result may have been due to inadequate drug levels in the retina or to intervention that was not initiated soon enough or continued long enough. Similar trials of another AR inhibitor, Tolrestat, are under way. (See further discussion of AR inhibition below under Basic Research.)

Sickle cell retinopathy. Patients with sickle cell disease may experience visual loss from sickle cell retinopathy. Peripheral retinal neovascularization, most commonly seen in patients with hemoglobin SC but also noted in patients with sickle cell anemia (hemoglobin SS) and sickle cell beta thalassemia, may cause vitreous hemorrhage or retinal detachment. Visual loss also may be caused by retinal arterial occlusions.

Recent work has demonstrated the value of laser photocoagulation for proliferative sickle cell retinopathy. Focal photocoagulation may diminish the incidence of vitreous hemorrhage and visual loss, but it is a difficult technique to master and may cause complications. Scatter photocoagulation, similar to that used for diabetic retinopathy, is being evaluated in the randomized trial that is nearing completion. Retinal vascular occlusions. It is now recognized that both branch and central retinal vein occlusions occur at about equal frequency, and together they represent the second most frequent cause of retinal vascular disturbance after diabetic retinopathy. Branch and central retinal artery occlusions are distinctly less common. Recently the Branch Vein Occlusion Study Group demonstrated the efficacy of laser photocoagulation for the management of neovascularization and macular edema as complications of branch retinal vein occlusion. Currently under study in the Central Vein Occlusion Study Group is the efficacy of laser photocoagulation for the management of iris neovascularization and macular edema secondary to central vein occlusion; it is hoped that this study will be completed by 1995. Systemic risk factors for venous occlusion are under study in a multicenter case-control study, and a pilot study is exploring the possible role of tissue plasminogen activator in lessening the complications of central vein occlusion.

Retinopathy of prematurity. Retinopathy of prematurity (ROP) is a disorder of retinal vascular maturation manifested by an abnormal proliferation at the developing ends of blood vessels in the immature retina of a prematurely born infant. Proliferation of new vessels into the vitreous may lead to circumferential traction and irreversible retinal detachment. Studies in the 1950s showed that therapeutic oxygen could, in excess, stimulate the development of this condition. In recent years there has been a growing concern that even levels of oxygen barely sufficient to sustain cerebral health can be enough to permit the development of ROP in infants with the lowest birth weights, who now are surviving with increasing frequency.

Continuous oxygen monitoring shows surprisingly little benefit in the prevention of ROP, and the role of vitamin E in preventing this disorder is still unclear. An important recent accomplishment is the demonstration, in a nationwide randomized trial, of the beneficial effect of peripheral retinal cryotherapy in reducing the risk of progression from the moderate "threshold" stage of ROP to more severe, sight-damaging stages.

Basic Research

Over the past 5 years there have been many exciting advances in our understanding of the retinal circulation and of the growth and metabolism of the retinal vascular cells, both *in vivo* and *in vitro*. These include advancements in the following areas:

- Biochemical mechanisms of the effects of hyperglycemia
- Retinal cell biology of cell-cell interaction and growth factors
- Basement membrane biochemistry and biology
- Retinal blood flow and vasoactive control
- Animal models.

Biochemical mechanisms of the effects of hyperglycemia. Clinical observations and studies of experimental diabetes in dogs leave little doubt that elevated blood glucose is a fundamental pathogenetic factor in diabetic retinopathy. Recent studies using cultured cells have found that elevated glucose levels affect the metabolism and growth of a variety of retinal cells, such as pericytes, capillary endothelial cells, and retinal pigment epithelial cells. This is not surprising since glucose and its metabolites are utilized by many pathways; however, the fundamental mechanism by which retinopathy is initiated remains unknown. Several theories currently under study are outlined below.

One theory relates to finding, in neural and vascular tissues, increased levels of intracellular sorbitol generated from glucose via the polyol pathway by the enzyme AR. Changes in sorbitol levels could affect important cellular metabolites such as myoinositol and enzymes such as sodium-potassium-activated adenosine triphosphatase (Na^+/K^+-ATPase). AR is present in many retinal cells including pericytes and endothelial cells of retinal capillaries, the Muller cells, ganglion cells, and the pigment epithelium, and an increased flux of glucose through the polyol pathway during hyperglycemia could initiate retinal damage.

A second but related theory postulates that hyperglycemia can activate an enzyme system called protein kinase C (PKC) in the retina.

Since PKC has been shown to affect vascular contractility, permeability, basement membrane synthesis, and vascular cell proliferation *in vitro*, the changes found in PKC activity during hyperglycemia may mediate some of the vascular abnormalities of diabetes.

Nonenzymatic glycation is initiated when the open-chain aldehyde form of glucose reacts with amino acid residues to form a Schiff base. Chemical rearrangements eventually result in ketoamine formation followed by stabilization of the cyclic hemiactal. Advanced glycation end products may be formed as a result of dehydration, chemical rearrangements, and cleavage. Nonenzymatic glycation occurs under normal glucose concentrations and is increased as a result of hyperglycemia. The physiological effect of this process is unclear even though nonenzymatic glaciation may alter the structure and function of macromolecules which react with glucose. It has been speculated that this process may compromise vascular barrier function, but the significance of nonenzymatic glaciation in the pathogenesis of diabetic vascular disease remains uncertain.

Lastly, there are suggestions that an increased glucose flux through the vascular cells could change the redox potential intracellularly and ultimately affect multiple cellular pathways such as PKC, DNA repair, and Na+/K+-ATPase. Reports that normalization of cellular redox potential can reverse hyperglycemia-induced vascular dysfunctions in animal models provide support for this possibility.

Retinal cell biology of cell-cell interaction and growth factors. The cells of the retinal capillaries are thought to be involved primarily in diabetic retinopathy. A notable decrease in pericytes is a classic early finding, and proliferation of endothelial cells is an essential step in the later development of proliferative retinopathy. One of the most important advances of the last several years has been the development of the ability to culture large quantities of these vascular cells from bovine and human retina. Specific antibodies have been identified for both pericytes and endothelial cells, and it has been shown that cultured vascular cells retain some of the same antigens as those expressed *in vivo*. Studies using cultured pericytes have demonstrated that elevated glucose levels can inhibit growth. A coculture model, which mimics the contact of endothelial cells and pericytes occurring *in vivo*, has provided insights into the role that cell-cell interactions may play in maintaining normal vascular function. In such a model the presence of pericytes inhibits the growth of capillary endothelial cells when the cells are in contact. This growth inhibition appears to be mediated through the activation of transforming growth factor p

(TGF-5) occurring when the cells are in contact. In another study using the coculture model, pericytes also have been shown to affect the ability of endothelial cells to form tight barriers.

Great advances also have been made in the identification and characterization of growth factors that may play a critical role in the etiology of proliferative retinopathy. The fibroblast growth factor (FGF) family, which includes acidic FGF and basic FGF, has made the most progress. The breakthrough in purification of these factors came from the observation that a tumor-derived endothelial cell mitogen binds with high affinity to heparin. Subsequently, the primary amino acid sequence and the genes for both terms of the FGF were determined, cloned, and sequenced. A variety of biologic activities has been associated with these factors. With respect to the study of diabetic retinopathy, the primary and most important activity is the finding that both acidic and basic FGF can stimulate the formation of new blood vessels in vivo. In cultured endothelial cells, FGF stimulates proliferation and migration and induces the production of proteases, events that are important in the process of angiogenesis. Although FGFs have been identified in both the retina and vitreous of control patients and diabetic patients, a causal role for these growth factors has not been conclusively demonstrated in any physiologic setting.

Insulin, insulin-like growth factor I (IGF-I), and their receptors also have been identified in the vitreous and retina. IGF-I levels may be increased in a subset of diabetic patients with severe proliferative retinopathy. Other new angiogenic factors, such as platelet-derived endothelial cell growth factor from alpha granules of platelet and vascular endothelia growth factor (VEGF), a growth factor isolated from sarcoma 180 cells, have been purified, but little is known about their distribution *in vivo*.

Basement membrane biochemistry and biology. The etiology of basement membrane thickening, the hallmark of the microvascular complications of diabetes, is not understood. Changes in the proportion or synthesis of the matrix components have been reported. Reduced synthesis of heparin sulfate proteoglycan has been found in kidneys of diabetic animal models. In addition, kidneys from diabetic patients have reduced levels of heparin sulfate proteoglycan and laminin, a component of the matrix. It has been reported that AR inhibitors prevent retinal (but not glomerular) capillary basement membrane thickening in galactosemic rats and also prevent the increases in type IV collagen and laminin observed in retinal capillary basement membrane of these animals. However, direct evidence in diabetic animals is needed before conclusions on the role of AR can be drawn. High glucose levels produce a variety of effects in cultured vascular endothelial cells or pericytes including synthesis of protein and collagen and increased mRNA levels for collagen IV and fibronectin. Altered turnover of matrix components may lead to basement membrane thickening, and the activity of enzymes such as collagenases or proteases or their inhibitors could be changed in diabetes.

Recent studies have shown that vascular cells adhere to basement membranes by binding to specific amino acid sequences with cell surface receptors and integrins that bind to fibronectin, collagens, and laminin. Basement membrane has been shown to affect cell attachment, migration, differentiation, and turnover of matrix components. These biologic processes are likely to play an important role in producing basement membrane thickening and microvessel leakiness.

Retinal blood flow and vasoactive control. Various retinal hemodynamic changes have been described in diabetic patients and animals. Several methods have been used to measure retinal blood flow and oxygenation. These methods include laser doppler velocimetry (LDV), computerized image processing of fluorescein angiograms, the entoptic blue field phenomenon, and retinal oximetry.

Recent LDV studies in diabetic patients with different levels of diabetic retinopathy have shown decreases in blood velocity and increases in diameter in the main retinal veins. Blood flow, however did not differ significantly from normal until the more advanced stages of retinopathy. Mean circulation times were increased in patients with advanced retinopathy, while conflicting results have been obtained for patients with early retinopathy.

In patients with poorly controlled diabetes, retinal flows were higher than normal, and normoglycemia achieved through insulin therapy decreased the flow toward normal. This regulatory decrease in flow in response to a decrease in blood glucose was present in patients with recently diagnosed diabetes but was less apparent in patients who had the disease longer. This suggests that regulatory response to retinal metabolic changes may be lost in the latter stages of the disease. In a recent study of the effect of improving glycemic control, patients in whom retinopathy underwent transient worsening following rapid improvement in control did not show the regulatory decreases in retinal blood flow that occurred in patients who did not show such worsening.

The normal vascular regulatory response to hyperoxia already may be impaired in patients with early diabetic retinopathy, and this response diminishes with the progression of the disease. This loss of regulatory response to hyperoxia may provide information on the metabolic state of the retina and the ability of the retina to respond to stress. A recent investigation of the effect of panretinal photocoagulation showed that the regulatory response to hyperoxia improved toward normal in those patients whose treatment resulted in regression of retinopathy. In patients who did not show regression, there was almost no improvement in the regulatory response, suggesting that the lack of such improvement may be related to abnormalities in retinal metabolism that persist in spite of photocoagulation. One of these abnormalities could be retinal hypoxia, which is thought to be present in diabetic retinopathy. Measurements of retinal oxygenation in eyes with diabetic retinopathy are needed to assess whether hypoxia of the retinal tissue is an important factor in the early development of diabetic retinopathy. The noninvasive technique of retinal vessel oximetry may offer a way to increase our knowledge of oxygen exchange in the retina of patients with diabetes.

Biochemical studies have demonstrated the presence of adrenergic hormones, reninangiotensin, vasopressin, and endothelin and their receptors in retinal vascular tissue and cells, but their role in the retinal circulation has not been quantitated.

Animal models. The development of animal models of diabetic retinopathy has been difficult and tedious, but information of great interest and importance has been produced. Long-term studies using dogs with chemically induced diabetes have shown that after 3 to 5 years of poorly controlled diabetes, these animals developed retinopathies and nephropathies very similar to those seen in diabetic patients. Good glycemic control instituted within a few weeks of the induction of diabetes prevented the appearance of retinal abnormalities, whereas secondary intervention with good control after 2% years of poor glycemic control was much less effective. This study suggests that irreversible biochemical changes that were not detected by available histologic methods may have occurred and/or that there may be a long lag period before the morphologic effects, if any, of improved control can be demonstrated.

An alternative model for diabetic retinopathy has been established by use of galactose-fed nondiabetic dogs. The rate of occurrence of retinal vascular changes is more rapid, possibly because of the accumulation of higher levels of galactitol than of sorbitol (galactitol, unlike sorbitol, cannot be further metabolized by this pathway) and perhaps also because of a higher affinity of AR for galactose than for glucose. Interestingly, galactosemic dogs have not developed nephropathy. This finding suggests that there may not be a single mechanism for vascular complications of diabetes.

The canine galactosemia model and a similar model in rats have been used to test the possible effect of AR inhibition on the development of retinopathy. In one study in dogs, the appearance of pericyte loss and microaneurysms was delayed, but in another study, there was no inhibition of retinopathy after 42 months of galactose feeding. In a group of rats, retinal vascular changes developing after 28 months of galactosemia were prevented by AR inhibition. AR inhibitors have a short plasma half-life in dogs, and their bioavailability in the retina is not known. Research in the design of AR inhibitors has been enhanced by the successful cloning and DNA sequencing of AR and by determining the crystal structure of this enzyme. The cloning of AR also has provided a tool for investigating its genetic expression.

The granulation tissue chamber model in the rat, which allows experiments to be conducted on vascular tissue *in vivo*, also has proved useful. This system allows rapid testing of the effect of various therapeutic agents on vascular functions such as flow and permeability. These studies have provided evidence that vascular pathologies are caused by alterations in multiple pathways.

Animal models for studying proliferative diabetic retinopathy or cicatricial ROP still have not been established. However, it has been reported that some strains of retinal-dystrophic rats develop retinal neovascularization. Further work is needed to characterize this promising model.

Important Research Questions to Be Addressed

The following research questions need to be addressed:

Are there important risk factors for the development and progression of retinopathy?

What factors determine why some diabetic persons develop macular edema and/or proliferative retinopathy and others do not? Epidemiologic studies of diabetic retinopathy similar to those conducted in Pima Indians and Mexican-Americans should continue in various groups. Case-control studies of individuals with severe proliferative retinopathy or macular edema can compare, among other things, blood levels of growth factors and other molecules that might alter the manifestations of the disease. What factors determine branch vein occlusion and central vein occlusion? What inventions can prevent the development of proliferative retinopathy?

What are the mechanisms by which photocoagulation produces its favorable effects? Why do some patients fail to respond favorably to photocoagulation? Can other therapeutic approaches be developed for these patients? At what stage of retinopathy should that coagulation be instituted? Attempts to collect post mortem ocular specimens from diabetic patients with varying degrees of treated and untreated retinopathy should continue and should be expanded. These specimens can be studied by anatomic, immunohistochemical, biochemical, or cell culture methods. Blood levels of growth factors should be studied in individuals whose severe proliferative disease does not respond to photocoagulation, for comparison to those individuals whose proliferative retinopathy was successfully treated.

Can better methods of treatment for retinopathies be developed?

This area of treatment might include laser photocoagulation, drugs, or surgery. Can methods for delivery of oxygen and other nutrients in the face of occlusive disease, both venous and arterial, be developed? Can methods for treatment or preventing ROP be refined to improve the effectiveness? What surgical techniques are most successful in dealing with vitreous hemorrhage and retinal detachment in these eyes? Given recent improvements in surgical techniques, is it necessary to continue the practice of giving blood transfusions before vitreous or retinal surgery to minimize the risk of surgical complications (anterior segment ischemia), or is the value of such transfusions outweighed by the risk of hepatitis or the transmission of HIV (human immunodeficiency virus)?

What can neonatologists do to reduce the risk of ROP? Could supplemental oxygen, supplied once ROP develops, curtail the progress of the retinopathy? What factors (other than oxygen), such as ambient light, affect the pathogenesis of ROP? What is the optimum strategy to permit the early detection and treatment of ROP? Can indications and techniques for therapy be refined to improve outcomes?

What are the mechanisms of the increased vascular permeability and progressive vascular occlusion that characterize diabetic retinopathy?

These may include improved drugs to inhibit AR or drugs that affect other metabolic pathways. The knowledge of the mechanisms of increased vascular permeability may be important in devising an effective preventive treatment for diabetic retinopathy.

What are the biochemical mechanisms involved in the pathogenesis of diabetic retinopathy?

Continued studies of cellular mechanisms should be pursued using (as appropriate) human tissues; animal models; or *in vitro* cultures of retinal vascular, neural, glial, or pigment epithelial cells. The role of growth factors in the pathogenesis of retinopathy needs further study. What are the effects on the retinal vasculature of the adrenergic hormones, renin angiotensin, vasopressin, endothelin, and of more recently discovered factors, such as endothelial cell-derived relaxing factor (EDRF)? Which factors are the most important regulators of retinal blood flow? Investigating those drugs that affect the metabolic pathways may be warranted.

What is the biochemical composition of the basement membrane of retinal microvessels? What changes occur in diabetes? What are the mechanisms of these changes, and what is their effect on capillary function? Appropriate biochemical analyses have been the classic approach to answering this question. However, the amount of retinal or other ocular basement membrane tissue available for such analyses, save in the case of the lens capsule, is likely to be small. Molecular and cellular biological approaches may be useful in defining the components and their function. Specific antibodies recently developed for subpopulations of major types of basement membrane macromolecules may be useful tools. What are the effects of these various basement membrane components on the metabolism and growth of retinal vascular cells?

What is the biochemical basis of the interaction between pericytes and endothelial cells? What interactions occur between vascular cells and neural and glial cells? Cell culture, light and electron microscopy, and immunocytochemistry may provide useful insights.

What effects do changes in the role of blood flow have in the progress of retinopathy in diabetic patients? Can retinal blood flow measurements and retinal vessel oximetry help develop a better understanding of the mechanism by which photocoagulation works and in guiding the initiation, location, and extent of photocoagalation treatment?

Chapter 66

Diabetes, Vision Impairment, and Blindness

Vision Impairment and Diabetes

Vision impairment is a common complication of diabetes mellitus, which is itself the leading cause of new cases of blindness among adults in the United States. Three percent of the country's 10 million diabetics have experienced severe vision loss as a result of the disease. This means that diabetics frequently have to face additional problems of impending loss of vision and blindness.

The purpose of this pamphlet is to explain the relationship between visual impairment and diabetes and to identify recent advances in treatment and rehabilitation to help diabetics and their families deal with the problems of vision loss. Diabetes and its complications are discussed here in a general way; no two cases of diabetes are exactly alike. Often, the person who has lived with this condition for a number of years knows more about his or her bodily responses than anyone else. Therefore, professionals and family members should listen to and work with blind diabetics, rather than do things "for" or "to" them.

Diabetes Explained

Diabetes mellitus is a serious chronic disease that occurs when the body cannot properly process carbohydrates (sugar and starches), protein, and fat to make energy. It is characterized by a relative lack of insulin action, which causes the blood glucose to rise. Insulin, a hormone produced by the pancreas, must be present in order for sugar circulating in the blood to pass through the wall of the blood vessels and reach the body tissues. In insulin-dependent diabetes mellitus (IDDM), Type I, the pancreas is unable to produce insulin, and daily injections of insulin are needed. In noninsulin-dependent diabetes mellitus (NIDDM), Type II, insulin is not present in sufficient amounts, or if it is, the individual cells of the body cannot accept it. Therefore, insulin and glucose remain in the blood. Both types of diabetes cause changes in the structure of the blood vessels, which appear to thicken and harden at a faster rate than normal. This damage, especially to the small blood vessels, results in poor circulation, and many body organs become damaged. Damage to the kidneys is called nephropathy; to the eyes, retinopathy; and to the nerve endings, neuropathy. Damage to the blood vessels in the feet and legs is described as peripheral vascular disease (PVD). It is suspected that the onset of these chronic complications can be delayed and their severity reduced with rigid control of blood glucose. Thus, treatment plans are designed to try to keep the blood sugars within normal ranges.

Diet, insulin, and activity are all considered to be integral parts of the treatment of diabetes and are interrelated. A change in any one of these three treatment components affects the other two components. Diet, insulin, and activity need ongoing monitoring by the diabetic person in order that a balance be maintained. Individual meal plans including food exchanges are developed and written for diabetics by a consulting dietitian. The amount of food varies according to body weight and lifestyle. Insulin by injection or pump is always prescribed as treatment for Type I diabetes; sometimes it is required in Type II. Ninety percent of people with Type II diabetes are obese. Weight reduction and diet are the treatments of choice. Oral medication (pills) may also be used to lower blood sugar. Activity (exercise) is encouraged for all people with either type of diabetes, for it burns blood sugar as well as improves blood circulation. Exercise should be a part of each day's routine but should never be too strenuous. It is best to exercise with the supervision and consent of a physician. Exercise should be avoided when blood sugar is not controlled.

On occasion, people with diabetes experience wide fluctuations in blood glucose levels. These extremes-hyperglycemia (high blood sugar) and hypoglycemia (low blood sugar)-are caused by different sets of circumstances, are identified by unique signs and symptoms, and require specific treatment.

Table 66.1. Acute Complications of Diabetes

Factor	Hyperglycemia (High blood sugar)	Hypoglycemia (Low blood sugar)
Onset	Gradual—days	Rapid—minutes to a few hours
Causes	Not enough insulin; too much food Illness—infection	Too much insulin action; not enough food Too much unplanned activity
Signs and symptoms	Tiredness; thirst; increased urination; hunger; ruddy skin color; headache; blurred vision; dry itchy skin	Dizziness; faintness; shakiness; instant hunger; cold, clammy sweat; paleness; irritability; double vision; stupor
Blood sugar	Over 250 mg*	Below 60 mg*
Urine sugar	Large amount	Usually negative
Treatment	Fluids Call doctor for increase of insulin dose	Sugar in some form, e.g., juice, milk, soft drinks, honey, commercially available concentrate glucose. Rest for 15 minutes. Repeat if necessary.

*Normal blood glucose levels fasting: 70 to 110 mg.

549

People with Type I diabetes may develop ketoacidosis if symptoms of high blood sugars are ignored. When the body cannot use blood glucose to make energy because of a lack of insulin, it begins to use stored body fat. This causes a buildup of ketones (acids). Ketoacidosis is a serious problem that can be effectively treated in a hospital. If symptoms are recognized in time, therapy can be initiated at home.

These acute complications are usually preventable by the initiation of appropriate responses to symptoms and the presence of glucose and ketones in the blood or urine. Checking urine for the presence of sugar and ketones and monitoring blood sugar levels on a regular schedule may identify problems before a crisis develops. Most products for testing urine sugars or ketones are simple to use, but their use requires good vision. Electronic devices have been developed to sense accurately the amount of sugar contained in a drop of blood. The monitors have a digital display of results. Now monitors are also available that audibly signal or announce blood glucose levels.

Recent advances in knowledge about diabetes and its management are encouraging. Through the use of an insulin pump, insulin can be delivered more like a normal pancreas does. People can monitor blood sugars more closely for good control of blood sugar levels. Pancreatic beta cell transplants for production of insulin also appear to be forthcoming in the near future.

Visual Complications of Diabetes

Diabetes mellitus has been known to be related to several abnormal conditions of the eye. They are blurred vision, retinopathy, cataracts, glaucoma, and occasionally neuropathy.

Blurred vision resulting from changes in the focusing power of the eye is often caused by hyperglycemia. It usually lasts until blood sugars return to normal ranges.

Diabetes for longer than five years' duration can affect both the tiny vessels and the nerve endings of the eyes, resulting in retinopathy, glaucoma, or cataracts. Occasionally, damage to the nerve endings, or neuropathy, paralyzes the muscles controlling the eyeball. This causes an inability to focus the eyes properly, which in turn results in double vision. Sometimes the eyelids are also paralyzed, causing dry, painful eyeballs. However, the paralysis is self-limiting and ceases within a few months.

Diabetic retinopathy, the most common cause of visual impairment in diabetics, occurs when blood vessels feeding the retina are damaged.

It develops gradually, with few early symptoms to warn that vision is threatened. During the early stage called background retinopathy, the vessels balloon outward and leak fluid. If fluid collects in the central part of the retina (macula), vision becomes blurred. (See Figure 66.1.) As the disease progresses, abnormal new blood vessels grow, and they may rupture and bleed into the clear gel that fills the center of the eye (vitreous humor). This blood may cause a reddish tint over the visual field. As blood collects, it prevents light from getting to the retina, and loss of vision develops. Scar tissue formations may contract and pull the retina from the back of the eye (detached retina). This stage of the condition is called proliferative retinopathy, and it may result in severe visual loss or permanent blindness.

Annual examination of the back of the eye (retina) by an ophthalmologist will identify retinopathy early. Fluorescein angiography, in which dye is injected into a vein and its progress in the eye is photographed, may be used as a diagnostic tool. If appropriate for a given individual, treatment is initiated as soon as possible. Powerful, precisely aimed beams of light from a laser are used to seal off leaking retinal blood vessels. This process, called photocoagulation, may reduce the chance of severe visual impairment in people with advanced retinopathy. Photocoagulation carries the risk of partial loss of central and side vision in some people. However, even though treatment might result in some visual loss, the benefits often outweigh the risks or side effects, especially in advanced diabetes retinopathy.

In cases where hemorrhages are large enough to cause blindness, a vitrectomy can be performed. During this procedure an ophthalmologist removes the blood, scar tissue, and vitreous humor from the center of the eye, replacing it with a clear saline solution. This procedure may increase the possibility that the retina will receive light. Occasionally, vision may be restored after a vitrectomy, at the level it was prior to the bleeding.

Cataracts are usually associated with the process of aging. However, diabetics seem to develop cataracts more frequently or more rapidly than nondiabetics. Cataracts are characterized by a gradual clouding of the transparent lens of the eye. During this early phase of development, the lens yellows, making it difficult to compare accurately the colors of various urine and blood test strips. This in turn makes it hard for the diabetic to monitor the test strips and thereby check his or her condition. As the lens becomes opaque, a progressive, painless loss of vision is experienced. Surgical removal of the cataract is usually successful if the retina is not damaged from retinopathy.

551

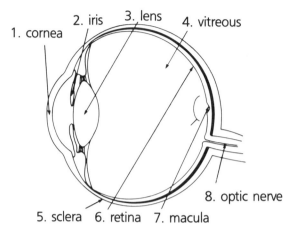

1. The cornea is the clear outer part of the eye. It protects the eye and primarily serves as a window.

2. The iris is the colored part of the eye. It controls the amount of light entering the eye through the pupil.

3. The lens, a clear structure made up of water and protein, focuses images.

4. The vitreous, a gelatinous substance that is about 99 percent water, is transparent and maintains the form of the eye.

5. The sclera is the protective white outer coating of the eye.

6. The retina is sensory tissue on which the lens focuses images. It contains the macula (7), the central area for detailed (reading) vision and visual acuity.

8. The optic nerve conveys the visual image from the retina to the brain, where it is "seen."

Figure 66.1. *The parts of the eye.*

Some vision is usually restored when the extracted lens is replaced with an implanted lens (intraocular lens) or when a contact lens or special eyeglasses are used.

Chronic glaucoma is a major cause of blindness in adults. It is thought to be more likely to develop in persons with diabetes than in members of the general population. Glaucoma is a disease in which the pressure of the fluid inside the eye is too high and causes destruction of the optic nerve. If chronic glaucoma remains undetected, gradual loss of vision occurs, beginning with side (peripheral) vision. The progress of the disease can be halted with proper treatment, but any loss of sight cannot be restored. Prescribed eye drops and, occasionally, oral medication can arrest the condition.

Hemorrhagic glaucoma caused by pressure from retinal hemorrhage is a severe and often painful form of the disease. It may occur in the diabetic who is already blind from retinopathy. This condition may require removal of the affected eye (enucleation) to eliminate the pain. The damaged eye is then replaced with an individually made prosthetic eye. It is also necessary for the patient to be under the care of an ophthalmologist.

Impact of Waning Vision on Diabetes Management

Excellent control of diabetes involves adherence to a fairly rigid routine of meals, medication, and exercise. The imposition of this regimen usually means that some aspect of the person's lifestyle has to be changed after the diagnosis of diabetes is made. Additional changes are needed as vision becomes increasingly impaired, and even more changes are required should blindness develop. The need to rely on others for assistance with many activities of daily living becomes an added stress.

Diabetics faced with the possibility of blindness often respond with depression and anger characterized by a refusal to follow established routines to control diabetes. These feelings may lessen in intensity when the patient discovers rehabilitation programs for visually impaired diabetics that make independence possible and provide interaction with others faced with the same difficulties. At this stage, new routines for diabetic management may be established for the visually impaired patient.

Fluctuations in blood sugar levels can also cause temporary emotional outbursts. For instance, the physical symptoms of low blood sugar are accompanied by nervousness, excitement, or hostility. High

Table 66.2. How to Manage Diabetes at Home with Blindness or Impaired Vision

Task	Impaired Vision	Blindness
Urine testing for sugar	Urine test reagent strips are sold over the counter under various proprietary brand names; with sighted assistance, these may be useful before consulting a physician.	Same as for impaired vision.
Blood glucose monitoring	Use magnifier to compare test strip with color chart. Use standard monitor together with timer, alarm system, and lighted display of results.	Assistance required. A monitor (Beta Scan™ Audio Model-Orange Medical Instrument) with audio report of results has been developed.
Medication	Ask pharmacist to put different medications in bottles of various sizes or shapes.	Label bottles with system of identifiable dots or textures.
Insulin	Use magnifier to check bottle label and dose in the syringe. Purchase a magnifier that clips onto disposable syringes. Use templet to stop the syringe at correct dose. An inexpensive one can be made with staples and tape.	Label bottles as above. Many devices (templets) are available that stop the plunger of the syringe at the correct dose. Use a needle guide (funnel shaped) to locate rubber stopper.

		To remove air bubbles from syringe, pull insulin into syringe and push it back into bottle three times. Use only 700 units of insulin from each 1,000-unit bottle to ensure that only insulin enters the syringe. Lay little finger of hand holding the syringe against the skin to act as a guide to the injection site.
Meals	Buy nested measuring cups and spoons. Use cookbooks for diabetics that are available in large print. Use low vision devices.	Buy nested measuring cups and spoons. Use braille cookbooks. Transcribe favorite recipes into braille or cassette tape.
Ambulation	Learn to use a cane. Have a sighted guide.	Learn to use a cane. Have a dog guide.
Foot care inspection	Have a family member inspect your feet frequently. Visit a podiatrist regularly.	
Shoes	Always feel inside your shoes with your hand to check for cracks, rough spots, or foreign objects before wearing the shoes.	
Socks	Wear clean socks or stockings to protect your skin from your shoes. Hose with holes or mends may cause an injury.	
Nails	Have a podiatrist or family member file, clip, or cut your toenails following the curve of the toe. Use emery boards with care to file nails between visits to the podiatrist.	

blood sugar can initially cause a happy or euphoric feeling that later develops into lethargy. Appropriate treatment to correct blood sugar levels helps stabilize these emotions.

Diabetics who experience either visual impairment or blindness often feel threatened by their loss of competency in diabetes management. Maintaining accuracy when taking medications and monitoring and interpreting blood and urine sugar tests and preventing problems with the feet and legs are some of the difficulties they face. New skills to improve competency in these tasks can be learned with help from rehabilitation teachers and diabetes educators. Aids and devices are developed each year to make these tasks easier. Catalogs and items for examination are available from various agencies.

Easing the Way

Diabetics who experience vision loss will need to adjust to their visual impairment. Frequently blind or visually impaired people are made to feel uncomfortable by sighted persons who are uneasy in their presence. This awkwardness can be eased if sighted people practice the following guidelines:

• Always make a blind person aware that you are talking to him by introducing yourself and gently touching his elbow.

• Meet a blind person at the door as she enters an office or room.

• When helping a blind person entering a room, briefly describe the area as you lead him to a chair and place his hands on the chair back so that he can seat himself.

• Tell a blind person if you must leave the room. Never let her wonder whether or not you are still there. Leave her in contact with some stationary object.

• During conversations, speak directly to a blind person in a normal tone of voice. Do not shout as if he were deaf. If a companion is present, do not use that person as an interpreter. Use the words you normally use; do not try to avoid words like "look" and "see" which are part of everyone's vocabulary.

- When offering to act as a guide, ask the person to take your arm just above the elbow and walk about half a step ahead of him. Never grab the person's cane. Do not insist upon helping someone who does not want assistance.

- If a dog guide is being used for travel, do not distract the dog from its job by petting or talking to it.

- When teaching or explaining something to a blind person, be explicit in giving directions, because she cannot watch what you are doing. Explain fully, and whenever possible, let the sense of touch substitute for vision. Break down procedures into a series of steps and teach one step at a time.

- When necessary to do something "to" or "for" a blind person, always explain what is going to happen. When using an instrument or a piece of equipment, allow him to touch it before it is used.

- Offer reassurance to a blind person who is in strange surroundings. Anxiety about unusual situations might lead to the loss of orientation and mobility skills, causing the person to be more dependent than usual. Be prepared to offer assistance if requested, but do not insist.

Family members and close friends of newly blinded diabetics may have as much difficulty facing the problem of vision loss as the diabetics themselves. They may either deny the existence of the vision loss or become overprotective and unaware of the degree of independence that is achievable with rehabilitation. Family attitudes may be changed by explanations and demonstrations of skills performed by blind persons. Counseling may also be beneficial.

The Future: Rehabilitation

Rehabilitation focuses on helping the individual adjust to vision loss as well as develop independent living skills. Many programs involve teams of professionals working with the diabetic person in different areas, and they may cover tips and training in:

- Daily living skills: personal management and home management
- Orientation and mobility training
- Communication skills: the use of braille, typing, writing, tape, and computers
- Vocational evaluation and skill development
- Use of leisure time
- Low vision evaluation and training
- Library of Congress Talking Book program
- Low vision devices and the use of remaining vision

In addition, special facilities are open to people who qualify for dog guides. The training for using a dog guide takes approximately one month at a residential training center.

Blind people with diabetes have the same capabilities and abilities to learn new skills that other blind people have. However, their training program schedules might have to be modified in order to accommodate diabetes management, and medical advice should be obtained as to the best time to begin or to pursue specific rehabilitation programs. Awareness of the following factors will be beneficial to counselors as well as diabetics involved in these programs:

- The person with diabetes should be asked to describe his or her daily living activities, diabetes maintenance routines, and symptoms of both hyperglycemia and hypoglycemia.

- The person's physician should be consulted to ascertain the individual's ability to participate fully in the program. Also, the person's physical condition and treatment plan should be discussed with the doctor.

- In residential programs, the diabetic person should have an opportunity to talk with the physician in charge and the dietician.

- Adequate time should be allotted for urine and blood testing, insulin injections, other medications, meals, and routine exercise.

- The more active classes, such as those in mobility, should be held shortly after a meal. It is wise to begin with less strenuous forms of exercise and gradually increase the amount and duration of activity.

- Everyone should recognize symptoms of hypoglycemia and hyperglycemia and respond accordingly.

- Injuries, especially to the extremities—hands and fingers, feet and legs—should be avoided.

- If peripheral neuropathy is present, problems with balance and coordination of foot and leg may affect mobility. An impaired sense of touch, if present, may make it harder to interpret information received from a cane and to perform some daily activities.

- Large-dot braille might be useful for people whose fingers lack sensitivity. A totally different system might be required for marking clothing and belongings.

- Some blind diabetics have fluctuating vision, which will influence both the desire and the ability to learn to perform functions.

The most common observation offered by blind diabetics who have attended rehabilitation programs is that they do not want to be treated too gently or to be overprotected. Encouraging independence and a realistic and positive attitude toward the illness is one of the most important benefits a rehabilitation program can give a blind or severely visually impaired diabetic.

Rehabilitation programs can help visually impaired people with diabetes to develop positive attitudes and skills for realistic independence in daily living. The blind person with diabetes works with a team of supportive professionals to plan goals and work toward achieving them. Quality of life for the person with diabetes can and should be fulfilling, whether the interests being pursued are in education, homemaking, a career, or the use of leisure.

Organizations and Resources

A wide range of government agencies and private organizations provide additional information and both free and priced publications about diabetes and blindness or visual impairment. The National Library Service for the Blind and Physically Handicapped of the Library of Congress (see list below) provides aid in assessing this information for blind or visually impaired persons. Check your telephone directory for local agencies, chapters, or affiliates.

American Diabetes Association
National Service Center
1660 Duke Street
P.O. Box 25757
Alexandria, VA 22313
(703) 549-1500 OR (800) 232-3472

Information and publications on diabetes, including the newsletter, Diabetes '89, are available.

American Foundation for the Blind
15 West 16th Street
New York, NY 10011
(212) 620-2000 OR (800) 232-5463

A wide range of publications are available, including the following:

AFB Directory of Services for Blind and Visually Impaired Persons in the United States. Contains names, addresses, and programs of most local, state, national, and federal agencies for visually handicapped people. Also includes schools, low vision services, dog guide schools, training programs, and information organizations.

Creative Recreation for Blind and Visually Impaired Adults. Contains useful hints for adapting a favorite leisure-time activity or choosing a new one.

How Does a Blind Person Get Around? Explains orientation and mobility training.

Low Vision Questions and Answers. Provides basic information about low vision and low vision services and devices.

Making Life More Livable by Irving R. Dickman. Describes simple, inexpensive adaptations that can be made in the homes of older people to allow them to continue everyday activities despite low vision.

Products for People with Vision Problems. Lists the products available from AFB, including syringes and other medical devices, kitchen utensils, tools, games, watches, and other helpful, everyday items.

Understanding Low Vision by Randall T. Jose, O.D. Examines the low vision field in depth through chapters by professionals who provide services to low vision patients.

Juvenile Diabetes Foundation
432 Park Avenue South
New York, NY 10016
(212) 889-7575

A series of free brochures is available on the following topics: Juvenile Diabetes Foundation, diabetes, the young diabetic child, infants with diabetes, pregnancy and diabetes, self-glucose monitoring, and insulin.

National Diabetes Information Clearinghouse
Box NDIC
Bethesda, MD 20892
(301) 468-2162

A free package of information is available, including bibliographies and brochures on diabetes and the eyes, diabetes Type I, diabetes Type II, managing diabetes, blood glucose testing, and the care of the feet. Also available is The Diabetes Dictionary which explains and defines terms that persons with diabetes and their families often hear and need to understand.

National Eye Institute
National Institutes of Health
Building 31, Room 6A32
Bethesda, MD 20892
(301) 496-5248

Information on medical developments such as laser surgery is available from this source.

National Institute of Diabetes and Digestive and Kidney Diseases
National Institutes of Health
Building 31, Room 9A04
Bethesda, MD 20892
(301) 496-3583

National Library Service for the Blind and Physically Handicapped
1291 Taylor Street, NW
Washington, DC 20542
(202) 287-5100 OR (800) 424-9100

Free library services are provided for any print-handicapped individual. Included are adult, young adult, and juvenile books and periodicals in braille and on Talking Book disks and cassette tape recordings. Eligible persons must register with the regional library serving their area. Regional library addresses are available from the Library of Congress, at the address above, or at local libraries.

National Society to Prevent Blindness
500 East Remington Road
Schaumburg, IL 60173
(312) 843-2020

Glossary

Cataract: a clouding of the lens of the eye. Cataract interferes with vision by blocking the passage of light rays to the back of the eye.

Diabetes: a serious chronic disease that occurs when the body cannot properly use carbohydrates (sugar and starch) as it should because of a lack of insulin or the inability to use insulin in the body.

Diabetic Retinopathy: a diabetes-caused disorder of the blood vessels in the retinal tissue at the back of the eye.

Fluorescein Angiography: a means of photographing the flow of blood in the retinal vessels of the human eye by tracing the progress of an injected fluorescein dye.

Glaucoma: an eye disease associated with increased pressure within the eye. Glaucoma can damage the optic nerve and cause impaired vision and blindness.

Insulin: a hormone produced by the pancreas. Insulin regulates the amount of glucose that circulates in the blood.

Laser: an intense, precisely aimed beam of light energy.

Macula: the area near the center of the retina that is responsible for fine or reading vision.

Pancreas: a major gland in the body that secretes insulin.

Photocoagulation: a surgical procedure using an intense beam of light to seal off or destroy leaking blood vessels and damaged tissue in the retina. Photocoagulation is used in the treatment of retinopathy.

Retina: the light-sensitive tissue that lines the inside of the back of the eye. The retina receives visual images and, via the optic nerve, sends messages to the brain, where "seeing" actually takes place.

Vitrectomy: surgical removal of the vitreous, the normally transparent gel that fills the center of the eye. When a diseased vitreous becomes clouded by blood and scar tissue, it can be removed with a special instrument. The vitreous is then replaced with a clear solution.

—by Allene Van Son, R.N.

Chapter 67

Diabetic Retinopathy

This chapter has been written to help people with diabetic retinopathy and their families better understand the disease. It describes the cause, symptoms, diagnosis, and treatment of diabetic retinopathy.

Diabetic retinopathy is a potentially blinding complication of diabetes that damages the eye's retina. It affects half of the 14 million Americans with diabetes.

At first, you may notice no changes in your vision. But don't let diabetic retinopathy fool you. It could get worse over the years and threaten your good vision. With timely treatment, 90 percent of those with advanced diabetic retinopathy can be saved from going blind.

The National Eye Institute (NEI) is the Federal government's lead agency for vision research. The NEI urges all people with diabetes to have an eye examination through dilated pupils at least once a year.

What is the retina?

The retina is a light-sensitive tissue at the back of the eye. When light enters the eye, the retina changes the light into nerve signals. The retina then sends these signals along the optic nerve to the brain. Without a retina, the eye cannot communicate with the brain, making vision impossible.

NIH Pub. No. 95–3252.

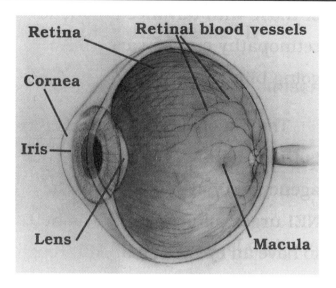

Retina   Retinal blood vessels

Cornea

Iris

Lens   Macula

Figure 67.1.

How does diabetic retinopathy damage the retina?

Diabetic retinopathy occurs when diabetes damages the tiny blood vessels in the retina. At this point, most people do not notice any changes in their vision.

Some people develop a condition called macular edema. It occurs when the damaged blood vessels leak fluid and lipids onto the macula, the part of the retina that lets us see detail. The fluid makes the macula swell, blurring vision.

As the disease progresses, it enters its advanced, or proliferative, stage. Fragile, new blood vessels grow along the retina and in the clear, gel-like vitreous that fills the inside of the eye. Without timely treatment, these new blood vessels can bleed, cloud vision, and destroy the retina.

Who is at risk for this disease?

All people with diabetes are at risk—those with Type I diabetes (juvenile onset) and those with Type II diabetes (adult onset).

During pregnancy, diabetic retinopathy may also be a problem for women with diabetes. It is recommended that all pregnant women with diabetes have dilated eye examinations each trimester to protect their vision.

What are its symptoms?

Diabetic retinopathy often has no early warning signs. At some point, though, you may have macular edema. It blurs vision, making it hard to do things like read and drive. In some cases, your vision will get better or worse during the day. As new blood vessels form at the back of the eye, they can bleed (hemorrhage) and blur vision. The first time this happens it may not be very severe. In most cases, it will leave just a few specks of blood, or spots, floating in your vision. They often go away after a few hours.

These spots are often followed within a few days or weeks by a much greater leakage of blood. The blood will blur your vision. In extreme cases, a person will only be able to tell light from dark in that eye. It may take the blood anywhere from a few days to months or even years to clear from inside of your eye. In some cases, the blood will not clear. You should be aware that large hemorrhages tend to happen more than once, often during sleep.

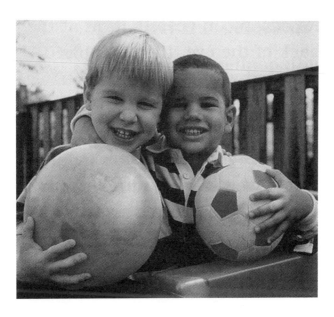

Figure 67.2. *View of boys by person with normal vision.*

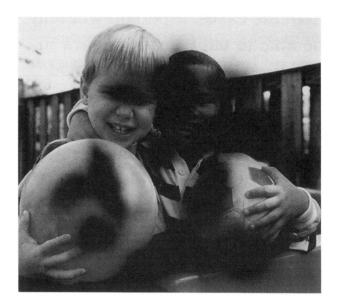

Figure 67.3. View of boys by person with diabetic retinopathy.

How is it detected?

Diabetic retinopathy is detected during an eye examination that includes:

- Visual acuity test: This eye chart test measures how well you see at various distances.

- Pupil dilation: The eye care professional places drops into the eye to widen the pupil. This allows him or her to see more of the retina and look for signs of diabetic retinopathy. After the examination, close-up vision may remain blurred for several hours.

- Ophthalmoscopy: This is an examination of the retina in which the eye care professional: (1) looks through a device with a special magnifying lens that provides a narrow view of the retina, or (2) wearing a headset with a bright light, looks through a special magnifying glass and gains a wide view of the retina.

- Tonometry: A standard test that determines the fluid pressure inside the eye. Elevated pressure is a possible sign of glaucoma, another common eye problem in people with diabetes.

Your eye care professional will look at your retina for early signs of the disease, such as: (1) leaking blood vessels, (2) retinal swelling, such as macular edema, (3) pale, fatty deposits on the retina—signs of leaking blood vessels, (4) damaged nerve tissue, and (5) any changes in the blood vessels.

Should your doctor suspect that you need treatment for macular edema, he or she may ask you to have a test called fluorescein angiography.

In this test, a special dye is injected into your arm. Pictures are then taken as the dye passes through the blood vessels in the retina. This test allows your doctor to find the leaking blood vessels.

How is it treated?

There are two treatments for diabetic retinopathy. They are very effective in reducing vision loss from this disease. In fact, even people with advanced retinopathy have a 90 percent chance of keeping their vision when they get treatment before the retina is severely damaged. These treatments are:

Laser Surgery: Doctors will perform laser surgery to treat severe macular edema and proliferative retinopathy.

Macular Edema: Timely laser surgery can reduce vision loss from macular edema by half. But you may need to have laser surgery more than once to control the leaking fluid.

During the surgery, your doctor will aim a high-energy beam of light directly onto the damaged blood vessels. This is called focal laser treatment. This seals the vessels and stops them from leaking. Generally, laser surgery is used to stabilize vision, not necessarily to improve it.

Proliferative Retinopathy: In treating advanced diabetic retinopathy, doctors use the laser to destroy the abnormal blood vessels that form at the back of the eye.

Rather than focus the light on a single spot, your eye care professional will make hundreds of small laser burns away from the center of the retina. This is called scatter laser treatment. The treatment shrinks the abnormal blood vessels. You will lose some of your side vision after this surgery to save the rest of your sight. Laser surgery may also slightly reduce your color and night vision.

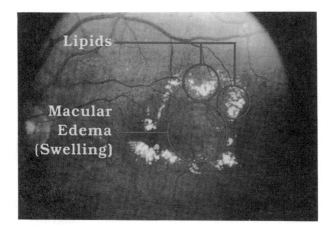

Figure 67.4. *The retina prior to focal laser treatment.*

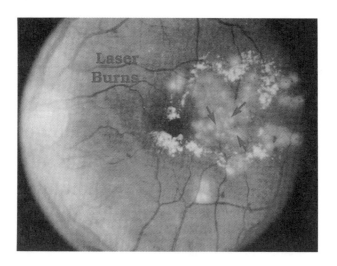

Figure 67.5. *The retina immediately after local laser treatment.*

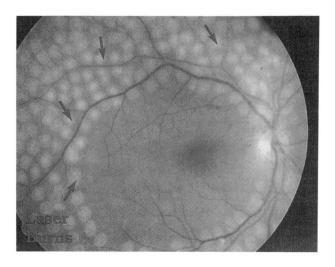

Figure 67.6. Scatter laser treatment.

Laser surgery is performed in a doctor's office or eye clinic. Before the surgery, your ophthalmologist will: (1) dilate your pupil and (2) apply drops to numb the eye. In some cases, the doctor also may numb the area behind the eye to prevent any discomfort.

The lights in the office will be dim. As you sit facing the laser machine, your doctor will hold a special lens to your eye. During the procedure, you may see flashes of bright green or red light. These flashes may eventually create a stinging sensation that makes you feel a little uncomfortable.

You may leave the office once the treatment is done, but you will need someone to drive you home. Because your pupils will remain dilated for a few hours, you also should bring a pair of sunglasses.

For the rest of the day, your vision will probably be a little blurry. Your eye may also hurt a bit. This is easily controlled with drugs that your eye care professional suggests.

Vitrectomy: If you have a lot of blood in the vitreous, you may need an eye operation called a vitrectomy to restore sight. It involves removing the cloudy vitreous and replacing it with a salt solution. Because the vitreous is mostly water, you will notice no change between the salt solution and the normal vitreous.

Studies show that people who have a vitrectomy soon after a large hemorrhage are more likely to protect their vision than someone who waits to have the operation. Early vitrectomy is especially effective in people with insulin-dependent diabetes, who may be at greater risk of blindness from a hemorrhage into the eye.

Vitrectomy is often done under local anesthesia (using drops to numb the eye). This means that you will be awake during the operation. The doctor makes a tiny incision in the sclera, or white of the eye. Next, a small instrument is placed into the eye. It removes the vitreous and inserts the salt solution into the eye.

You may be able to return home soon after the vitrectomy. Or, you may be asked to stay in the hospital overnight. Your eye will be red and sensitive. After the operation, you will need to wear an eyepatch for a few days or weeks to protect the eye. You will also need to use medicated eye drops to protect against infection.

Although laser surgery and vitrectomy are very successful, they do not cure diabetic retinopathy. Once you have proliferative retinopathy, you will always be at risk for new bleeding. This means you may need treatment more than once to protect your sight.

What research is being done?

The National Eye Institute (NEI) is currently supporting a number of research studies in both the laboratory and with patients to learn more about the cause of diabetic retinopathy. This research should provide better ways to detect, treat, and prevent vision loss in people with diabetes.

For example, it is likely that in the coming years researchers will develop drugs that turn off enzyme activity that has been shown to cause diabetic retinopathy. Some day, these drugs will help people to control the disease and reduce the need for laser surgery.

What can you do to protect your vision?

The NEI urges all people with diabetes to have an eye examination through dilated pupils at least once a year. If you have more serious retinopathy, you may need to have a dilated eye examination more often.

A recent study, the Diabetes Control and Complications Trial (DCCT), showed that better control of blood sugar level slows the onset and progression of retinopathy and lessens the need for laser surgery for severe retinopathy.

The study found that the group that tried to keep their blood sugar levels as close to normal as possible, had much less eye, kidney, and nerve disease. This level of blood sugar control may not be best for everyone, including some elderly patients, children under 13, or people with heart disease. So ask your doctor if this program is right for you.

For more information about diabetic retinopathy or diabetes, you may wish to contact:

American Academy of Ophthalmology
655 Beach Street, P.O. Box 7424
San Francisco, CA 94109-7424
(415) 561-8500

American Optometric Association
243 Lindbergh Boulevard
St. Louis, MO 63141
(314) 991-4100

American Diabetes Association
1660 Duke Street
Alexandria, VA 22314
(703) 549-1500

Juvenile Diabetes Foundation International
432 Park Avenue South
New York, NY 10016
(212) 889-7575

National Eye Institute
2020 Vision Place
Bethesda, MD 20892-3655
(301) 496-5248

National Diabetes Outreach Program
National Institute of Diabetes and Digestive and Kidney Diseases
1 Diabetes Way
Bethesda, MD 20892-3560
1-800-GET-LEVEL

Chapter 68

Eye Facts about AIDS, HIV and the Eye

What is AIDS?

AIDS stands for Acquired Immunodeficiency Syndrome. It is a disease of the body's immune system, which helps us to fight off sickness.

What is HIV?

AIDS is caused by a virus called the Human Immunodeficiency Virus (HIV), which attacks many cells in the body. HIV especially attacks white blood cells called lymphocytes. One special kind of lymphocyte is known as the T-cell.

You can be infected with HIV but not get sick with AIDS until many years later. You are considered to have AIDS when:

- Your T-cells drop below a certain level (under 200 T-cells per cubic millimeter) in a blood test;
- Your immune system is no longer able to keep you healthy.

How do you catch HIV and AIDS?

Anyone can catch HIV. It can be spread by:

American Academy of Ophthalmology ©1993. Used by permission.

- Having sex with an infected person, man or woman;
- Sharing hypodermic needles;
- Being born to a mother who has HIV;
- Receiving transfusions with infected blood.

Blood banks in the United States now test blood for HIV. It is very rare to get AIDS from blood transfusions.

What about HIV in the tears?

While the HIV virus can be found in tears of people with AIDS, no cases of AIDS have ever been reported from tear contact. Ophthalmologists are especially careful in cleaning their lenses and instruments which come in contact with the tears.

How does AIDS affect the eye?

Cotton Wool Spots—The most common eye problem from AIDS doesn't threaten vision. Your eye has an inner layer called the retina, which sends images to the brain and helps us see.

AIDS can cause tiny amounts of bleeding and white spots in the retina. These white spots are called "cotton wool spots" because of the way they look.

CMV Retinitis—A serious eye infection of the retina is caused by CMV, the cytomegalovirus (CMV). About 20-30% of people with AIDS have CMV. Most infections happen when the number of T-cells gets dangerously low, usually under 40.

The T-cell count can rise and fall quickly. If you have HIV, you should have an examination by an ophthalmologist every 3 months when your T-cell count is under 250.

CMV can harm your vision permanently. Call an ophthalmologist right away if you see:

- Floating spots or "spiderwebs;"
- Flashing lights;
- Blind spots or blurred vision.

Red Eye—People with AIDS sometimes have red eyes, infections which last for a long time. A disease called shingles can occur more commonly in people with HIV.

Detached retina—Sometimes CMV causes the retina to separate from the back of the eye. A detached retina can cause a serious vision loss. The only way to attach it again is to have an eye operation.

Kaposi's sarcoma—Kaposi's sarcoma (KS) is a kind of tumor that looks like purple-red spots. In the eyes, it can look like a bump on the eyelid or a spot on the white part of the eye. KS can look frightening, but it grows slowly and does not harm the eye.

What are the treatments for AIDS eye problems?

There are two drugs to fight CMV infections: Ganciclovir®(DHPG) and Foscarnet®. These drugs don't kill CMV but slow it down. You must go to your ophthalmologist for regular eye exams in case CMV flares up.

The earlier your ophthalmologist finds CMV, the better the odds your vision can be helped. If only one eye is infected, you can protect the other eye by taking anti-CMV medicines.

Kaposi's sarcoma (KS) can be treated with radiation, laser surgery, freezing or surgery.

There are other eye infections with AIDS. The symptoms are the same as CMV: floaters, flashes or blind spots. But each disease has its own treatment and only your ophthalmologist can tell which you need.

When people are very sick with AIDS, the brain can also become affected. As a result a person's vision can be blurry or double. Treatment can sometimes help.

Regular eye exams are important in HIV infection

It's very important to know if you are HIV+ at an early stage. If you get treatment before you are sick, you can stay well longer.

If your T-cell count falls under 250, it is more likely that you will get a serious eye infection. If your T-cell count drops or if your vision changes, you need to call your ophthalmologist.

Regular eye exams by an ophthalmologist may help to discover CMV early, before you lose much vision.

Chapter 69

Studies of the Ocular Complications of AIDS

Purpose

In order to address issues related to eye involvement in patients with the acquired immune deficiency syndrome (AIDS), the National Eye Institute has funded the Studies of Ocular Complications of AIDS (SOCA), a multicenter clinical trials group. SOCA's major activities involve evaluating treatments and treatment strategies for cytomegalovirus (CMV) retinitis, the most frequent ocular opportunistic infection in patients with AIDS. SOCA's initial clinical trial, the Foscarnethanciclovir Cytomegalovirus Retinitis Trial (FGCRT) was completed in October 1992. SOCA's current trial is the CMV Retinitis Retreatment Trial (CRRT).

The purpose of the CMV Retinitis Retreatment Trial (CRRT) is:

* To compare the relative merits of three therapeutic regimens in patients with AIDS and CMV retinitis, who have been previously treated but whose retinitis is either nonresponsive or has relapsed. These three therapeutic regimens are: 1) foscarnet; 2) high-dose ganciclovir; and 3) combination foscarnet and ganciclovir.

* To compare two treatment strategies in patients with relapsed or nonresponsive CMV retinitis: 1) continuing with the same anti-CMV drug; or 2) switching to the alternate drug.

NIH Pub. No. 93–3960. *Clinical Trials Supported by the National Eye Institute*, pp.45-48.

Background

CMV retinitis is the most common intraocular infection in patients with AIDS, affecting an estimated 20 percent to 25 percent of patients. Untreated, CMV retinitis is a progressive disorder, the end result of which is total retinal destruction and blindness. Given current projections for the AIDS epidemic, it is estimated that there may be as many as 30,000 to 50,000 patients with CMV retinitis in the United States in 1993.

Two drugs are now approved by the United States Food and Drug Administration for the treatment of CMV retinitis: ganciclovir (Cytovene®) and foscarnet (Foscavir®). Both drugs are currently approved only as an intravenous (IV) formulation. Each drug is given in a similar fashion, consisting of an initial 2-week high-dose treatment (induction), followed by long-term lower-dose (maintenance) treatment. All patients with CMV retinitis relapse when anti-CMV therapy is discontinued, generally within 2 to 3 weeks; therefore, maintenance therapy is required.

Despite the use of continuous maintenance therapy, given enough time, all patients with CMV retinitis on maintenance therapy eventually relapse. Furthermore, the time to relapse progressively shortens with each successive relapse. While relapse can often be controlled by reinduction with the same drug followed by continued maintenance therapy, with each relapse, additional retina is destroyed. Therefore, treatment strategies designed to prolong the time to relapse are needed.

Current therapy with foscarnet is to begin with an induction dose of 60 mg/kg every 8 hours followed by a maintenance dose of 90 mg/kg/day. After the first relapse, the maintenance dose of foscarnet is generally increased to 120 mg/kg/day. Conversely, current practice for patients on ganciclovir is to use an induction of 5 mg/kg every 12 hours and maintenance dose of 5 mg/kg/day for each induction and maintenance course, whether or not there has been a previous relapse. One of the regimens to be tested in the CRRT is higher maintenance dose ganciclovir, 10 mg/kg/day. Pilot data from small, uncontrolled case series have suggested that combination therapy with both ganciclovir and foscarnet may be effective in controlling rapidly relapsing CMV retinitis, when therapy with a single agent alone has not been effective. Therefore, combination therapy will also be evaluated. Finally, because of a potential beneficial effect on the development of resistant CMV for patients with relapsed retinitis, it may be that switching to the alternate drug will significantly prolong the time to relapse.

Description

Approximately 300 patients will be enrolled in the CRRT. Eligible patients will have AIDS, CMV retinitis, have been previously treated for their retinitis with either ganciclovir or foscarnet, and have active disease despite previous therapy (nonresponsive or relapsed). Patients will be randomized to one of three treatments: 1) foscarnet; 2) high-dose ganciclovir; or 3) combination ganciclovir and foscarnet. Randomization will be stratified for prior drug therapy.

Patients randomized to the foscarnet arm will receive induction foscarnet at a dosage of 90 mg/kg every 12 hours for 2 weeks, followed by maintenance foscarnet at a dose of 120 mg/kg/day.

Patients randomized to high-dose ganciclovir will receive induction ganciclovir at a dosage of 5 mg/kg every 12 hours for 2 weeks, followed by maintenance ganciclovir at a dosage of 10 mg/kg/day. Patients randomized to the combination arm will continue on standard maintenance therapy with the drug they currently receive (either ganciclovir or foscarnet) and receive induction therapy with the other drug at standard doses, followed by maintenance therapy with both ganciclovir at 5 mg/kg/day and foscarnet at 90 mg/kg/day. Patients who relapse while on the assigned therapy will be reinduced and treated according to standardized treatment algorithms.

Because of the differences in drug administration methods, treatment will not be masked. However, evaluation of retinitis progression will be performed in a masked fashion by the Fundus Photograph Reading Center. Outcome measures of this trial include survival, retinitis progression, changes in visual function (visual acuity and visual fields), drug toxicity, and quality of life. Patients will be followed until death or common study closeout.

Patient Eligibility

Males and females eligible for the CRRT must be age 18 years or older and have AIDS and CMV retinitis. They must have active CMV despite a minimum of 28 days of previous treatment with an anti-CMV drug. Furthermore, they must have an absolute neutrophil count >500 cells/ l, platelet count >20,000 cells/ l, and a serum creatinine <2.5 mg/dl in order to tolerate the drug regimens.

Patient Recruitment Status

Ongoing. Recruitment began in December 1992.

Current Status of Study

Ongoing.

Results

None.

Publications

Foscarnet-Ganciclovir Cytomegalovirus Retinitis Trial

Studies of Ocular Complications of AIDS (SOCA) Research Group in collaboration with the AIDS Clinical Trials Group (ACTG): Studies of Ocular Complications of AIDS Foscarnet-Ganciclovir Cytomegalovirus Retinitis Trial: 1) rationale, design, and methods. *Controlled Clin Trials* 13:22–39,1992.

Studies of Ocular Complications of AIDS Research Group, in collaboration with the AIDS Clinical Trials Group: Mortality in patients with the acquired immunodeficiency syndrome treated with either foscarnet or ganciclovir for cytomegalovirus retinitis. *N Engl J Med* 326:213–220,1992.

CMV Retinitis Retreatment Trial

None.

Clinical Centers

California

Gary N. Holland, M.D.
Jules Stein Eye Institute
University of California, Los Angeles
100 Stein Plaza
Los Angeles, California 90024-7003
Telephone: (310) 825-9508

William R. Freeman, M.D.
Shiley Eye Center, 0946
University of California, San Diego
La Jolla, California 92093-0946
Telephone: (619) 534-3513

James O'Donnell, M.D.
Beckman Vision Center
University of California, San Francisco
Box 0730, Room K-301
10 Kirkham Street
San Francisco, California 94143
Telephone: (415) 476-1921

Florida

Janet Davis, M.D.
Bascom Palmer Eye Institute
University of Miami
900 N.W. 17th Street
Miami, Florida 33136
Telephone: (305) 326-6377

Illinois

David Weinberg, M.D.
Department of Ophthalmology
Northwestern University
222 East Superior Street
Chicago, Illinois 60611
Telephone: (312) 908-8040

Louisiana

Bruce A. Barron, M.D.
LSU Eye Center
Louisiana State University Medical Center
2020 Gravier Street, Suite B
New Orleans, Louisiana 70112
Telephone: (504) 568-6700 ext.307

Maryland

Douglas A. Jabs, M.D.
Wilmer Ophthalmological Institute
The Johns Hopkins Medical Institutions
Maumenee 119
600 North Wolfe Street
Baltimore, Maryland 21287-9217
Telephone: (410) 955-2966

New York

Murk-Hein Heinemann, M.D.
Department of Ophthalmology
Memorial Sloan-Kettering Cancer Center
1275 York Avenue, Suite A325
New York, New York 10021
Telephone: (212) 639-7237

Alan Friedman, M.D.
Department of Ophthalmology
Mount Sinai School of Medicine
Box 1183
One Gustave L. Levy Place
New York, New York 10029-6574
Telephone: (212) 241-6241

Dorothy Friedberg, M.D.
Department of Ophthalmology
New York University Medical Center
310 Lexington Avenue
New York, New York 10016
Telephone: (212) 687-0265

Texas

Richard Alan Lewis, M.D., M.S.
Cullen Eye Institute
Baylor College of Medicine
6501 Fannin Street, NC-200
Houston, Texas 77030
Telephone: (713) 798-6100

Resource Centers

Chairman's Office

Douglas A. Jabs, M.D.
Wilmer Ophthalmological Institute
The Johns Hopkins University and Hospital
550 North Broadway, Suite 700
Baltimore, Maryland 21205
Telephone: (410) 955-1966

Coordinating Center

Curtis L. Meinert, Ph.D.
Department of Epidemiology
School of Hygiene and Public Health
The Johns Hopkins University
615 North Wolfe Street, Room 5010
Baltimore, Maryland 21205
Telephone: (410) 955-8198

Fundus Photograph Reading Center

Matthew D. Davis, M.D.
Department of Ophthalmology
University of Wisconsin
610 North Walnut Street, Room 417
Madison, Wisconsin 53705-5240
Telephone: (608) 263-6071

Drug Distribution Center

Gary Stewart, M.S., R.Ph.
Ogden Bioservices Corporation
625 C Lofstrand Lane
Rockville, Maryland 20850
Telephone: (301) 762-0069

NEI Representative

Richard L. Mowery, Ph.D.
National Eye Institute
Executive Plaza South, Suite 350
6120 Executive Boulevard
Rockville, Maryland 20892
Telephone: (301) 496-5983

Chapter 70

Ganciclovir Implant Study for Cytomegalovirus Retinitis

Purpose

To determine the therapeutic efficacy of a sustained-release in-traocular drug delivery system for ganciclovir therapy of cytomega-lovirus (CMV) retinitis in patients with AIDS.

Background

CMV retinitis occurs in 20–30 percent of patients with AIDS and is the leading cause of visual loss in these patients. At present, Ganciclovir and Foscarnet are the only two drugs that have been ap-proved by the Food and Drug Administration for the treatment of CMV retinitis. The therapeutic regimen for each drug consists of a 2-week induction period followed by daily maintenance intravenous infusions. Unfortunately, CMV retinitis usually progresses despite daily main-tenance therapy, and both drugs are associated with significant sys-temic toxicity that often limits their therapeutic usefulness. As an alternative to intravenous administration, direct intravitreal injec-tions of ganciclovir have been studied and have been shown to be ef-fective in delaying the progression of CMV retinitis. The short half-life of the drug, however, necessitates one to two intraocular injections a week to maintain therapeutic levels. Widespread adoption of this tech-nique has been limited due to the logistical difficulties and inherent risks associated with numerous intravitreal injections.

NIH Pub. No. 93–3960. *Clinical Trials Supported by the National Eye Insti-tute*, pp. 35-36.

A drug delivery system capable of continuous delivery of ganciclovir into the vitreous cavity has recently been developed. The device consists of a 6-mg pellet of ganciclovir that is coated with a series of polymers with variable permeability to ganciclovir. The device is surgically implanted through the pars plana At present, two devices are under study: one that releases ganciclovir at a rate of 2 µg/hr and another that releases ganciclovir at a rate of 1 µg/hr. Results from phase I studies have been encouraging. The purpose of this study is to determine the therapeutic efficacy of each of the devices in a randomized, controlled clinical trial.

Description

Approximately 45 patients will be enrolled. All patients must have non-sight-threatening CMV retinitis (>3,000 µm from fovea and >1,500 µm from the optic disc) and not have been previously treated with ganciclovir or foscarnet. Patients with unilateral non-sight-threatening CMV retinitis will be randomly assigned to one of three groups: 1) immediate therapy with a device designed to release ganciclovir into the vitreous cavity at a rate of 2 µg/hr over approximately a 4-month period, 2) immediate therapy with a device designed to release ganciclovir into the vitreous cavity at a rate of 1 µg/hr over approximately an 8-month period, or 3) delayed therapy. In patients with bilateral non-sight-threatening CMV retinitis, one eye will be randomly assigned to receive a ganciclovir implant with the other eye assigned to deferral. The eye assigned to immediate treatment will be further randomized to receive either a 2 µg/hr or 1 µg/hr device. The primary endpoint will be time to retinitis progression, defined as the time (days) from initiating therapy until advancement of 750 µm over a 750 µm front of any border of any lesion is observed. Standardized nine field photographs will be taken at 2-week intervals and analyzed in a masked fashion by the Fundus Photograph Reading Center to determine evidence of CMV retinitis progression.

Patient Eligibility

All patients must have AIDS as defined by the Centers for Disease Control and non-sight-threatening CMV retinitis (>3,000 µm from the fovea and >1,500 µm from the optic disc). Patients cannot have been previously treated with systemic ganciclovir or foscarnet and must not have evidence of other organ involvement with CMV. Patients must have an absolute neutrophil count (ANC) greater than 1,000 cells/ml and a platelet count greater than 25,000/mm.

Patient Recruitment Status

Ongoing. Recruitment began November 1992.

Current Status of Study

Ongoing.

Results

None.

Publications

None.

Clinical Centers

Maryland

Daniel F. Martin, M.D.
Robert B. Nussenblatt, M.D.
National Eye Institute
National Institutes of Health
Warren Grant Magnuson Clinical Center
Building 10, Room 10N202
Bethesda, Maryland 20892
Telephone: (301) 496-3123

Texas

Rajiv Anand, M.D.
Department of Ophthalmology
University of Texas
Southwestern Medical Center
5323 Harry Hines Boulevard
Dallas, Texas 75235-9057
Telephone: (214) 688-3838

Resource Centers

Chairmen's Office

Daniel F. Martin, M.D.
Robert B. Nussenblatt, M.D.
National Eye Institute
National Institutes of Health
Warren Grant Magnuson Clinical Center
Building 10, Room 10N202
Bethesda, Maryland 20892
Telephone: (301) 496-3123

Fundus Photograph Reading Center

Matthew D. Davis, M.D.
Department of Ophthalmology
University of Wisconsin
610 North Walnut Street, Room 417
Madison, Wisconsin 53705-5240
Telephone: (608) 263-6071

Data and Safety Monitoring Committee

Susan Ellenberg Ph.D.
Food and Drug Administration
Rockville, MD

Frederick L. Ferris III, M.D.
National Eye Institute
Bethesda, MD

Douglas A. Jabs, M.D.
The Johns Hopkins University
Baltimore, MD

Marvin Podgor, Ph.D.
National Eye Institute
Bethesda, MD

Ex Officio Members

Wiley A. Chambers, M.D.
Food and Drug Administration
Rockville, MD

Emily Y. Chew, M.D.
National Eye Institute
Bethesda, MD

Robert B. Nussenblatt, M.D.
National Eye Institute
Bethesda, MD

Chapter 71

Thyroid Eye Disease

Thyroid disease and its effects on the eye became better known when former President George Bush and his wife, Barbara, developed disorders of the thyroid gland. The function of the thyroid gland is to secrete, or form, hormones that control a wide range of the body's metabolic processes. Not enough hormone secretion results in hypothyroidism, which may cause fatigue, intolerance to cold, weight gain and dry skin. Too much secretion of hormone results in hyperthyroidism. Hyperthyroid persons may have heat intolerance, nervousness, weight loss and heart palpitations.

What is thyroid eye disease?

Although the thyroid gland is located in the neck, problems in the gland's function may lead to changes in the eye and orbit (eye socket). The combination of thyroid dysfunction and eye changes is called *Graves' disease* or thyroid eye disease. The eye symptoms usually appear when thyroid hormone levels are too high but can occur when these levels are normal or below normal. The most obvious eye abnormality in Graves' disease is proptosis (protrusion of the eyeballs).

Who gets Graves' disease?

Graves' disease is five times more likely to affect females than males. It most commonly occurs in women during their 20s and 30s.

UIC Department of Ophthalmology, unnumbered publication, March/April 1993.

The disease is unpredictable in severity and duration but generally lasts months or years. In children with Graves' disease, the eye problems tend to be less severe.

What causes thyroid eye disease?

The cause of the eye changes in Graves' disease is unknown. However, the immune system is involved in the development of the signs and symptoms. The immune system not only fights disease but also participates in inflammation. In persons with Graves' disease, the tissues around the eye, including the orbital fat and eye muscles, become swollen and inflamed.

What are the symptoms and signs of thyroid eye disease?

Patients with Graves' disease may have a variety of eye symptoms that are not always recognized right away as features of a thyroid disorder:

- Protrusion of one or both eyeballs.
- Puffy, swollen eyelids.
- Gritty, burning, irritated eyes that frequently water.
- Diplopia (double vision).
- Decreased vision, often following reduced brightness of colors.
- Redness and swelling of the conjunctiva, the thin layer covering the white part of the eye.
- Difficulty in completely closing the eyelids, especially while sleeping.

The most common eye sign in Graves' disease is proptosis, in which the eyes appear to bulge outward. This finding is present in 70 to 90 percent of cases of thyroid eye disease. The swelling that causes proptosis is due to collections of fluid, fat and inflammatory cells.

The muscles that move the eyes may also become congested and stiff. This leads to double vision, since the muscles are unable to move the eyes together. As the disease gets worse, scarring of these muscles may occur, resulting in permanent limitation of eye movements.

Proptosis may gradually increase to the extent that the cornea (the transparent tissue covering the front of the eye) becomes exposed. This exposure leads to drying and inflammation, which can progress to severe infections and ulcers of the cornea in extreme cases. Also, the orbital swelling may be so severe that the pressure within the eye increases leading to glaucoma. The optic nerve, which is responsible for sending information received from the eye to the brain, may become strangled, resulting in severe or total vision loss.

How is thyroid eye disease diagnosed?

The characteristic eye signs often make an eye doctor suspicious that Graves' disease is present. Also, blood testing frequently shows abnormal levels of thyroid hormones. Magnetic resonance imaging (MRI), computed tomography (CT)of the orbits and eyes or ocular ultrasound (sound waves) may also be sued to diagnose the disease. These imaging methods can reveal swelling of the eye tissues and muscles in a pattern consistent with thyroid eye disease.

What is the treatment of thyroid eye disease?

Medical control of the thyroid disorder often does not eliminate the eye problems, which may last one to two years longer. It is not possible to predict which patients will develop advanced eye disease. Mild corneal exposure may be treated with eye drop lubricants (tear supplements) and pressure dressings to cover the eye. Some patients tape their eyes closed when they sleep to prevent further exposure. Severe cases of corneal exposure may need a lateral tarsorrhaphy, an operation that involves stitching part of the eyelids together. In some severe cases of corneal exposure, the muscles that raise the upper eyelids are surgically weakened to cause ptosis (eyelid droop) so the eyelids more adequately cover the eyes.

Infection and ulceration of the cornea may require frequent use of antibiotics to prevent perforation of the cornea.

Double vision may be corrected with the use of prisms attached to glasses, which partly compensate for limited eye movements. Surgery to reposition the eye muscles is recommended for repair of eye muscle imbalance only after Graves' disease stabilizes.

For advanced disease with severe corneal exposure and strangulation of the optic nerve, different treatments may be used, including steroid medications, radiation and/or surgery. Steroid medication decreases the inflammation in the eye muscles and orbital tissue. Steroids usually are given orally, although the intravenous route is sometimes used. Often high doses are needed. The dosage is gradually decreased, and a low dosage is maintained until symptoms improve. Unfortunately, steroids have many possible adverse side effects.

Radiation therapy targeted to the tissue behind the eyeball is sometimes used to decrease orbital inflammation. Some physicians use combinations of radiation and steroids.

Surgical orbital decompression is an important method of relieving severe pressure on the optic nerve, which threatens vision. Various surgical procedures are used to make room in the eye socket for the swollen and thickened orbital tissue. This allows the bulging eye to relax back to its normal position.

Follow up with an eye physician is an important part of preventive care for patients with Graves' disease.

—by Jeffrey Nichols, M.D.

Index

Index

600

607

V

varicella zoster virus (VZV)
  ocular complications due to 241
  recent accomplishments 245–46
  treatment of 245–46
venule(s), description of 25
VEPs
  see visually evoked potentials
vestibulo-ocular reflex (VOR), in visual pursuit of objects 93
vimentin, following retinal detachment 255
vinculin(s), in corneal wound healnig 225
viral retinitis 181
vision
  binocular, breakdown in 123
  central
    see visual acuity
  child's testing at home 137–38
  cloudiness of, cataracts as cause of 363–70
  explanation of 91
  halo, definition of 326
  importance of cornea in 204
  improvement in, vitrectomy for 502, 505
  loss of
    age-related macular degeneration as cause of 457–58
    lasers for 157–63
    prevention of 121
  low
    see low vision
  normal
    development of 117–18
    view of *567*
  peripheral
    definition of 5
    loss following glaucoma *311*
  poor, eye's focusing ability and 22
  protection of 461
    methods of 572
  scotoma effects on *452*
  testing of, importance of 118
  tunnel, definition of 327
Vision Foundation, Inc. 86

vision testing
  in eye examination 22–23
  potential, for cataracts 391
Visions 82
visual acuity
  definition of 6
  normal 22
visual acuity test, in diabetic retinopathy detection 568
visual defects, correction of, prescription for 22–23
visual disorders, prevalence of 91
visual fluid, definition of 6
visual function
  MEG in 94
  MRI in 94
  PET in 94
  VEPs in 94
Visual Impairments 76–77
visual impairments
  age-related 30
  aids for 514
  causes of 30
  and diabetes 547
  prevalence of 30
  resources for 514–15
  severe, functional behaviors associated with 33
  see also low vision
visual information, processing of, by eye and brain 94
visual neuroscience, research related to 92
visual system, disturbances in
  effects of 91
  research related to 92
visually evoked potentials (VEPs), in visual function assessment 94
vitamin(s), for macular degeneration 463, 465
vitamin A
  for cicatricial diseases of conjunctiva 225
  11-"cis" retinaldehyde form of, for macular degeneration 471
vitamin A supplements, for retinitis pigmentosa 267–69
vitamin E supplements, effects on retinitis pigmentosa 267–68